Diabetic Foot Ulcer

Mohammad Zubair • Jamal Ahmad
Abida Malik • Mallikarjuna Rao Talluri
Editors

Diabetic Foot Ulcer

An Update

Springer

Editors
Mohammad Zubair
Department of Medical Microbiology
Faculty of Medicine
University of Tabuk
Tabuk
Kingdom of Saudi Arabia

Jamal Ahmad
Consultant, Diabetes & Endocrinology
Superspeciality Center
Aligarh
Uttar Pradesh
India

Abida Malik
Ex-Chairperson-Department of Microbiology, Former Dean-Faculty of Medicine, J N Medical College & Hospital
Faculty of Medicine
Aligarh Muslim University
Aligarh
Uttar Pradesh
India

Mallikarjuna Rao Talluri
Research Associate
Bioanalytical Department
AXIS Clinicals
Hyderabad
Telangana
India

ISBN 978-981-15-7638-6   ISBN 978-981-15-7639-3 (eBook)
https://doi.org/10.1007/978-981-15-7639-3

This Springer imprint is published by the registered company Springer Nature Singapore Pte Ltd.
The registered company address is: 152 Beach Road, #21-01/04 Gateway East, Singapore 189721, Singapore

Preface

Diabetes mellitus (DM) is a chronic disorder (an excess of glucose levels in blood) because insulin is no longer produced in the pancreas (type I DM) or the body is unable to utilize produced insulin in the body properly (type II DM). DM is the world's most endemic and mortality causing disease affecting more than 6% of the adult population. The growth rate of DM patients has been increasing rapidly due to different factors such as genetic, environmental, lifestyle, increased calorie intake, and less body exercise. But the development of medication is not as much as the growth rate of DM and its complications. Type I DM has no preventive medicine, but type II can be prevented and controlled by maintaining a healthy lifestyle. However, their complications can be delayed by taking insulin therapy.

The complications of DM have more impact on different metabolisms in the body and are not specific to any particular disease, because insulin is the principal hormone responsible for the uptake of glucose from blood to different cells of the body. DM mainly damages the blood vessels and leads to the preliminary complications in the eyes, kidneys, and nerves. All these complications are interlinked to each other because glucose is the principal fuel for cellular functions. The damage of nerves due to DM is known as diabetic neuropathy (DN); its main symptoms are numbness and tingling that lead to skin damage.

Skin damage due to DM is because of peripheral arterial damage, i.e., lower blood circulation. Diabetic foot ulceration/diabetic foot ulcer (DFU) is one of the foremost DM complications associated with it and sometimes may cause amputation.

The availability of information on DFU prevalence, major symptoms, pathogenesis, complications, treatments, and management was very less. This book provides updated knowledge on the prevalence of DFU around different parts of the world, its development, pathophysiology, major complications, and new methodologies in its treatment. The editors sincerely acknowledge the efforts of authors in manifesting their perspectives about DFU.

Shamina Begum et al. describe the occurrence of DM, its complications, and the current scenario about prevalence, risk factors, and different strategies and policies to control DFU around Asia and European continents.

Zulfiqarali G. Abbas explains the common causes of DFU, in relation to peripheral neuropathy, and analyzes over the last two decades conditions of DFU complications and prevention and control programs in Africa and Antarctica.

Kanakamani Jeyaraman presents the implications of DFU in relation to clinical, social, and economic problems because of endemic type II DM and the annual outlay on DM and its complications including DFU in American and Australian continents.

Ayman Faisal Foad explains the pathophysiology of wound healing with respect to different control factors and importance of proteins and vitamin C in wound healing.

Hyder O. Mirghani describes the different approaches for image (scanning) models to differentiate harm at various tissue levels for providing the remedial approaches to different foot inflammation including DFU due to DM.

Mohammad Zubair and Farha Fatima demonstrates the various complications due to DM, mainly focused on development of DFU, and explains the risk factors for DFU development and approaches for timely diagnosis to overcome complications of DFU.

Ahmad Faraz et al. explain the major healthcare challenges in the twenty-first century and how DM and its complications impact the mortality rate around the globe and also elucidate the association of diabetic neuropathy with the diabetic foot abnormalities.

Tarek Kabil describes the association of inflammation wounds with different microbes (aerobic and anaerobic) and their involvement in DFU and its complications.

Fohad Mabood Husain et al. illustrate the DFU and DN contribution for the development of different pathogenic microorganisms at infectious sites and how these microbial infections lead to tissue and bone injury.

M. Oves et al. illustrate the hidden role of fungus in infection management.

Thomas Thanyath demonstrates the risk factors for DFU, and evaluation of DFU at appropriate stages in different diabetic patients using various identification methods.

Hamid Ashraf et al. explain the management of different microbial infections associated with DFU using different antibiotics.

Vijay Viswanathan and Sai Prathiba A. explain the recent circumstances about the DFU and its treatments in the Indian subcontinent.

Zulfiqarali G. Abbas elucidates complications, its prevalence, and management strategies to control and prevent DFU in developing countries.

Deepti Singh and Hifzur R. Siddique discuss about the role of different growth factors, their usage in control and prevention, and future prospects in DFU management.

Rashid Mir et al. expound the current approaches in the control, prevention, and treatment of DFU and also explain the role of stem cell therapy in different wound healing infections including DFU management.

M. Ahmed Mesaik et al. explain the importance of alternative medicine (AM) against the rising of global DM patients and the management of AM in the DM and its complications including DFU and diabetic foot infections (DFIs).

Mohamed Ali-Seyed and Ayesha Siddiqua enlighten the role of phytomedicine (traditional medicine) and herbal formulations in the treatment of DM and

DFU. They also explain the possible mechanism of action of important medicinal plants against DM and their future scope in identification of different phytocompounds against DM, DFU, and other complications.

Sumbul Rehman explains the common complications including DFU due to prolonged high blood glucose levels and the management of bloodletting by leeching therapy using *Hirudo medicinalis.*

Mohammad Azam Ansari et al. describe the prevalence of DM and DFU complications and emphasize the delayed wound healing because of DFU, possibly employing nanotechnology in the management of DM and DFU treatment using nanoformulations.

Tabuk, Saudi Arabia Mohammad Zubair
Aligarh, India Jamal Ahmad
Aligarh, India Abida Malik
Hyderabad, India Mallikarjuna Roa Talluri

Contents

Part I World Preview

1 **Diabetic Foot Complications in Asia and European Continents** 3
Shamina Begum, Mohammad Zubair, Marai M. Alamri, Fohad Mabood Husain, Farha Fatima, Mohammad Oves, Mohammad Azam Ansari, and Iftekhar Hassan

2 **Diabetic-Foot Complications in African and Antarctica Continents** 29
Zulfiqarali G. Abbas

3 **Diabetic-Foot Complications in American and Australian Continents** 41
Kanakamani Jeyaraman

Part II Complications and Treatments Updates

4 **Acute and Chronic Wound Healing Physiology** 63
Ayman Fisal Ahmed Foad

5 **Screening of Foot Inflammation in Diabetic Patients by Noninvasive Imaging Modalities** 77
Hyder O. Mirghani

6 **Molecular Mechanism and Biomechanics of the Diabetic Foot: The Road to Foot Ulceration and Healing** 87
Mohammad Zubair and Farha Fatima

7 **Foot Pressure Abnormalities, Radiographic, and Charcot Changes in the Diabetic Foot** 121
Ahmad Faraz, Hamid Ashraf, Saifullah Khalid, and Razeen Fatima

8 **Aerobic and Anaerobic Bacterial Infections and Treatment Strategies** 135
Tarek Hassan M. Kabil

9 MRSA, EBSL, and Biofilm Formation in Diabetic Foot Ulcer Infections 149
Fohad Mabood Husain, Mohammad Shavez Khan, Mohammad Zubair, Altaf Khan, Saba Noor, Iftekhar Hassan, Mohammed Arshad, Mohd Shahnawaz Khan, Faizan Abul Qais, and Salman Al-Amery

10 Fungal Infection: The Hidden Enemy? 161
Mohammad Oves, Mohd Ahmar Rauf, Fohad Mabood Husain, Mohammad Zubair, Iqbal M. I. Ismail, and Arun Iyer

11 Diabetic Foot Syndrome: Risk Factors, Clinical Assessment, and Advances in Diagnosis 177
Thomas Antony Thaniyath

Part III Developments, Future Prospective, New Possible Treatments

12 Advances in Prevention and Empirical Treatment of Diabetic Foot Infection 201
Hamid Ashraf, Jamal Ahmad, and Anees Akhtar

13 Prevention of Diabetic Foot: Indian Experience 215
Vijay Viswanathan and A. Sai Prathiba

14 Low-Cost Management of Diabetic Foot 221
Zulfiqarali G. Abbas

15 Role of Growth Factors in the Treatment of Diabetic Foot Ulceration 233
Deepti Singh and Hifzur R. Siddique

16 Stem Cells in the Treatment of Diabetic Foot Ulcers 251
Rashid Mir, Imadeldin Elfaki, Ajaz Ahmad Waza, and Faisel M. AbuDuhier

17 Alternative Medicine in the Management of Diabetic Foot Ulcers/Infections 269
M. Ahmed Mesaik, Hyder O. Mirghani, and Fakhralddin Elfakki

18 Modern Phytomedicine in Treating Diabetic Foot Ulcer: Progress and Opportunities 281
Mohamed Ali Seyed and Siddiqua Ayesha

19 Management of Diabetic Foot Ulcer by *Hirudo medicinalis*, the "Healing Leech" 315
Sumbul Rehman

20 Nanotechnology and Diabetic Foot Ulcer: Future Prospects 331
Mohammad Azam Ansari, Khursheed Ali, Zeba Farooqui, Hanan A. Al-Dossary, Mohammad Zubair, and Javed Musarrat

Correction to: Nanotechnology and Diabetic Foot Ulcer: Future Prospects C1

About the Editors

Mohammad Zubair is an Assistant Professor at the Department of Medical Microbiology, Faculty of Medicine, University of Tabuk, Kingdom of Saudi Arabia. He completed his PhD and post-doctorate research on diabetic foot infections and has extensive teaching and research experience in the field of medical science. His research focuses on the extended spectrum beta-lactamase gene (CTX, TEM & SHV), pro and anti-inflammatory cytokines, healing proteins and their clinical correlations. He has published more than 35 papers in international, peer-reviewed journals, and has presented his work at various international conferences. He is also the recipient of the prestigious "Marvil Levin" research awards presented by the American Diabetes Association (ADA) at the 72nd Scientific Session held at Philadelphia, USA.

Jamal Ahmad is a former Professor of Endocrinology; ex Dean of the Faculty of Medicine, J.N. Medical College; and ex Director of the Rajiv Gandhi Centre for Diabetes & Endocrinology, Faculty of Medicine, Aligarh Muslim University, India. He has made a significant contribution toward determining the role of protein glycation in diabetes and its associated complications. He has published more than 240 research articles in various international and national journals, was Principal Investigator or Co-Investigator in a number of research projects, and has completed 9 phase III international, multi-centre, multicounty new drug trials in diabetes mellitus. He is a former President of the Endocrine Society of India, and the recipient of the prestigious RSSDI fellowship-2015 and a Lifetime Achievement Award by Diabetes India 2019.

Abida Malik is a former Professor and Chairperson of the Department of Microbiology, and the former Dean of the Faculty of Medicine, Jawaharlal Nehru Medical College, Aligarh Muslim University. A leading Indian microbiologist, she has over 41 years of teaching and research experience and authored more that 185 publications. She established the Virology Lab in 1976, Mycology lab in 1980 and was founded and responsible for the AIDS Surveillance Centre for 20 years. She is the former president of the Indian Association of Microbiologists, and received the Dr U. C. Chaturvedi Life Time achievement Award for her services to microbiology in 2011.

Mallikarjuna Rao Talluri is currently a Research Associate at AXIS Clinicals Limited, Hyderabad, India, where his work focuses on development methods and the quantification of new drugs and their bioavailability and bioequivalence. He is an expert on the evaluation of the biological activities of natural products (bio-guided extraction), and scientific writing, and has experience in instrumental handling, such as LC-MS/MS, HPLC, column chromatography, and TLC. He has worked extensively in the field of phytopharmacology, and has published more than 50 papers in peer-reviewed, international and national journals.

Contributors

Zulfiqarali G. Abbas Abbas Medical Centre, Dar es Salaam, Tanzania

Muhimbili University of Health and Allied Sciences, Dar es Salaam, Tanzania

Faisel M. AbuDuhier Vice-Rector for Academic Affairs; Director, Prince Fahd Bin Sultan Research Chair & Department of Medical Lab Technology, Faculty of Applied Medical Sciences, University of Tabuk, Tabuk, Kingdom of Saudi Arabia

Jamal Ahmad Retired Professor & Former-Director Rajiv Gandhi Center for Diabetes & Endocrinology, Faculty of Medicine, J N Medical College & Hospital, Aligarh Muslim University, Aligarh, India

Consultant- Diabetes & Endocrinology Super Specialty Centre, Aligarh, India

Anees Akhtar Department of Microbiology, Faculty of Medicine, J N Medical College & Hospital, Aligarh Muslim University, Aligarh, India

Salman Al-Amery Department of Biochemistry, College of Science, King Saud University, Riyadh, Kingdom of Saudi Arabia

Marai M. Alamri Department of Surgery, Faculty of Medicine, University of Tabuk, Tabuk, Kingdom of Saudi Arabia

Hanan A. Al-Dossary Department of Epidemic Disease Research, Institute for Research and Medical Consultations (IRMC), Imam Abdulrahman Bin Faisal University, Dammam, Kingdom of Saudi Arabia

Khursheed Ali Department of Agricultural Microbiology, Faculty of Agricultural Sciences, Aligarh Muslim University, Aligarh, Uttar Pradesh, India

Mohamed Ali Seyed Department of Clinical Biochemistry, Faculty of Medicine, University of Tabuk, Tabuk, Kingdom of Saudi Arabia

Mohammad Azam Ansari Department of Epidemic Disease Research, Institute for Research and Medical Consultations (IRMC), Imam Abdulrahman Bin Faisal University, Dammam, Kingdom of Saudi Arabia

Mohammed Arshad Department of Clinical Laboratory Sciences, College of Applied Medical Sciences, King Saud University, Riyadh, Kingdom of Saudi Arabia

Hamid Ashraf Rajiv Gandhi Center for Diabetes & Endocrinology, Faculty of Medicine, J N Medical College & Hospital, Aligarh Muslim University, Aligarh, India

Shamina Begum Department of Medical Microbiology, Faculty of Medicine, University of Tabuk, Tabuk, Kingdom of Saudi Arabia

Imadeldin Elfaki Department of Biochemistry, Faculty of Sciences, University of Tabuk, Tabuk, Kingdom of Saudi Arabia

Fakhralddin Elfakki Department of Family & Community Medicine, Faculty of Medicine, University of Tabuk, Tabuk, Kingdom of Saudi Arabia

Ahmad Faraz Department of Physiology, Faculty of Medicine, J N Medical College & Hospital, Aligarh Muslim University, Aligarh, India

Zeba Farooqui College of Pharmacy, University of Houston, Houston, TX, USA

Farha Fatima Department of Zoology, Faculty of Life Science, Aligarh Muslim University, Aligarh, India

Razeen Fatima Department of Medicine, Faculty of Medicine, J N Medical College & Hospital, Aligarh Muslim University, Aligarh, India

Ayman Fisal Ahmed Foad Department of Pathology, Faculty of Medicine, University of Tabuk, Tabuk, Kingdom of Saudi Arabia

Orotta College of Medicine & Health Sciences, Asmara, Eritrea

Iftekhar Hassan Department of Zoology, College of Science, King Saud University, Riyadh, Kingdom of Saudi Arabia

Fohad Mabood Husain Department of Food Science and Nutrition, College of Food and Agriculture Sciences, King Saud University, Riyadh, Kingdom of Saudi Arabia

Riyadh, Kingdom of Saudi Arabia

Iqbal M. I. Ismail Department of Chemistry, King Abdulaziz University, Jeddah, Kingdom of Saudi Arabia

Arun Iyer Use-Inspired Biomaterials & Integrated Nano Delivery (U-BiND) Systems Laboratory, Department of Pharmaceutical Sciences, Eugene Applebaum College of Pharmacy and Health Sciences, Wayne State University, Detroit, MI, USA

Kanakamani Jeyaraman Royal Darwin Hospital, Darwin, NT, Australia

Northern Territory Medical Program, Flinders University, Darwin, NT, Australia

Tarek Hassan M. Kabil Department of Medical Microbiology & Immunology, Faculty of Medicine, University of Tabuk, Tabuk, Kingdom of Saudi Arabia

Saifullah Khalid Department of Radio-diagnosis, Faculty of Medicine, J N Medical College & Hospital, Aligarh Muslim University, Aligarh, India

Altaf Khan Department of Pharmacology and Toxicology, Central Laboratory, College of Pharmacy, King Saud University, Riyadh, Kingdom of Saudi Arabia

Mohammad Shavez Khan Department of Agricultural Microbiology, Aligarh Muslim University, Aligarh, India

Mohd Shahnawaz Khan Department of Biochemistry, College of Science, King Saud University, Riyadh, Kingdom of Saudi Arabia

M. Ahmed Mesaik Department of Medical Microbiology, Faculty of Medicine, University of Tabuk, Tabuk, Kingdom of Saudi Arabia

Rashid Mir Prince Fahd Bin Sultan Research Chair, Division of Molecular Biology, Department of Medical Lab Technology, Faculty of Applied Medical Sciences, University of Tabuk, Tabuk, Kingdom of Saudi Arabia

Hyder O. Mirghani Department of Internal Medicine, Faculty of Medicine, University of Tabuk, Tabuk, Kingdom of Saudi Arabia

Javed Musarrat Faculty of Agricultural Sciences, Department of Agricultural Microbiology, Aligarh Muslim University, Aligarh, Uttar Pradesh, India

School of Biosciences and Biotechnology, Baba Ghulam Shah Badshah University, Rajouri, Jammu & Kashmir, India

Saba Noor National Institute of Cancer Prevention and Research, Noida, Uttar Pradesh, India

Mohammad Oves Department of Biological Science, Faculty of Science, King Abdulaziz University, Jeddah, Kingdom of Saudi Arabia

Center of Excellence in Environmental Studies, King Abdul Aziz University, Jeddah, Kingdom of Saudi Arabia

Faizan Abul Qais Department of Agricultural Microbiology, Aligarh Muslim University, Aligarh, India

Mohd Ahmar Rauf Use-Inspired Biomaterials & Integrated Nano Delivery (U-BiND) Systems Laboratory, Department of Pharmaceutical Sciences, Eugene Applebaum College of Pharmacy and Health Sciences, Wayne State University, Detroit, MI, USA

Sumbul Rehman Department of Ilmul Advia (Unani Pharmacology), Faculty of Unani Medicine, Aligarh Muslim University, Aligarh, Uttar Pradesh, India

A. Sai Prathiba M. V. Hospital for Diabetes and Prof. M. Viswanathan Diabetes Research Centre (WHO Collaborating Centre for Research, Education and Training in Diabetes), Chennai, India

Siddiqua Ayesha School of Public Health SRM University, Chennai, Tamil Nadu, India

Hifzur R. Siddique Molecular Cancer Genetics and Translational Research Lab, Section of Genetics, Department of Zoology, Aligarh Muslim University, Aligarh, India

Deepti Singh Molecular Cancer Genetics and Translational Research Lab, Section of Genetics, Department of Zoology, Aligarh Muslim University, Aligarh, India

Thomas Antony Thaniyath Faculty of Medicine, University of Tabuk, Tabuk, Kingdom of Saudi Arabia

Vijay Viswanathan M. V. Hospital for Diabetes and Prof. M. Viswanathan Diabetes Research Centre (WHO Collaborating Centre for Research, Education and Training in Diabetes), Chennai, India

Ajaz Ahmad Waza Centre of Research for Development, University of Kashmir, Srinagar, Kashmir, India

Mohammad Zubair Department of Medical Microbiology, Faculty of Medicine, University of Tabuk, Tabuk, Kingdom of Saudi Arabia

Part I

World Preview

Diabetic Foot Complications in Asia and European Continents

1

Shamina Begum, Mohammad Zubair, Marai M. Alamri, Fohad Mabood Husain, Farha Fatima, Mohammad Oves, Mohammad Azam Ansari, and Iftekhar Hassan

1.1 Introduction

Diabetic Foot Ulcer (DFU) is a major global concern accounting for costly complications. Its prevalence is gaining momentum particularly in Asia and European Continents. The intent of this chapter is to provide an overview of diabetic foot ulcer both globally and regionally. It also provides insights on the social and economic burden along with the factors that cause it. Different ways of diagnosis of DFU are also described followed by the management strategy which can be implemented for achieving improved health outcomes. This chapter focuses on the regional wise

S. Begum · M. Zubair (✉)
Department of Medical Microbiology, Faculty of Medicine, University of Tabuk, Tabuk, Kingdom of Saudi Arabia

M. M. Alamri
Department of Surgery, Faculty of Medicine, University of Tabuk, Tabuk, Kingdom of Saudi Arabia

F. M. Husain
Department of Food Science and Nutrition, College of Food and Agriculture Sciences, King Saud University, Riyadh, Kingdom of Saudi Arabia

F. Fatima
Department of Zoology, Faculty of Life Science, Aligarh Muslim University, Aligarh, India

M. Oves
Center of Excellence in Environmental Studies, King Abdul Aziz University, Jeddah, Kingdom of Saudi Arabia

M. A. Ansari
Department of Epidemic Disease Research, Institute for Research and Medical Consultations (IRMC), Imam Abdulrahman Bin Faisal University, Dammam, Kingdom of Saudi Arabia

I. Hassan
Department of Zoology, College of Science, King Saud University, Riyadh, Kingdom of Saudi Arabia

M. Zubair et al. (eds.), *Diabetic Foot Ulcer*,
https://doi.org/10.1007/978-981-15-7639-3_1

comparison of Asia and European Continents concerning the adequate treatment and prevention of DFU. As per the International Diabetes Federation [1], the annual estimation of the foot ulcer ranged from 9.1 million to 26.1 million people, globally. The diabetic proportion and the foot ulcer history are understandably higher as compared to the individual ratio of an active ulcer, i.e., 3.1–11.8%. This percentage accounts for the global population of about 12.9 million to 49 million [2]. The foot ulcer lifetime incidence is predicted to be 15–25% among diabetes. The complication of diabetic food includes Charcot neuroarthropathy (CN), amputation, and ulceration. The complications of the foot are substantially increasing, which is predicted to be more than 5% of the diabetic patients will have foot ulcer history, while the overall lifetime concerning the risk of foot ulceration might exceed 25%. Given that the overall amputation ratio is preceded by foot ulcers, it can be safely presumed that the success in the mitigation of the incidence concerning foot ulcers would reduce the occurrence of amputation.

1.1.1 Foot Ulceration Pathogenesis

The ulcer of the foot occurs rarely due to a single pathology, instead, its major occurrence is due to its interaction with either two or more contributory causes that cause a high-risk foot breakdown. For instance, the neuropathic foot ulceration does not lead to spontaneous ulceration. It occurs due to insensitivity combination including in either extrinsic (such as barefoot walking, step on the sharp object, and inadequate fit of the shoes) or intrinsic factors (such as insensitivity and callus among the patients, who walks and which leads to the ulcer development), leading to ulceration [3]. The most significant contributory cause in the ulceration pathway is neuropathy.

1.1.2 Neuropathy

For the past many years, the link between the autonomic and somatic neuropathy as well as foot ulceration has been identified. The prospective follow-up researches in the previous decades have confirmed the somatic neuropathy causative role. The risk is sevenfold among the patients that suffer from a loss in the sensory ability, leading to the development of the ulcer in the foot in contrast to the patients with non-neuropathic diabetes. The inadequate balance, as well as instability, are substantially recognized as the challenging peripheral neuropathy, which is presumably secondary for the proprioceptive loss [4].

The dysfunction of the peripheral autonomic (sympathetic) makes the skin dry along. It, in the peripheral vascular disease, results in a warm foot with distended dorsal foot veins. This increases the difficulties concerning the education of the patient given the recognized fact that each foot problem develops as a result of vascular disease. This makes it challenging for the patients to identify that their warm feet, which is pain-free are at an increasing unperceived trauma risk, which subsequently results in foot ulceration [5]. In case, the preventive programs concerning the education of being planned, it is necessary to dedicate substantial attention to the effective and careful neuropathy development, leading to understandable terms.

Practically, the simple clinical examination can lead to easy documentation of the peripheral neuropathy for obtaining the neuropathy evidence. In it, the most significant process is to remove the socks and shoes of the patients and examine the feet closely. The tools, for instance, the neuropathy disability scorecard or the monofilament can be used to assists in the identification of the neuropathic foot [3] that can be used for the neuropathic evidence. Also, to identify the increased risk of the foot, there is no need to conduct comprehensive testing through a survey or using electrophysiology.

1.1.3 Peripheral Vascular Disease

The peripheral ischemia, which occurs from the disease of proximal arterial, is identified as a component that occurs in the pathway for the foot ulceration, accounts for the third in all patients [3]. Whereas, the details concerning the ischemic foot are that the feet are dry, red, as well as neuropathic. These characteristics further increase its susceptibility to its pressure resulting from the footwear type.

1.1.4 Other Risk Factors

The deformity of the foot, primarily the claw toes and the prominent metatarsal heads, which is a well-recognized ulceration risk factor. Likewise, the accumulation of the plantar callus is linked with the sevenfold risk increase in a cross-sectional study, while the patients' follow-up increase showed it occurrence for only callus sites for the neuropathic feet, leading to an infinite increase in the risk. The other risk factors concerning the complication of the diabetic feet include microvascular complications that increase the diabetes duration, plantar foot pressure, peripheral edema, as well as the foot ulcer history or the amputation [3].

The foot ulcer prevention for the identified risk factors is integral, in case, a decrease in the ulcer incidence is required. It is suggested that enhancement of the educational programs and provision of podiatric care on a regular basis can improve early diagnosis of the patients and helps provide the treatment at an initial level. Accordingly, different psychosocial factors are also identified to lead to ulceration incidence. The patient's behavior concerning the ulceration and its risk factors are not based on the risk abstraction definition, but on the risk, a perception held by the patients. Thereby, in case, the patient does not believe that the foot ulcer lies in the neuropathy path to amputation, there lie low prospects concerning following their educational device, leading to an increased risk of developing a foot ulcer. This necessitates introducing different interventions for ensuring adequate care as well as preventive measures. This includes a proper examination of the patient's feet and collecting information concerning neuropathy, vascular disease, deformities, edema, and more.

1.1.5 Ulceration Pathway

The ulceration pathway refers to the combination of one or two risk factors that lead to the development of the foot ulcer among the diabetic patients. Various studies have accounted for the commonest triad of components leading to the diabetic foot breakdown such as trauma (footwear), peripheral neuropathy (insensitivity), deformity (toes clawing, metatarsal head prominence), and more. Mechanical trauma (standing on the nail), as well as neuropathy or the thermal trauma (insensate feet of the patient who use a heating pack), are the common examples of the two-component pathway leading to the ulceration among the diabetic patients [6]. Another common example includes "corn cures" which refers to inadequate chemical use.

1.1.6 Sensory Loss Among the Patients

The neuropathy foot problems can only be reduced, when the clinicians give consideration to the fact that patients who have insensitive feet have lost their ulcer warning signs, such as pain, which requires the patient to make a visit to the doctor [6]. The sensitivity to the pain is integral for the patient to lead to various medical consultations, including the training and healthcare-oriented toward the deliverance of relief from the foot ulcer. Therefore, the training should be integrated for the clinicians to help assist in providing treatment to the patient with no pain sensation.

1.1.7 Charcot Neuroarthropathy

The occurrence of Charcot neuroarthropathy (CN) is reported for the patients who are at a loss concerning the sensation, autonomic dysfunction (i.e., increase in the blood flow as well as the dry skins) following by the trauma (unperceived by the patient) [6, 7]. The common risk factor indicated CN is the warm foot which has bounding pulses though there exists sensation loss. The patient presents with a swollen foot, unilateral warm, either with or without pain symptoms, as well as discomfort with proper circulation, is required to be assessed for Charcot neuroarthropathy. Its risk can be reduced with proper care and instigation of educational interventions.

1.2 Overview of the Diabetic Foot Ulcer (DFU)

Primarily, diabetic foot ulcer is identified as the most prevalent problem among the diabetic patients, with an annual incidence percentage of 2.2% on average [8]. Despite taking all the corrective measures for preventing the DFU, the occurrence of DFU can cause substantial complications in the form of infection, amputations, as well as death. Prompers [9] stated that the occurrence of infection among the diabetic foot ulcer is present among the 58% of the patients who present a new foot ulcer. An earlier European study of Prompers [10] showed that about 5% of the diabetic patients had DFU, where a major amputation was required in 1 year. Another research on the European states presents that the mortality rates for the next 5 years concerning the diabetic foot ulcer, which is 45% high for the neuropathic ulcers, along with 55% high for the ischemic ulcers [8].

The predicted and actual percentage concerning the diabetic foot ulcer showed similar and at times worst statistics for various common tumor types, which include the breast, prostate, and colon [11–13]. The incidence of the diabetic foot ulcer is prevalent across the world, leading to severe economic consequences for not only patients but their families as well as the society at large. Boulton et al. [14] presented The Lancet article and wrote that the occurrence of the diabetic foot ulcer is probably of neuropathic origin. Since a major part of the occurred foot ulcer is the potential of neuropathic origin, these are extremely preventable for the developing regions, which frequently report the incidence of Type 2 diabetes for the next 20 years. Boulton et al. [14], in his paper, stated that "*Individuals that are at an increasing ulceration risk could be identified easily through the instigation of careful examination, education as well as the frequent follow-up.*" It is stated that the foot care problem continues to prevail for the former Soviet countries, though the development of the multidisciplinary foot clinic is becoming more commonplace. Figure 1.1 presents the pathway concerning the physical foot ulcers and the different factors associated with it.

Understanding the economic impact and burden of the diabetic foot ulcer, it is necessary to study the recurrence rates of foot ulcers. The present recurrent rates, as presented by Boulton et al. [14], are less than 50% subsequent to 3 years. This recurrence rate is substantial for the determination of the economic impact posed by the foot ulcer [15]. The cost associated with the diabetic foot disease does not only comprise of the immediate cost but also cost in the form of home care and ulcers (subsequently). For understanding the total resource required, a broader view should

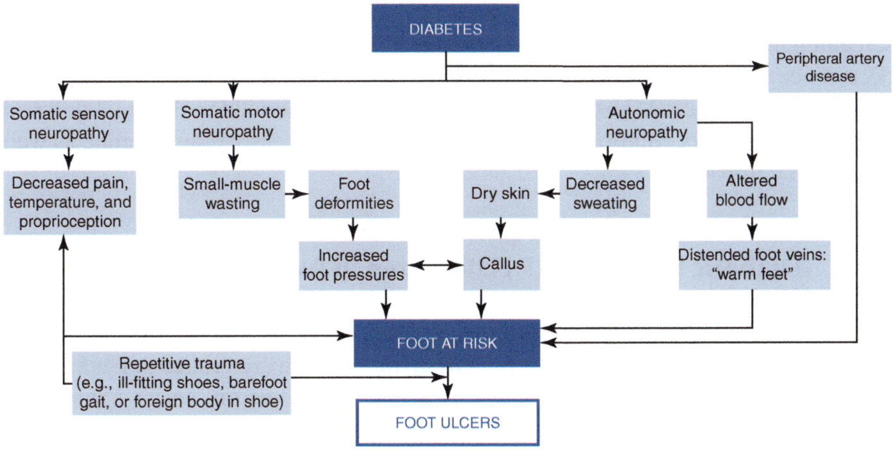

Fig. 1.1 Pathways to diabetic foot ulceration [15]

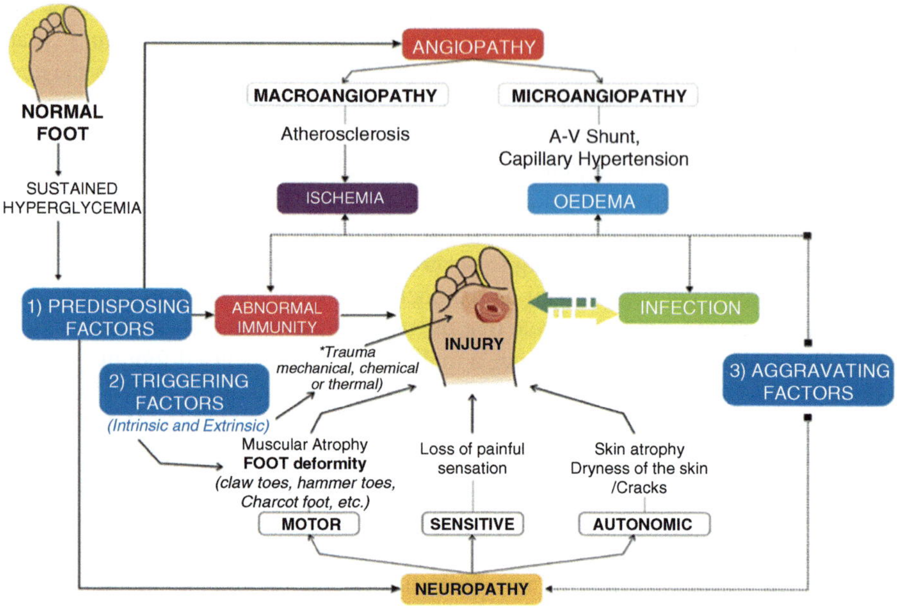

Fig. 1.2 **Diabetic foot ulcer common pathway for occurrence and recurrence**: *Risk factors and predisposing factors for the development of diabetic foot ulcers (DFUs). There are two main protagonists among the risk factors and/or predisposing factors of DFUs: angiopathy and neuropathy, whose presence, together with intrinsic (foot deformity) and/or extrinsic triggers, such as trauma (mechanical, chemical, or thermal), causes the loss of skin integrity. Aggravating factors, such as ischemia, abnormal immunity, and neuropathy, favor the development of DFU infections* [16]

be gathered comprising of the increasing quality of life and the ultimate outcome. This recurrence rate can be reduced through the instigation of the frequent screening as well as patient education which leads to a decrease in the expenditure and the screening healthcare costs. Figure 1.2 presents the overall procedure involved in the occurrence and reoccurrence of the diabetic foot ulcer. Majorly, the occurrence of the diabetic foot ulcer is based on the different factors that lead to the breakdown of the skin. The factors comprise of the sequelae related to sensory, autonomic, as well as motor neuropathies.

1.2.1 Diabetic Foot Ulcer (DFU) Burden in Asia

The data concerning the problems of diabetic foot ulcers in Asia are scarce. Such as the report of the International Working Group on the footcare clinics in China show that there are only five specialist foot care clinics in the region, where none offers podiatry services. The increase in the amputations remains a major and interesting area in the diabetic foot ulcer. Accordingly, another country such as India comprises of the more diabetic population as compared to other countries, where the occurrence of amputations is quite frequent [14]. The most primary cause of foot ulceration is its late diagnosis and is generally associated with gross infection and neuropathy. Concerning a wide overview of the continent, diabetic foot problems are substantially scared. Other causes related to the increasing cost of diabetic patients is related to the barefoot gait, which is quite frequent, where the traditional healer or the elders in the village are contacted for help.

In contrast to the other Asian countries that have a link with the Europeans, a small degree of inclination is observed for education and training. For instance, the Netherland team comprising the podiatrist's teams, surgeons, and diabetologists help deliver information as well as care concerning the diabetic foot ulcer patients in Jakarta. Another study in Canada, which used the diabetes population risk tool showed that diabetes development is at a higher risk in South Asia as compared to any other region. Another research further showed that the diabetic disease rate of prevalence for the South Asian patients is predicted to be four times high as compared to any other ethnic group [17]. Similarly, across the globe, the number of patients with diabetes is estimated to have escalated from 171 million in the year 2000 to 366 million until the year 2030 [18]. These figures are further expected to increase by 2030, which for India is expected to be 46 million, for Pakistan it is 14 million, whereas, for Bangladesh, it is 11.1 million [19].

1.2.2 Diabetic Foot Ulcer (DFU) Burden in European Continents

Despite the implementation of various international guidelines for the prevention of diabetic foot ulcers along with the establishment of the substantial multidisciplinary foot clinics, the disparity in clinical care is evident [4]. For instance, there are only a few countries in East Europe which have foot clinics or podiatry services. Also, in the UK, a community-based study showed that its patients that are at risk of ulceration are predicted to be further diagnosed as a result of a simple clinical test, which includes screening strategies implication for the developing countries. In the Soviet countries, difficulties related to the care are also present, although the multidisciplinary foot clinic is further becoming a common part of the large cities across different European countries. Boulton et al. [14] have reported that the provision of the best foot care is available at the Baltic state.

The provision of adequate care for the European countries is also integral given the increasing cases of diabetes with about 55 million people, where the risk of developing diabetic ulcers prevails in about eight million people. The burden of the diabetic ulcer on the European countries because of the unsuccessful DFU treatment which causes about 450,000 lower limb amputations that account for health authorities' costs of about EUR 2–2.5 billion [20]. The diabetic foot ulcer management is substantially costly for the countries. For instance, Marion Kerr carried out a detailed investigation concerning the care cost associated with the foot complication in diabetic patients. The report findings stated that diabetic patients with low risk of ulcers require the regular change in the dressing as well as visits to the orthotics, podiatry, as well as the hospital in case the condition becomes worst. The cost computed in England for managing such conditions is found to be £325 million. In case, the condition becomes worst, and patient's hospitalization is required then the annual cost is about £213 million, where the cost of amputation is more, which ultimately leads to the total cost of management to vary across £639 to £662 million in England.

Various collaborative studies in the European countries such as one from Manchester, Athens, Antwerp, and Rome have shown no substantial difference for the patients at the hospitals and diabetic clinics concerning the determination of the foot lesion risk factors including neuropathy prevalence as well as of the peripheral vascular disease [15]. These findings highlight that foot prevention similar strategies should be instigated for the delivery of effective care across the European countries. Likewise, another research on the three districts of the UK supported that active foot ulcer is found among type 2 diabetic patients along with 5% of the population that have had an ulcer. Another research on the large community-based report endorsed that incidence rate concerning the foot ulcer is 2% on an annual basis, which is comparable to the primary care delivery of the foot ulcer in the Netherlands. A significant finding of the community study is that the simple tests help identify the ulceration risk, where the modified neuropathy disability score, i.e., a dichotomous variable composite score, is the best for prediction of the ulcer risk.

Concerning the ethnic minority in the region, the data is found to be interesting. For instance, the risks for the diabetic foot ulcer among the Asian and African Caribbean's is much lower as compared to the other minorities [15]. The findings in France also report an increase for the diabetic foot ulcer, where the clinic in Paris reported the inpatient's stays of the patients decline following the multidisciplinary foot care team establishment. The difference in the amputation rates is observed to vary across Europe, which generally shows a reduction in the success of the amputation rates. Despite the unchanged increase in Germany, the diabetic foot ulcer reports provide an optimistic result for the Netherland as well as Italy. This amputation reduction might be associated with the International Consensus implementation consequences for the diabetic foot in Tuscany. The podiatry service increase might also be linked to the amputation reduction in the Netherlands.

1.3 Factors for Diabetic Foot Diseases in Asia and European Continents

1.3.1 Poverty and Hygiene

Another factor that leads to the occurrence of diabetic foot ulcer is poverty. Most studies reported that the link of poverty with the unhygienic conditions lead to infectious sequelae. The other primary factors include the occurrence of diabetic foot ulcers which comprise walking barefoot or late diagnosis of the diabetic foot for initial clinical assessment. For the developing countries such as Asia, the difference in urban–rural life continues to prevail, where the Western lifestyle is being deployed along with the change in the behavior concerning the rural conditions.

Such as reflecting on the Asian countries, for instance, Sri Lanka, Nepal, India, Samoa, Thailand, the Solomon Islands, and more, where more than 50% of the national population in the rural areas has diabetes [21]. Accordingly, recent statistics, for instance, in India and China [22–24] the prevalence of diabetes is found to be greater for the rural area as compared to the urban area. Another research concerning the Hwang et al. [25] through its multiple surveys has shown that the diabetes prevalence was fivefold more from 1985 to 2010, among the developing countries' rural population [26].

Barefoot walking is a common practice across different rural areas in Asia. Such as in the rural areas, the outhouses are located at a substantially considerable distance at the dwelling places, leading to foot injuries due to walking barefoot. Similarly, the lack of hygiene leads to other factors which cause diabetic foot ulcer. For instance, these individuals have a lack of awareness concerning the risk factor or the preventive measures which can be achieved through a better education level. Precisely, in the rural areas of the region, foot injuries often occur due to the house rate and other rodents [14]. For the peripheral neuropathy diabetic patients, these injuries are often not noticed until the patient starts observing symptoms [27]. These patients then present such injuries to the clinics for foot care with the injury or ulcer that has been progressed to fulminating foot sepsis.

Another care that must be taken care of includes occlusive footwear, which causes sweating and can lead to the occurrence of the fungal infection [28], especially for tropical countries. Dorresteijn et al. [29] writes that to prevent foot ulcer occurrence, the individuals must wear the prescribed footwear which does not usually wear at home, where these individuals are more active. Messenger et al. [30] report that the mortality ratio for the low-income countries is substantially high with increased hospitalization ratio. Therefore, in order to reduce the occurrence ratio, it is integral that caregivers must provide the patients with the information necessary for meeting the adequate level of hygiene along with the proper procedure for ensuring its adequate care. One primary thing that the diabetic patients need to ensure, in the words of Boulton et al. [14], is:

> *The two golden rules of prevention are regular foot inspection and not walking barefoot.*

1.3.2 Sociocultural Practices

Different sociocultural practices continue to affect the foot ulceration prevalence across different countries. For instance, the sociocultural practices, i.e., walking barefoot, religious practices, improper use of footwear, and inadequate knowledge concerning foot care can lead to an increase in the foot complications prevalence across Asia [31]. Other causes of the foot ulcer include stress, smell leading social isolation, as well as decreased mobility of the patients. Accordingly, the awareness concerning adequate foot care is also lacking among the Asian countries, with incomplete information of the foot care, including foot protection, and limited self-care practices. Various Asian studies have expressed that most of the patients do not refer to healthcare due to fear and related healthcare factors. This includes the fear of contact with the healthcare nurses and professionals who are consulted for determining the glucose level in the blood, dressing of the wounds, and procedure for collecting the data. These fairs could be overcome through the provision of a better and organized diabetic clinic focused on providing adequate health education, availability of cheap drugs, as well as accessibility and opening hours [32].

Other sociocultural factors that serve as a risk include believes which the people hold, generally in the developing countries, toward illness and health. These beliefs are generally related to individual as well as nature-related factors infused together with the social factors, and few cases related to the supernatural factors. Whereas, in the European countries, the healthcare sectors were referred to when required. This indicates the stark difference among the population of the two regions [33, 34]. Studies suggest that the focus of the non-westerners is mainly on the social and supernatural spheres, where the first contact point includes family, friends, relatives, and traditional healers. Whereas, in comparison to the western countries, particularly Europeans, the focus is on the individual characteristics as well as nature, following the consultation with the profession [33, 34].

1.3.3 Ignorance

Lack of awareness of the diabetic foot ulcer refers to another factor for its occurrence. Particularly in the developing countries of Asia, various diabetic foot burden is observed, where the prevalence of other socioeconomic factors leads to its hindrance. This also includes the lack of integration of their foot care into their lives. Such as the finding of the earlier study showed that diabetic patients who do not practice foot care are at a 2.52% increased risk of developing foot ulcers as compared to those who do. Similar findings are observed across different countries in Asia, including Kenya, Ethiopia, Arbaminch, India, Mekele, and more [35, 36]. The self-care practice can also lead to a reduction in diabetic foot ulcer development because of the benefits it provides. This includes washing of the feet on the regular basis, following by the drying of feet appropriately, status evaluation of the foot on a regular basis, adequate circulation as well as proper management of the abnormality at an earlier age that can occur on the foot. Thereby, for the prevention of the diabetic patient foot ulcer, preventive measures, and proper care of the feet should be maintained.

1.3.4 Environment and Other Related Factors

There are various environments as well as other related risk factors that can lead to the development of foot ulcers among diabetic patients. Different factors are found to be associated with the increase in the ulceration risk, which are generally linked to the economic development in the region, along with urbanization [37]. Different dietary patterns, individuals' sedentary behavior, as genetic background, epigenetic susceptibility, as well as obesity, are found to increase the prospects of foot complications among the diabetic patients. Concerning the history of the Asians and the studies conducted on them, it is found that the majority had undergone some sort of nutritional transition, increase in the refined carbohydrates consumption, animal fats, meats, as well as low intake of the dietary fibers as well as vegetables [38]. Similar practices are observed in terms of intake of the sugar-sweetened beverages in China as well as European countries, as provided by the recent statistics and behavior [39]. Various risk factors concerning the diet can be significantly related to Asians. For instance, the diet of the South Asians, substantially depends on the increased carbohydrate consumptions, along with saturated fats and Trans fats [40], which is substantially conducive to the development of the foot complications. For instance, early studies in China have shown that the people who consume the extensive amount of white rice have increased level of glycemic load, linked with the diabetes risks [40, 41]. The similar findings are noted for the diabetic care of the patients who consume white rice in India [41]. Despite rice being recognized as the staple food item for centuries, however, the shift is observed to occur among the traditional rice types (such as polished rice), which increase the glycemic excursion as compared to the offering of a traditional rice type. Conclusively, it is found that increased glycemic excursion exists for Asians as compared to other population groups.

Another factor identified includes physical inactivity. In many populations, the risk factor in T2DM is physical inactivity [42]. Specifically, in the occupational setting, the decline has been observed in physical activity because of increasing urbanization [43], along with the sedentary behavior, which has also risen. To prevent diabetes in large communal areas such as Asia and the Pacific, this research highlights the significance of encouraging physical activities and minimizes sedentary behavior. In this study, the researchers examined the multiethnic cohorts and observe the relationship between diabetes and adiposity, researchers comparing with Europids, Asian develop diabetes with lower BMI [22, 44]. In the Asian population, this is assumed to visceral adiposity [45]. As a result, lower BMI cutoffs in Asians are being used to describe obesity [46]. Central obesity is defined by the circumference of the lower waist [46, 47]. According to the two observational studies, there is an association between diabetes with increasing adiposity. This condition does not differ between Asian populations and Europid [48]. Thus, there is a traditional difference in the relationship between adiposity-diabetes is probably characterized as a chance for diabetes at each and every level of BMI (waist circumference) or diabetes with a lower level of BMI.

It is seen that diabetes risk in all ages of Asian populations is quite high. Studies highlighted other factors related to age or obesity that raised the awareness regarding diabetes in Asian Population. Many novel putative risk factors have appeared recently as a significant environmental determinant and behavioral for T2DM. Environmental risk due to toxic waste, other chemical, and sleep disturbance are also included. Many developing countries are suffering from pollution issues, during adult life it has the potential to contribute to the diabetes epidemic or sometimes in utero exposure.

According to the observations made by Hales and Barker [49] on the association between the metabolic disturbance and risk of diabetes in adult age with the lower birth weight. The essential role of utero environments in physiology and customized developmental trajectory and this is highly appreciated, thereby modifying the obesity's risk, other chronic diseases, and T2DM in adult age [26]. Likewise, a hypothetical study designed for adulthood utero nutritional deprivation may predispose a person to T2DM [26]. During early life, in some parts of China, it exposed to some serious famine, therefore it becomes the cause to increase the risk of diabetes in adults as compared to those who do not face the extreme nutritional deprivation in utero development.

During midlife, the risk of diabetes is higher among the generations unprotected by utero low nutrition and who are later exposed to the richest diet [50]. The phenomena concerning the condition of undernutrition at the early life followed by environmental exposure to a "metabolically challenging" along with a diet that is highly energizing may lead to the high occurrence of diabetic patients [26]. The emergency rate in Cambodia about T2DM is at the same rate as those developed countries [17]. In 1975, Cambodia faced a severe shortage of food because of the upheaval condition of socioeconomic and politics. Nauruans were exposed to famine conditions during World War II on another Pacific Island and on Nauru such as Truk, where they were relocated. After three-decade, the rate of diabetes prevalence was high in Nauru in the entire world [51]. Due to war and famine, these are unexpected health issues, which were later pursued by overnutrition. Moreover, Yajnik study [52] suggested that India is experiencing the burden of diabetes due to the early developed health issues and epigenetic. In addition, according to the epidemiological studies, there is a link between the offspring risks and utero undernutrition, among the Pima Indians specifically. Exposed to maternal obesity and diabetes there is a high risk of T2DM and obesity in offspring [26, 53]. Comparing with USA and Europe, Asia is also having a high risk of prevalence of GDM and young-onset diabetes [54]. In future generations, there is an increase in the risk of diabetes; therefore, Asia may operate the intergenerational cycle [26].

1.4 Evaluation of Diabetic Foot Infections (DFI)

The understanding of DFI is significant due to its reporting of 1–5% of the foot ulcer among diabetic patients. Countries across the world dedicate a substantial amount of time as well as resources to reduce its occurrence [8]. This requires the patients to be reviewed on a routine basis along with the community podiatry foot protection to provide primary care and nursing. The evaluation of this care is substantially critical as it helps in prevention against the diabetic foot ulcer patient's emergency admission to the hospital, prevention against avoidable amputations, and care delivery.

1.4.1 Evaluation: Physical Examination

The DFI management incepts by examining the medical history of the patients along with their physical examination using laboratory as well as imaging findings. The diabetic patients with foot infection might not integrate the general symptoms and signs of the infection (such as vomiting, nausea, malaise, fever, and anorexia) due to the modifications in the leukocytic immune response [8]. The earliest sign concerning the patient with diabetic foot ulcers is unexplainable hyperglycemia. The physical examination of the patients, either in Asia or Europe, may present the “diabetic flu” symptoms including the anorexia, vomiting, fevers, chills, and nausea, which should prompt close inspection for the ulcer foot or infectious signs. This examination should be closely linked to the ulcer size, its depth, odor, drainage, or the margins. The suspiciousness concerning the osteomyelitis should occur based on a close examination of the erythrocyte sedimentation rate of below 70 mm/h, ulcer >2 cm^2, positive probe for testing the bone, and the abnormal radiographic findings including the cortical disruption. The presence of osteomyelitis and its high sensitivity and specificity are based on the bone test probe [8]. The accurate osteomyelitis diagnosis is based on the positive predictive values which range from 53% to 89% along with a positive probe to bone test. Substantially, the probe to bone inability is linked with a negative predictive value of about 98%. The elevation of the extremity should occur for determination of the extremity as to whether the Charcot sets as a base for the erythema stems or the infection. Among the patient’s supine for about 5–10 min, the low extremity should be elevated, while simultaneously observing the erythema resolution, which provides the noninfectious injury. The infection can be clinically diagnosed due to the purulent drainage, or at least the presence of two inflammation signs (i.e., warmth, swelling, erythema, induration, pain, or tenderness).

1.4.2 Evaluation: Laboratory Testing

The evaluation of the patients through laboratory testing is integral to present the infection severity in the quantifiable form, following a response to the treatment. The laboratory finding is required to include the information concerning the patients’ blood count, metabolic panel, C-reactive protein, as well as erythrocyte sedimentation rate. Also, the patient’s nutritional status should also be assessed by collecting prealbumin and albumin. The level of the glucose should also be assessed, as the glycemic control loss occurs at the initial stage of the infection. Also, the imaging modalities are used for the characterization of the bony involvement and the degree of soft tissues affected [8]. For the initial workup of the foot infection in diabetic patients, the plain radiographs are also useful. The radiographic abnormalities should be paid special attention, which includes soft tissue gas, radiopaque foreign bodies, cortical erosion, and periosteal reactions. Also, for assessing the progressive signs, the repetition of the plain radiographs can be held. However, these radiographs are not very sensitive and should be combined with the different modalities for better characterization of the suspected infection [8]. The osteomyelitis evaluation through magnetic resonance imaging (MRI) is found to present good specificity as well as sensitivity. Similarly, in the absence of the MRI, nuclear medicine scans can be used.

1.4.3 Evaluation: Microbiology

Following infection identification, antibiotic therapy requires culture. For this, deep tissue cultures should be attained. It is because these will present more reliable detection of the causative organism as compared to the superficial swabs. The use of these tissues is more reliable for deriving the causative organism in comparison to the superficial swabs. Despite bone cultures being ideal, these assessments of deep soft tissue culture might be beneficial in the detection of the osteomyelitis offending organism [8]. Following its proper evaluation, the IDSA system can be used for the classification of the infection which assists in the selection of the best treatment for improving communication among providers.

1.5 Strategy for Prevention of Diabetic Foot Management

Preventive strategies concerning the management of the diabetic foot are integral. This requires healthcare financers and decision-makers to optimize the resource allocation in an effective way of delivering adequate care quality. This involves funding as well as investing in different programs that help prevent diabetes as well as prevent foot complications among the diabetic patients. The diabetic patient's organization, as well as other advocating the diabetic care change, need to provide arguments that help devise decision for adequate care of the patients reducing the diabetic foot ulcer occurrence. These strategies should be centered on improving the patient's awareness level, where the diabetic ulceration prevention is prioritized, which serves as a substantial healthcare agenda. The preventive strategies also require the partnership of the different industry players, which is not only linked to their valuable contribution for improvement toward their therapeutic care but also facilitates education, research, as well as diabetes awareness programs. From an epidemic perspective, there exists a need for professionals to find a new way of organizing the delivery of the care program and for managing the extensive workload. These preventive strategies require effective working such as shared responsibility, better work management, and improved team work.

1.5.1 Education

For preventing the occurrence of diabetic foot problems, the primary prevention strategy is education. Although this might be particularly targeted for the providers and the patients, the professionals are initially required to understand the significance which the patient's education holds. Once these professionals are educated and trained, they are able to deliver effective patient education. However, the efficiency of the patient's education concerning the education of the treatment and its condition is found to be controversial for diabetic patients with an ulcer. In order to prevent the below-knee amputation and ulceration, the education provision is found to have a low rate of amputation as compared to the patients who are not provided with the education [55]. Delivering education is found to be substantially involved in end-stage renal failure, with substantial self-knowledge improvement [56]. The deliverance of education to the patients makes them aware of the complications, signs, and symptoms of the patients.

This is found by a randomized controlled trial, where the instigation of education as a part of the intervention provided to be extremely beneficial as compared to the control group that was not provided with any education. The reasons highlighted include that the intervention group was involved in practicing foot care as compared to the control group who did not [57]. However, this intervention is not always effective such as Lincoln et al. [58] study using an observer-blinded randomized control design, showed that no difference exists for the two groups in terms of the ulcer incidence at the 6 months along with the amputation rate. Though the difference or no difference might be based on the patient's education that is being delivered or the pedagogical approaches used [59]. Although Kruger and Guthrie [60] reported that didactic teaching produced better results for the hands-on teaching experience.

Another research by Lam et al. [13] indicated that the teaching following the group discussion pattern is also not ideal. Although, diversified findings continue to prevail for the patient's education, various guidelines have prompted the use of the education as an intervention for providing adequate foot care to the patients and the use of adequate footwear [26]. It has strongly been recommended by the international working group to educate the diabetic patients of the footwear and promote self-foot care practices [26]. Similarly, education is required by the professionals comprising of the general practitioners, nurses, doctors, and allied health professionals in the health care sector. Different education materials can be used for improving the education level of the professionals, which help in providing necessary training to the professionals. Table 1.1 below provides information about the sources that could be used for training and teaching the students. This includes the use of different websites, guidelines, as well as books, which can easily be accessed by professionals. However, the primary focus of this education should be on the patients and their caregivers, who are at risk of developing a foot ulcer. This education can be provided into three domains related to care for the foot, care for diabetes mellitus, and lastly the footwear choice. It is because earlier researches in the same domain have found that the aspect concerning diabetes mellitus is not well understood as well as well managed.

Often, the level of glycated hemoglobin (HbA1c) is high among the patients, i.e., at about 10.0% or more. Previous research in 2014 on the multidisciplinary team effectiveness on its efficiency to treat the diabetic foot found that about 45% of the

Table 1.1 Materials for professional education

Professional education	Patients education
Books • Clinical care of the diabetic foot, Armstrong [62] • Diabetic foot problems, Nather • Levin and O'Neal's the diabetic foot, Bowker and Pfeifer [63] • The diabetic foot, Nather [64] • Surgery for diabetic foot: a practical operative manual, Nather [65] *Websites* • International Diabetes Federation (https://www.idf.org) • American Diabetes Association (http://www.diabetes.org) • Centers for Disease Control and Prevention (https://www.cdc.gov/diabetes) *Guidelines* • IWGDF guidance on the management and prevention of foot problems in diabetes 2015 • Diabetic foot problems: prevention and management, NICE guideline 2015 • Best practice guideline for ASEANPlus: management of diabetic foot wounds • 2012 Infectious Diseases Society of America clinical practice guideline for the diagnosis and treatment of diabetic foot infections	*Books* Type 2 diabetes basics, International Diabetes Center [61] Websites American Diabetes Association DiabetesPro Patient Education Library (https://professional.diabetes.org/content/patient-education-library) diabetic living (http://www.diabeticlivingonline.com)

patient among the total of 206 patients found that the HbA1c level of the patients was more than 10.0% [26]. Thus, the education initiatives introduced should first be centered on providing necessary awareness and education to the patients related to the management of diabetes, foot care, exercise, diet as well as medication. This should be followed by foot hygiene awareness and knowledge. Accordingly, patients must be educated on adequate footwear use. These materials generally include online reading material, as well as books [26, 66]. Other materials that could be used for the education of the patient include the offering of the education pamphlets. These pamphlets should include information concerning the "Happy Feet," "Knowing Diabetes," as well as "Patients" Guide for "Footwear."

1.5.2 Foot Care and Screening

The basics of care for the good foot in the individuals affected with diabetes include sufficient observation and the chances to apply the messages for the self-care and routine observation of foot [67]. The observation of Foot by physicians must emphasize the existence of peripheral arterial disease (PAD), peripheral neuropathy, former ulceration and unusual anatomy of the foot, all of this can forecast individuals at higher chances to develop the foot ulcers [67]. For instance, the routine checkups of the diabetic foot by an expert and professionally trained person must involve the following steps, i.e., foot examination, which includes the observation of the sensation of foot by the help of a tuning fork or a10-g monofilament, foot pulses' palpation, assessment of the deformity of foot along with the footwear. It realizes aspects which predispose the complexities of foot complications to offer the knowledge and, if needed, to intervene for the prevention of these issues. Realization of pre-existing complexities that can need the cure. Focus on the significance of observation of the foot and spreading awareness for the examination of your own feet. Identification of common medical issues, for example, the existence of PAD that will highlight more common vascular pathology.

It is controversial to say that the effect of foot screening may reduce the risk of foot wounds in diabetic patients. Lavery et al. [68] the combinations of education and foot screening try to minimize the frequency of amputation by 47.4% ($p < 0.05$), and also minimizes the length of stay of inpatient by 21.7% ($p < 0.05$). however, according to the retrospective case-control study, in which 61 Pima Indians were included with prior amputation, and 183 were included without Prior amputation. Mayfield et al. [69] the risk of amputation cannot be minimized by taking one of more foot care screening ($p = 0.31$), more relevant researches are required. Moreover, outcomes may affect the frequency of foot screening. More researches are required to examine the effect of different occupied frequencies. In our clinic every diabetic patient has to go through the foot and eye screening test on a yearly basis, heart, and kidney screening as well [70]. According to the primary health care level, in Singapore, a strategy is planned by the Ministry of Health about the diagnosis of diabetes as early as possible.

1.5.2.1 Patient Care Pathway for a Screening of Patients for Diabetic Foot Complications

All diabetic patients attending diabetes clinics are referred for screening tests for feet. The nurse who is running the clinic will ensure that the screening takes place and GP is assigned to patients accordingly [6].

1.5.2.1.1 Screening Level 1: Initial Assessment

By podiatrists, all the patients are gone through by vascular and neurological assessments using the Doppler ultrasound and monofilament, in specific form DH 140 findings are recorded. If the patient is clear with diseases and certified normal then the patient has referred again to the diabetes clinic with a yearly appointment.

1.5.2.1.2 Screening Level 2: Further Assessment

In Floriana Health Center, patients who have done their level one screening are having vascular and neuropathic problems, such patients are recommended for further in-depth screening. More tests were done to identify pathological issues with afoot. The follow-up will be continued in Floriana Health center and advise is given to patients by experts. On the other hand, patients are referred for third level screening when they are diagnosed with vascular pathology.

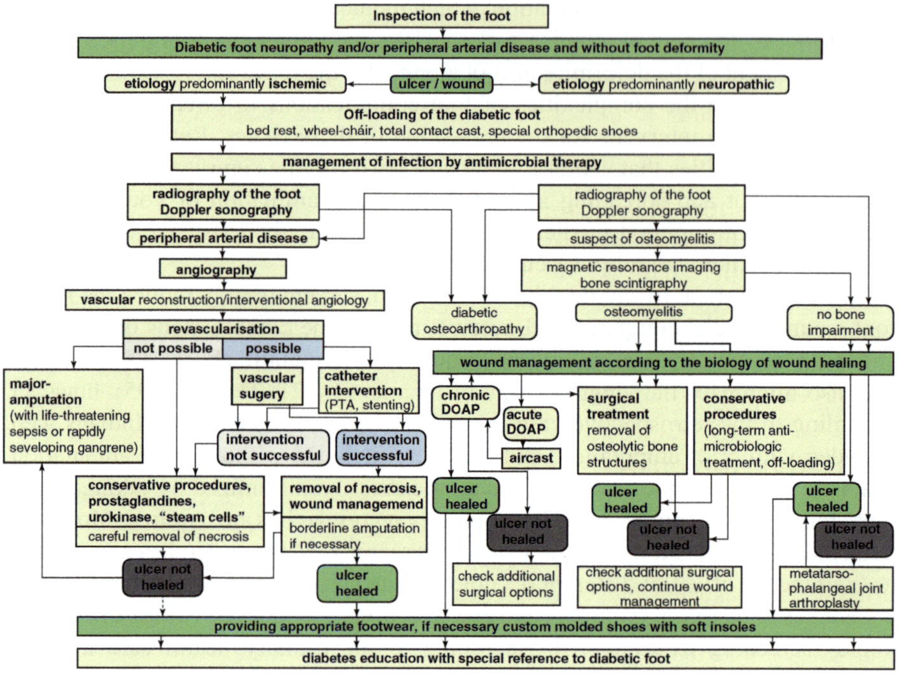

Fig. 1.3 Clinical pathway of diagnosis and treatment of diabetic foot in the structured health care group [71]

1.5.2.1.3 Screening Level 3: Assessment with Vascular Surgeon

This level of screening is generally held at the hospital where a vascular surgeon is present, who is approached for providing consultation.

The algorithm that is used for the education of the diabetic foot complication is presented in Fig. 1.3.

1.5.2.1.4 Algorithm for Diabetic Foot Complications Screening

This clinical pathway presented in Fig. 1.3 is used for the clinical audit. This pathway is found to be effective for the identification of the early cases concerning the vascular and neuropathic pathology. This accounts for the early treatment of the patients using different intervention tools. This pathway enables the practitioners to improve the patient's quality of life, which also assists them to sustain an adequate glycaemia control.

1.5.2.2 Clinical Screening Tests

1.5.2.2.1 Sensation

The two basic methods for the detection of sensory loss linked with foot ulcer risk are the 10-g monofilament, vibration perception having a tuning fork of 128-Hz and the Ipswich Touch Test. The most commonly used is the 10-g monofilament [72, 73]. By the use of a 128-Hz tuning fork or a 10-g monofilament is not without the restrictions, usually, the error in the operation or poor methods, for example hard hit of the tuning fork, means that it will be heard and will alert the receiving person.

1.5.2.2.2 The 10-g Monofilament

The 10-g monofilament was basically created to test the loss of sensors in the hands of individuals affected by leprosy. Monofilaments friendly in use yet there are a few aspects for the wrong usage; a 10-g monofilament that is inserted against the skin will call up the coarse light touch [67]. It is essential to understand that not all accessible 10-g monofilaments will provide a 10-g force.

1.5.3 Government Intervention

The prevention of diabetic foot ulcers can occur across different regulatory channels in both developing and developed countries. For instance, across Asia and Europe, different national campaigns, and funding programs can be introduced for reducing the diabetic foot ulcer. The program DESMOND (Diabetes Education and Self-management for Ongoing and Newly Diagnosed) has been executed in the UK to provide care since 2003 [74]. The instigation of such a program has substantially affected the glycemic control, along with the provision of a better understanding concerning the patient's diabetes mellitus. Several studies have emphasized the significance of government intervention as a national scale preventive tool, which enables improved foot care status among diabetic patients reducing foot complications. For instance, the efforts of the Ministry of Health in Singapore are noteworthy, where they declared war on diabetes [26]. In its efforts, it introduced two different ministerial task forces, where the first task was related to Diabetes Prevention and Care, while the second task was more focused on promoting a healthy lifestyle. These initiatives are required to be long and sustainable. These government interventions are not only required to cater to the diabetes problem but also assist mitigating the complication as well as other related chronic diseases, including ischemic heart disease, stroke, hypertension, as well as renal impairment.

1.5.4 Cost-Effectiveness of Prevention

The preventive measures central at reducing the complication are not only integral for improved foot health but also for reducing the economic burden. It has been emphasized by the Markov model that the cost-utility analysis is critical [14]. It emphasizes that the instigation of the intensive preventions could assist in reducing the occurrence probability for the amputations and foot ulcers by 25%. This strategy would be effective in terms of cost-effectiveness for all the diabetic patients unless they comprise of specific risk factors. It is because these prevention measures would then be focused on those specific risk factors. Various other researches also confirm these findings. For instance, diabetes foot ulcer's treatment along with its related infections, the amputations below the knee, and the surgeries need the lower limbs revascularize, which account for a substantial diabetic treatment cost [14]. Although, these complications are found to frequently occur, vary few researchers have provided the division of the care in the primary prevention or the secondary preventive measures, which are generally infused together in a single term called secondary preventive measures. This is done for ensuring adequate health and lower incidence of ulceration [75]. However, the use of the primary prevention measures is integral for ensuring adequate health of the patients.

The use of the Markov model for predicting the transition of the patient from one condition to another is observed, with an understanding that this transition is based on the present condition and not the past, where these exist for a continuum. The transition example includes the change in the state of the patient from that of an untreated patient, to treated and then the final outcomes (such as cure, amputation, or death, where the last is an unescapable outcome). There is a need to apply both secondary as well as primary preventive measures at all levels which help reduce the risk among the patients (ranging from low to high), which helps reduce the overall cost. Such as the diabetic foot ulceration is decreased with the 10% (0.90 RR), which cost an individual about $50 per person and would require a greater than 90% probability for amputation reduction (i.e., about $39K) for the diabetic patients. This cost is either equal or lower than that of the standard care, in comparison to the provision of no preventive care. This also provides a reduction of patient's risk from the previous care costs which cost a patient about $125.

The small number of projects are formulated to eradicate or decrease the troubles of DFUs. This is rather due to the acknowledged effects of DFUs on the needs of disconnections, enhancing the expenses of healthcare, and the total lifestyle quality. The scarcity of these projects, even in huge centers of academic healthcare, can be associated with the idea of an exact shortcoming of advantages in the economic aspects. The researchers are in between the far and few, and former models of Markov have not elaborated on the chances for the total savings, where the cost efficiencies are not been represented. The variance in the research from the prior offerings is that one observed the varying levels of success (risk elimination which ranges from 5% to 25%) and allocating the expenses to all and determine a potential threshold of rates to determine the requirement for the measures of prevention. One significant restriction defined by the writers was splitting the patients of low risk from the patients of moderate-to high-risk that can be the reason behind the population having a higher risk to overlook the favor because of the enhanced preventing expense. A complete assessment of the total population will have been warranted to facilitate and support the best usage to prevent diabetic foot ulcers and the following complexities. There is a definite requirement to motivate preventive projects as a way to decline the higher expenses of care.

Several serious and expensive complexities influence the patients of diabetes. It includes the diseases of heart, failure of kidney, blindness, and complexities of the foot. The issues of the foot are usual, threats the life of an individual, and place a higher burden in the financial aspects on the industry of healthcare, individuals with diabetes along with the families, and the community as well. Each year, greater than one million individuals suffer from lower limb amputation as a result of diabetes. This shows a remarkable issue from the aspect of the economy, specifically if the outcomes of amputation in the extended hospitalization, healing, and an enhanced requirement for the social facilities and home care. In developed states, the long-term (3 years) expenses linked with the starting amputations are anticipated to be as greater as almost approximately US$64,000. This anticipation does not include the indirect expenses as a result of the loss of efficiency, any incurred expenses by an individual affected with diabetes and the person in their family providing the care, and involves no computation to overlook the quality of life. The decline of these expenses, as well as the improved quality of life of individuals affected with diabetes, will need intense care and knowledge to make the results for the health. To invest in the foot care of diabetes and the prevention projects might be one of the most cost-efficient types of the expense of healthcare, offering the project which is target-oriented and applied appropriately. There are a number of reasons for the issues of diabetic foot problems.

1.6 Geographic Differences in Clinical Outcome

A substantial difference exists concerning the clinical outcome of the patients across similar countries [76–78]. Several studies have suggested that few patients are being managed considerably well as compared to the others in different countries. This might be because of the lack of emphasis on the clinical space in a certain region as compared to the others [76, 79]. This lack of emphasis might be in the form of training and education intervention introduced for adequate health care and management for the patients as well as a medical staff [76]. This necessitates the need to employ the internationally recognized care components, as well as standard pathways for the referral in general care practices as well as specialized. These principles are generally published by institutes such as National Institute for Health and Care Excellence [80], and International Working Group on the Diabetic Foot [81], though the monitoring of the professional adherence to these practices is not ensured.

1.7 Conclusion

The prevalence of diabetic foot ulcers is found across the world, with substantial economic consequences on a small scale (patients and family) as well as on the large scale (society). When the use of the resource is assessed, the broader use of the resource includes estimating the quality of life along with the final outcome. The primary preventive measure concerning the reduction in the foot complication for diabetic patients across Asia as well as Europe includes the use of aggressive glycemic control for the peripheral neuropathy concerning ulceration in the lower limb or infection. Although at the time, the foot ulceration prevention might not be possible, the prevention of the small ulcer prevention is likely to be feasible, along with sepsis, gangrene, or osteomyelitis.

The chapter also provides insights that education serves as the primary tool for ensuring prevention of the foot ulcer among the patients and is an integral component for the preventive programs. Another potential benefit for using education is it is simple, repetitive as well as dual targeted, for instance, to the patients as well as healthcare workers. Accordingly, the screening of the foot also substantially contributes to the prevention of diabetic foot ulcers. Though, for the prevention to be effective, the government needs to introduce different, effective, prolonged as well as sustainable practices. Similarly, when an education program for the prevention purpose is being formulated, the associated personnel or the healthcare must be considerate toward the fact that individuals are not able to understand the terms such as neuropathy or the foot ulcer.

For instance, the provided education should be tailored as per the understanding of the patient and the social background. Similarly, the focus and the proliferation of the foot care service is required for employing an integrated approach to improve the patient's care outcomes, including disability, mobility, disability as well as mortality. This is necessary for each and every kind of community, such as India and China, where the prevalence of diabetes is found, where the majority of the people reside in rural areas. For this, foot screening practices can be devised, which are not only effective but are also cost-effective for the current healthcare system. Similarly, the chapter provides insights on the issue's guidelines which can help motivate the patients for adequate health of the foot, along with a different educational recommendation.

References

1. Armstrong DG, Boulton AJ, Bus SA (2017) Diabetic foot ulcers and their recurrence. N Engl J Med 376(24):2367–2375
2. Zhang P, Lu J, Jing Y, Tang S, Zhu D, Bi Y (2017) Global epidemiology of diabetic foot ulceration: a systematic review and meta-analysis. Ann Med 49(2):106–116
3. Aumiller WD, Dollahite HA (2015) Pathogenesis and management of diabetic foot ulcers. J Am Acad PAs 28(5):28–34
4. Boulton AJ, Kirsner RS, Vileikyte L (2004) Neuropathic diabetic foot ulcers. N Engl J Med 351(1):48–55
5. Vileikyte L, Rubin RR, Leventhal H (2004) Psychological aspects of diabetic neuropathic foot complications: an overview. Diabetes Metab Res Rev 20(S1):S13–S18
6. Boulton AJ (2006) Diabetic foot complications. Eur Endocrinol (1):51–52. https://doi.org/10.17925/EE.2006.00.01.51
7. Safavi PS, Jupiter DC, Panchbhavi V (2017) A systematic review of current surgical interventions for Charcot neuroarthropathy of the midfoot. J Foot Ankle Surg 56(6):1249–1252
8. Del Core MA, Ahn J, Lewis RB III, Raspovic KM, Lalli TA, Wukich DK (2018) The evaluation and treatment of diabetic foot ulcers and diabetic foot infections. Foot Ankle Orthop 3(3):2473011418788864
9. Prompers L, Huijberts M, Apelqvist J, Jude E, Piaggesi A, Bakker K, Edmonds M, Holstein P, Jirkovska A, Mauricio D, Tennvall GR (2007) High prevalence of ischaemia, infection and serious comorbidity in patients with diabetic foot disease in Europe. Baseline results from the Eurodiale study. Diabetologia 50(1):18–25

10. Prompers L, Schaper N, Apelqvist J, Edmonds M, Jude E, Mauricio D, Uccioli L, Urbancic V, Bakker K, Holstein P, Jirkovska A (2008) Prediction of outcome in individuals with diabetic foot ulcers: focus on the differences between individuals with and without peripheral arterial disease. The EURODIALE Study. Diabetologia 51(5):747–755
11. Jemal A, Ward EM, Johnson CJ, Cronin KA, Ma J, Ryerson AB, Mariotto A, Lake AJ, Wilson R, Sherman RL, Anderson RN (2017) Annual report to the nation on the status of cancer, 1975–2014, featuring survival. J Natl Cancer Inst 109(9):djx030
12. Jupiter DC, Thorud JC, Buckley CJ, Shibuya N (2016) The impact of foot ulceration and amputation on mortality in diabetic patients. I: From ulceration to death, a systematic review. Int Wound J 13(5):892–903
13. Lam K, Van Asten SA, Nguyen T, La Fontaine J, Lavery LA (2016) Diagnostic accuracy of probe to bone to detect osteomyelitis in the diabetic foot: a systematic review. Clin Infect Dis 63(7):944–948
14. Boulton AJ, Vileikyte L, Ragnarson-Tennvall G, Apelqvist J (2005) The global burden of diabetic foot disease. Lancet 366(9498):1719–1724
15. Boulton AJ, Armstrong DG, Kirsner RS, Attinger CE, Lavery LA, Lipsky BA, Mills JL Sr, Steinberg JS (2018) Diagnosis and management of diabetic foot complications. American Diabetes Association, Arlington, VA
16. Ramirez-Acuña JM, Cardenas-Cadena SA, Marquez-Salas PA, Veloz IG, Favila AP, Cid-Baez MA et al (2019) Diabetic foot ulcers: current advances in antimicrobial therapies and emerging treatments. Antibiotics 8(4):193
17. Rosella LC, Mustard CA, Stukel TA, Corey P, Hux J, Roos L, Manuel DG (2012) The role of ethnicity in predicting diabetes risk at the population level. Ethn Health 17(4):419–437
18. Wild S, Roglic G, Green A, Sicree R, King H (2004) Global prevalence of diabetes: estimates for the year 2000 and projections for 2030. Diabetes Care 27(5):1047–1053
19. Waisundara VY, Shiomi N (2018) Diabetes mellitus in South Asia. In: Diabetes and its complications. IntechOpen, London
20. Cordis (2019) Device for diabetic foot ulcers. 2019. Available from: https://cordis.europa.eu/article/id/92892-device-for-diabetic-foot-ulcers
21. Atlas D. International Diabetes Federation (2015) IDF diabetes atlas, 7th edn. Brussels, Belgium, International Diabetes Federation
22. Ramachandran A, Mary S, Yamuna A, Murugesan N, Snehalatha C (2008) High prevalence of diabetes and cardiovascular risk factors associated with urbanization in India. Diabetes Care 31(5):893–898
23. Ramachandran A, Ma RC, Snehalatha C (2010) Diabetes in Asia. Lancet 375(9712):408–418
24. Ma RC, Chan JC (2013) Type 2 diabetes in East Asians: similarities and differences with populations in Europe and the United States. Ann N Y Acad Sci 1281(1):64
25. Hwang CK, Han PV, Zabetian A, Ali MK, Narayan KV (2012) Rural diabetes prevalence quintuples over twenty-five years in low-and middle-income countries: a systematic review and meta-analysis. Diabetes Res Clin Pract 96(3):271–285
26. Nanditha A, Ma RC, Ramachandran A, Snehalatha C, Chan JC, Chia KS, Shaw JE, Zimmet PZ (2016) Diabetes in Asia and the Pacific: implications for the global epidemic. Diabetes Care 39(3):472–485
27. Mishra SC, Chhatbar KC, Kashikar A, Mehndiratta A (2017) Clinical updates: diabetic foot. BMJ 359
28. Thomas J, Jacobson GA, Narkowicz CK, Peterson GM, Burnet H, Sharpe C (2010) Toenail onychomycosis: an important global disease burden. J Clin Pharm Ther 35(5):497–519
29. Dorresteijn JA, Kriegsman DM, Assendelft WJ, Valk GD (2012) Patient education for preventing diabetic foot ulceration. Cochrane Database Syst Rev 10:CD001488
30. Messenger G, Taha N, Sabau S, AlHubail A, Aldibbiat AM (2019) Is there a role for informal caregivers in the management of diabetic foot ulcers? A narrative review. Diabetes Ther 10:2025–2033
31. Mariam TG, Alemayehu A, Tesfaye E, Mequannt W, Temesgen K, Yetwale F, Limenih MA (2017) Prevalence of diabetic foot ulcer and associated factors among adult diabetic patients

who attend the diabetic follow-up clinic at the University of Gondar Referral Hospital, North West Ethiopia, 2016: institutional-based cross-sectional study. J Diabetes Res 2017:1
32. Hjelm K, Beebwa E (2013) The influence of beliefs about health and illness on foot care in Ugandan persons with diabetic foot ulcers. Open Nurs J 7:123
33. Helman C (2007) Culture, health and illness. CRC press, Boca Raton
34. Kleinman A (1980) Patients and healers in the context of culture: an exploration of the borderland between anthropology, medicine, and psychiatry. University of California Press, Berkeley
35. Deribe B, Woldemichael K, Nemera G (2014) Prevalence and factors influencing diabetic foot ulcer among diabetic patients attending Arbaminch Hospital, South Ethiopia. J Diabetes Metab 5(1):1–7
36. Gebrekirstos K, Solomon KG, Fantahun A (2015) Prevalence and factors associated with diabetic foot ulcer among adult patients in Ayder Referral Hospital Diabetic Clinic Mekelle, North Ethiopia, 2013. J Diabetes Metab 6(8)
37. Hu FB (2011) Globalization of diabetes: the role of diet, lifestyle, and genes. Diabetes Care 34(6):1249–1257
38. Ma RC, Lin X, Jia W (2014) Causes of type 2 diabetes in China. Lancet Diabetes Endocrinol 2(12):980–991
39. Misra A, Khurana L, Isharwal S, Bhardwaj S (2008) South Asian diets and insulin resistance. Br J Nutr 101(4):465–473
40. Hu EA, Pan A, Malik V, Sun Q (2012) White rice consumption and risk of type 2 diabetes: meta-analysis and systematic review. BMJ 344:e1454
41. Mohan V, Radhika G, Sathya RM, Tamil SR, Ganesan A, Sudha V (2009) Dietary carbohydrates, glycaemic load, food groups and newly detected type 2 diabetes among urban Asian Indian population in Chennai, India (Chennai Urban Rural Epidemiology Study 59). Br J Nutr 102(10):1498–1506
42. Chan JC, Malik V, Jia W, Kadowaki T, Yajnik CS, Yoon KH, Hu FB (2009) Diabetes in Asia: epidemiology, risk factors, and pathophysiology. JAMA 301(20):2129–2140
43. Ng SW, Howard AG, Wang HJ, Su C, Zhang B (2014) The physical activity transition among adults in China: 1991–2011. Obes Rev 15:27–36
44. Nyamdorj R, Pitkäniemi J, Tuomilehto J, Hammar N, Stehouwer CD, Lam TH, Ramachandran A, Janus ED, Mohan V, Söderberg S, Laatikainen T (2010) Ethnic comparison of the association of undiagnosed diabetes with obesity. Int J Obes 34(2):332–339
45. Lear SA, Humphries KH, Kohli S, Chockalingam A, Frohlich JJ, Birmingham CL (2007) Visceral adipose tissue accumulation differs according to ethnic background: results of the Multicultural Community Health Assessment Trial (M-CHAT). Am J Clin Nutr 86(2):353–359
46. Who EC (2004) Appropriate body-mass index for Asian populations and its implications for policy and intervention strategies. Lancet (London, England) 363(9403):157
47. King GL, McNeely MJ, Thorpe LE, Mau ML, Ko J, Liu LL, Sun A, Hsu WC, Chow EA (2012) Understanding and addressing unique needs of diabetes in Asian Americans, native Hawaiians, and Pacific Islanders. Diabetes Care 35(5):1181–1188
48. Cameron AJ, Sicree RA, Zimmet PZ, Alberti KG, Tonkin AM, Balkau B, Tuomilehto J, Chitson P, Shaw JE (2010) Cut-points for waist circumference in Europids and South Asians. Obesity 18(10):2039–2046
49. Hales CN, Barker DJ (2013) Type 2 (non-insulin-dependent) diabetes mellitus: the thrifty phenotype hypothesis. Int J Epidemiol 42(5):1215–1222
50. Li Y, He Y, Qi L, Jaddoe VW, Feskens EJ, Yang X, Ma G, Hu FB (2010) Exposure to the Chinese famine in early life and the risk of hyperglycemia and type 2 diabetes in adulthood. Diabetes 59(10):2400–2406
51. King H, Keuky L, Seng S, Khun T, Roglic G, Pinget M (2005) Diabetes and associated disorders in Cambodia: two epidemiological surveys. Lancet 366(9497):1633–1639
52. Yajnik CS (2009) Nutrient-mediated teratogenesis and fuel-mediated teratogenesis: two pathways of intrauterine programming of diabetes. Int J Gynecol Obstet 104(Suppl):S27–S31
53. Ma RC, Tutino GE, Lillycrop KA, Hanson MA, Tam WH (2015) Maternal diabetes, gestational diabetes and the role of epigenetics in their long term effects on offspring. Prog Biophys Mol Biol 118(1–2):55–68

54. Tutino GE, Tam WH, Yang X, Chan JC, Lao TT, Ma RC (2014) Diabetes and pregnancy: perspectives from Asia. Diabet Med 31(3):302–318
55. Malone JM, Snyder M, Anderson G, Bernhard VM, Holloway GA Jr, Bunt TJ (1989) Prevention of amputation by diabetic education. Am J Surg 158(6):520–524
56. McMurray SD, Johnson G, Davis S, McDougall K (2002) Diabetes education and care management significantly improve patient outcomes in the dialysis unit. Am J Kidney Dis 40(3):566–575
57. Litzelman DK, Slemenda CW, Langefeld CD, Hays LM, Welch MA, Bild DE, Ford ES, Vinicor F (1993) Reduction of lower extremity clinical abnormalities in patients with non-insulin-dependent diabetes mellitus: a randomized, controlled trial. Ann Intern Med 119(1):36–41
58. Lincoln NB, Radford KA, Game FL, Jeffcoate WJ (2008) Education for secondary prevention of foot ulcers in people with diabetes: a randomised controlled trial. Diabetologia 51(11):1954
59. Gershater AM, Pilhammar E, Apelqvist J, Alm-Roijer C (2011) Patient education for the prevention of diabetic foot ulcers: interim analysis of a randomised controlled trial due to morbidity and mortality of participants. Eur Diabetes Nurs 8(3):102-7b
60. Kruger S, Guthrie D (1992) Foot care: knowledge retention and self-care practices. Diabetes Educ 18(6):487–490
61. International Diabetes Center (2014) Type 2 diabetes basics. IDC Publishing, Minneapolis
62. Armstrong DG, Lavery LA (eds) (2015) Clinical care of the diabetic foot. American Diabetes Association, USA
63. Levin ME, Bowker JH, Pfeifer MA (2008) Levin and O'Neal's the diabetic foot. Elsevier Health Sciences, Amsterdam
64. Nather A, Cao S, Chen JL, Low AY (2018) Prevention of diabetic foot complications. Singap Med J 59(6):291
65. Nather A (ed) (2016) Surgery for diabetic foot: a practical operative manual. World Scientific Publishing Company, Singapore
66. Nather A, Soegondo S, Adam JM, Nair HK, Zulkilfly AH, Villa MA, Tongson LS, Yeng BC, Wijeyaratne M, Somasundaram N, Mutirangura P (2015) Best practice guidelines for ASEANPlus: management of diabetic foot wounds. Sri Lanka J Diabetes Endocrinol Metab 5(1)
67. Baker N, Kenny C (2014) Prevention, screening and referral of the diabetic foot in primary care. Diabetes Prim Care 16:307–316
68. Lavery LA, Wunderlich RP, Tredwell JL (2005) Disease management for the diabetic foot: effectiveness of a diabetic foot prevention program to reduce amputations and hospitalizations. Diabetes Res Clin Pract 70(1):31–37
69. Mayfield JA, Reiber GE, Nelson RG, Greene T (2000) Do foot examinations reduce the risk of diabetic amputation? J Fam Pract 49(6):499
70. Nather A, Voon ASL (2012) Foot screening. In: Nather A (ed) The diabetic foot. World Scientific, Singapore, pp 157–166
71. Weck M, Slesaczeck T, Paetzold H, Muench D, Nanning T, von Gagern G et al (2013) Structured health care for subjects with diabetic foot ulcers results in a reduction of major amputation rates. Cardiovasc Diabetol 12:45. https://doi.org/10.1186/1475-2840-12-45
72. Mayfield JA, Sugarman JR (2000) The use of the Semmes-Weinstein monofilament and other threshold tests for preventing foot ulceration and amputation in persons with diabetes. J Fam Pract 49(11 Suppl):S17–29
73. Miranda-Palma B, Sosenko JM, Bowker JH, Mizel MS, Boulton AJM (2005) A comparison of the monofilament with other testing modalities for foot ulcer susceptibility. Diabetes Research and Clinical Practice 70(1):8–12. https://doi.org/10.1016/j.diabres.2005.02.013
74. Davies MJ, Heller S, Skinner TC, Campbell MJ, Carey ME, Cradock S, Dallosso HM, Daly H, Doherty Y, Eaton S, Fox C (2008) Effectiveness of the diabetes education and self management for ongoing and newly diagnosed (DESMOND) programme for people with newly diagnosed type 2 diabetes: cluster randomised controlled trial. BMJ 336(7642):491–495

75. Rauner MS, Heidenberger K, Pesendorfer EM (2004) Using a Markov model to evaluate the cost-effectiveness of diabetic foot prevention strategies in Austria. In: Proceedings of the western multiconference, international conference on health sciences simulation, Jan 18, pp 63–68
76. Jeffcoate WJ, Vileikyte L, Boyko EJ, Armstrong DG, Boulton AJ (2018) Current challenges and opportunities in the prevention and management of diabetic foot ulcers. Diabetes Care 41(4):645–652
77. Wrobel JS, Mayfield JA, Reiber GE (2001) Geographic variation of lower-extremity major amputation in individuals with and without diabetes in the Medicare population. Diabetes Care 24(5):860–864
78. Margolis DJ, Hoffstad O, Nafash J, Leonard CE, Freeman CP, Hennessy S, Wiebe DJ (2011) Location, location, location: geographic clustering of lower-extremity amputation among Medicare beneficiaries with diabetes. Diabetes Care 34(11):2363–2367
79. Margolis DJ, Jeffcoate W (2013) Epidemiology of foot ulceration and amputation: can global variation be explained? Med Clin 97(5):791–805
80. National Institute for Health and Care Excellence. Diabetic foot problems: prevention and management. Available from: www.nice.org.uk/guidance/ng19
81. International Working Group on the Diabetic Foot. Guidance documents. Available from: www.iwgdf.org/guidelines/

Diabetic-Foot Complications in African and Antarctica Continents

2

Zulfiqarali G. Abbas

2.1 Introduction

Continent of Africa is the second biggest on the earth, it is almost three times the size of Europe, 1000 ethnic groups live in 54 countries and speak more than 1000 dialects. As of now with 1.1 billion population, Africa is anticipated to increment and reach 2.4 billion in 2050. A great part of the expansion will occur in Sub-Saharan Africa (SSA), which incorporates 46 of African's 54 nations huge numbers of the world's least fortunate nations [1, 2]. Antarctica is the fifth-biggest mainland as far as absolute territory (it is bigger than both Oceania and Europe). Antarctica is an extraordinary mainland in that it does not have a local populace. There are no nations in Antarctica, albeit seven countries guarantee various pieces of it. Antarctica is the main landmass with no perpetual human home. There are, however, human settlements, where researchers and supporting staffs live piece of the year on turning premise [3]. The rate of diabetes mellitus is expanding in the populace over the world. Africa is encountering a quick increment in the commonness of diabetes. In December 2019, it was reported that people with diabetes in Africa are 19 million and if present patterns proceed with the general commonness is anticipated to be 29 million by 2030 and 47 million by 2045, which is increment of 143% [4]. There is currently considerable proof affirming that diabetes has arrived at pestilence extents in many creating or recently industrialised countries, and is relied upon to turn into the dominating medical issue in new developing countries [1]. Diabetes stays a main source of dismalness and mortality in both developed and developing world and force an overwhelming weight on their health services [5–21].

As the prevalence of diabetes is increasing along with it in parallel complications of diabetes will also increase. Among all the complications caused by diabetes, the

Z. G. Abbas (✉)
Abbas Medical Centre, Dar es Salaam, Tanzania

Muhimbili University of Health and Allied Sciences, Dar es Salaam, Tanzania
e-mail: zabbas@cats-net.co.tz

M. Zubair et al. (eds.), *Diabetic Foot Ulcer*,
https://doi.org/10.1007/978-981-15-7639-3_2

most serious and dreadful complication will be diabetic foot, which will be associated with the highest morbidity and mortality [5–21]. Data across the world are reporting that 40–60% of all lower limb non-traumatic amputation are directly related to diabetes [21–25]. Up to 85% of amputation done in the people with diabetes are due to foot ulcer. There is a 50% risk of developing a serious lesion in the second limb in those people with diabetes who had a previous lower limb amputation within 2 years [21–25]. It has been shown in the literatures from Africa that patients with diabetic foot are associated with peripheral neuropathy compared to peripheral arterial disease (PAD) [5–20].

African continent is developing very fast and becoming more affluent due to urbanisation. At the same time, we report in the literatures increase rates of peripheral arterial diseases in people with diabetes in past two decades, which can be critical and costly [26]. Amputations are expensive, devastating on the people with diabetes and their families, leading to loss of independency and livelihood [26]. Complications of lower limb are associated with high rates of morbidity and mortality [5–21].

Time is tissue, which implies that therapeutic help for diabetic foot ulcers ought to be looked for as fast as could be allowed and intervention should be taken as a medical emergency [21–25]. Time is not tissue, which implies that a patient presenting with a diabetic foot ulcer, with a history of days, weeks or months, means it becomes difficult to save a toe, or a foot or a leg or even prevent death due to delay presentation [21–25]. Ideally these patients with diabetic foot ulcers should not delay to report at health centre.

In African setup reasons for late presentations have been reported by Abbas et al. and are mostly associated with cultural, traditional and customary behaviours [5–9, 13, 14, 19–21]. In the African continent, it is very common to go through many stages before patients actually lands in the health centre. First of all, patient will try to treat a foot lesion at home using a razor blade called bathroom surgery or herbal solution [5–8, 21]. Procedures are performed by relatives or patients themselves. If treatment at home fails then patients would be advised by relatives to see herbalist, faith healer or traditional healer. After going through herbalist, traditional or faith healer and if it fails then patients and relatives will decide to go to nearest primary health care centre or district or regional hospitals where unfortunately we cannot find a health care worker dealing with diabetic foot problems. All these journey delays treatment of diabetic foot ulcer and foot deteriorates. By the time patient is referred to a specialised centre or referred hospital it could be too late to salvage a foot and sometimes even to prevent death of the patient [6–9, 13, 14, 21]. In some community's delay in getting an expert opinion in the hospital is because of fear losing a limb, as according to culture losing a limb in African patients is considered a worse outcome than having a disease. Among health care workers at grass root level can lead to worse outcomes due to lack of knowledge. Awareness and education among health care workers are extremely important specially at the grass root level who are the first to see these patients [6–9, 13, 14, 21].

2.2 Pathophysiology of Foot Ulcers

The pathophysiology of diabetic foot lesions is complex and multifactorial. Contributory factors include peripheral neuropathy (sensory, motor, autonomic) peripheral arterial disease, neuro-ischemia, infection, biomechanics, social-economic factors, non-ulcerative lesions of ulcers and local trauma. The pattern of foot ulcer occurrence depends on the varying degree of contribution of each of these factors. For example, an ulcer may be secondary to both ischemia and neuropathy so-called neuro-ischaemic ulcer.

2.3 Diabetic Foot Complications

Diabetic foot ulcer is a major public health problem in many African countries [1, 2, 5–22]. It is the main cause of prolonged hospital admission due to late presentation and can lead to high morbidity and mortality [1, 2, 5–22].

2.3.1 Peripheral Neuropathy (PN)

Published literature from the Western world reports that PN is the foremost common complication of diabetes, happening in 5–80% of patients with diabetes [27, 28]. Peripheral neuropathy is one of the most common diabetic foot complications affecting patients with diabetes in both developed and less developed world [8, 9, 16–21, 29–48] (Table 2.1).

Diabetic peripheral neuropathy commonly presents as bilateral symmetrical glove and stocking distribution predominately sensory neuropathy. Foot with peripheral neuropathy is classical numb, warm, dry and painless, but pulses are palpable. Typical patient will present with numbness of feet, pins and needles sensation, burning feet, feeling like walking in the sand, stabbing pain, fatigue or weakness of feet. Due to the loss of protective sensation in the feet patient can easily sustain injury.

The resulting loss of sensation in the feet invariably leads to sequelae that include callosities, cracked soles, breakdown of skin or non-discernible injuries, such as burn or rat bite. These complications can result in foot ulcers, which in our set leads to infection, gangrene, amputation or even death [8, 9, 16–21, 29–48]. This is the main reason that peripheral neuropathy with foot ulcers are admitted in the hospital, leads to prolonging stay in and are associated with amputation [8, 9, 16–21, 29–48]. Peripheral neuropathy also remains the most common initiating factor for diabetic foot ulcer (DFU). The prevalence of PN rates across Africa in last two decades has been documented [8, 9, 16–21, 29–48] (Table 2.1).

In a major study performed in Tanzania, Abbas et al. found no differences in the rates of PN among African and Asians diabetic patients with ulcers [17, 18]. In another comparative study, Abbas and colleagues found no significant differences in

Table 2.1 Prevalence of diabetic peripheral neuropathy (PN) across the African continent in last two decades

Publication year	Author	Ref. No.	Country	Prevalence of PN (%)
2020	Abbas	[19]	Tanzania	84.7
2019	Garoushi	[29]	Libiya	42.2
2019	Khalil	[30]	Egypt	20
2018	Chahbi	[31]	Morroco	15
2018	Khalifa	[32]	Egypt	69
2017	Kisozi	[33]	Uganda	24.9
2017	Awadalla	[34]	Sudan	68.2
2015	Assaad-Khalil	[35]	Egypt	29.3
2015	Olamoyegun	[36]	Nigeria	69.6
2015	Ogbera	[37]	Nigeria	37
2015	Kuate-Tegueu	[38]	Cameroon	77.4
2012	Owolabi	[39]	Nigeria	71
2011	Jarso	[40]	Ethiopia	48.2
2009	Abbas	[17]	Tanzania	81
2009	Oguejiofor	[41]	Nigeria	69.2
2009	Mugambi-Nturibi	[42]	Kenya	42
2008	Gill	[43]	Ethiopia	41
2006	Ndip	[44]	Cameroon	27.3
2006	Ugoya	[45]	Nigeria	75
2005	Abbas	[20]	Tanzania	100
2004	Morbach	[18]	Tanzania	82
2003	Moulik	[46]	Zambia	61
2000	Abbas	[16]	Tanzania	25.5
2000	Benotmane et al.	[47]	Algeria	84.4
1999	Kadiki et al.	[48]	Libiya	45.7

the prevalence of neuropathy in patients with foot ulcers from Tanzania, Germany and India [18]. There is no difference across the world in the rates of PN [18]. Published data from the last two decades across Africa have shown wide difference in the occurrence of PN [8, 9, 16–21, 29–48] (Table 2.1).

2.3.2 Peripheral Arterial Diseases (PAD)

Peripheral arterial disease is defined clinically in patients with a history of intermittent claudication, rest pain, absence of pedal pulses abnormalities on non-invasive arterial assessment indicates disturb or impaired lower limb circulation [21, 22]. There are no specific diabetes-related peripheral arterial lesions, but the distribution of arteriosclerosis in patients with diabetes is different compare to what is seen in non-diabetes patients. In patients with diabetes, it is more frequently, younger age groups are affected more, no differences in gender, progression rate is faster, it is multisegmented and more distally [21–22]. It is general to see that ischemic foot is associated with pain at rest, increase risk of foot ulcers, digital necrosis or gangrene and absent pulses. This in turn increases the risk of localised or widespread infection of the lower limbs.

PAD is very common in the industrialised world, but was not that common in Africa and Asia [8, 10, 14, 16–19, 30, 32, 35, 37, 44, 46, 49–56]. Now across Africa and Asia rates of PAD are increasing [8, 10, 14, 16–19, 30, 32, 35, 37, 44, 46, 49–56] (Table 2.2). More people in Africa are adopting the Western style of life as are becoming more urbanised, sedentary lifestyle, lack of exercise, changing diet, etc. Abbas et al. established that rates of PAD in Tanzania are not different by ethnicity as it was in the past [18]. PAD is now playing a more substantial role in the causation of foot ulcer in Africa than was previously thought. Likely, reasons for this include increased urbanisation and adoption of behaviours and diet from the west. Prevalence rates of PAD are increasing across Africa seen in last two decades [8, 10, 14, 16–19, 30, 32, 35, 37, 44, 46, 49–56] (Table 2.2).

Peripheral arterial diseases are underdiagnosed and treated in Africa and we need to conduct more measurements of Ankle Brachial Index [17, 21, 22]. Computer tomography scan angiography of lower limbs are quite comparable in visualising vessels. It is done to evaluate the extent of arterial block and help in the feasibility of revascularization [22].

Table 2.2 Prevalence of peripheral arterial disease (PAD) across the African continent in last two decades

Publication year	Author	Ref. No.	Country	Prevalence of PAD (%)
2020	Abbas	[19]	Tanzania	27.2
2019	Khalil	[30]	Egypt	20
2018	Khalifa	[32]	Egypt	12
2016	Codjo	[49]	Benin	42
2015	Ogbera	[37]	Nigeria	40
2015	Assaad-Khalil	[35]	Egypt	11
2014	Konin	[50]	Ivory Coast	22
2014	Mwebaze	[51]	Uganda	39
2014	Okello	[52]	Uganda	24
2014	Oyelade	[53]	Nigeria	52
2013	Umuerri	[54]	Nigeria	35.6
2009	Abbas	[17]	Tanzania	26
2007	Kumar	[55]	South Africa	29
2006	Ndip	[44]	Cameroon	21.3
2004	Morbach	[18]	Tanzania	12
2003	Moulik	[46]	Zambia	41
2002	Abbas	[14]	Tanzania	21
2000	Abbas	[16]	Tanzania	12.5
1997	Levitt	[56]	South Africa	8.2

2.3.3 Diabetic Foot Ulceration (DFU)

Diabetic peripheral neuropathy in Africa is still the main underlying risk factor in the causation of diabetic foot ulcers [8, 10, 12, 13]. In one of the studies conducted in Tanzania it showed that 15% of admitted cases were of diabetic foot ulcer and out of this 80% were first-time ulcer [14]. Across African continent prevalence of DFU ranges from 12% to 24% [34, 44, 57–61]. It further showed in the study that the amputation rate was found 33% as a frequent outcome in people with DFU and associated with neuro-ischemic lesions and/or progressive infection [14]. Mortality rate was as high as 54% who presented late with severe foot ulcers Wagner score ≥4 [14]. It has been reported the same with high rates of morbidity and mortality from other parts of Africa [10, 14, 62–67]. It is difficult to obtain consent from patients for surgery due to severe DFU, which can reflect low amputation rates than what is actually expected [14]. Some patients discharge themselves against medical advice with severe DFU and thus risk severe sepsis and may be death [14].

Major factors contributing to development of the DFU in rural Africa are walking bare foot. In particular, farmers walking barefoot, or due to religious obligations people have to walk barefoot and, in some cultures, entering the house we need to take out of footwear. This could be due to culture or may be low income [8, 10, 11, 21]. People with diabetes living below poverty line could be difficult for them to buy appropriate footwear. Flip flop slippers are very cheap and rubber made commonly used in the developing world and rural Africa it is common to produce footwear from worn out motor car tyres [8, 10, 21]. Poverty can lead to unhygienic condition, which is in turn prone to DFU [11–15, 21]. Patients with peripheral neuropathy sustain injuries but presents with DFU when they become symptomatic and by that time foot ulcer has already progressed to fulminating foot sepsis. Most of the time it has been noticed and reported that these patients do not have access to basic education on foot care at primary, district or regional health centre are most at risk developing infected ulcers [12, 13].

2.3.4 Diabetic Foot Infection

In Africa first presentation to health centre is usually too late when patient has already developed localised gangrene or full foot gangrenous with severe sepsis. This may not respond to supportive treatment with intravenous antibiotics, intravenous fluids and insulin, this progress to serious systemic infection and high risk of mortality [1, 5–21]. First presentation at health centre is late with severe infected DFU and already has acute limb-threatening conditions leading to foot or leg amputation in 25–50% for patients with diabetes [22–25]. Fungal infection in between the toes is also common and dryness of the feet seen in patients with diabetes develops cracks and fissures on the sole of the feet [16–21]. All these open lesions in the skin lead to secondary bacterial infection [16–21]. We can start with antibiotics initial empirically and then can be changed after the results of culture and sensitivity [68]. According to the International Working Group of Diabetic Foot superficial swabs are not recommended for culture [22–25]. Obtain specimens of superficial swabs are not useful due to give polymicrobial growth. Deep tissue biopsy is recommended by IWGDF to give proper and useful data [22–25]. Unfortunately, in Africa majority of laboratory services do not have resources to provide or maintain microbiology routine services. Microbiology services are only available in the university tertiary level of the hospitals [68]. Reports of the utility of Gram staining has been published is equally sensitive compare to cultures in the management of diabetic foot ulcer [68].

Infection is the immediate cause of amputation and this varies widely by geographic regions. True rates of amputation following foot infection in Africa remain underestimated [1, 6–21]. There are many cited reasons for amputation in patients with diabetes, but gangrene and infection are common and occur simultaneously [16–21]. Medical health care workers always think (Incorrectly) that a degree of self-neglected among the patients with DFU. This happens because foot with infected ulcers frequently feel no pain due to peripheral neuropath. Developing countries need treatment planning for the prevention and management of diabetic foot infections.

Diabetic foot ulceration, infection and amputation are preventable through organised foot care programmes. Education is the only tool in the developing world that can prevent diabetic foot complications. Education should be targeted to health care workers, patients and relatives and it has shown to reduce complications by 85%.

DFU and infections are very common where services are scarce especially as in Africa, for example, Chiropody services are almost non-existing in Africa. Foot lesions once sustained by the patient are either ignored or detected relatively late. During this process, the patient starts treatment himself at home by home therapy such as socking in herbal medications, applying the herbal medication, etc. This leads to further deterioration of the foot with high risk of morbidity and even mortality due to sepsis [9–16, 21].

2.3.5 Amputation

Gangrene and infection appear to be most common cited indications for foot amputation in patients with diabetes [8, 10]. High rates of amputation are seen across Africa from 16% to 55% [8, 10, 61–63, 65–67]. However the true lower limb amputation rate resulting from foot infections in Africa remains underestimated. About 10% of patients who needed and agreed to undergo surgery died due to severe sepsis in Africa before the surgical procedure [8].

2.3.6 Mortality

Mortality rates are high in African patients with diabetic foot ulcers [8, 10, 61–63, 65–67]. Abbas and colleagues ascertained clinical correlates for mortality of patients with diabetic foot ulcers in Tanzania. They found that the overall mortality rate was high in the patients with foot ulcer was 29% and was significantly higher among patients with PAD, neuro-ischaemic, late presentation, or non-healing ulcers [8, 10, 14]. The mortality rate was 54% who presented when gangrene has set [8, 10, 14]. The highest mortality rate has been documented in those patients who did not undergo amputation of the affected limb [8, 10, 14].

2.4 Prevention

It is important that it should be directed to people with diabetes and health care workers.

Education is the only tool we have in Africa, which is free of charge for the patients and effective if implemented. Several educations have been conducted and were successful in both the developing and developed world [5, 6, 69–74].

2.4.1 Step by Step (*SbS*) Foot Project

Step by step foot project was first and the unique project started from the developing world. It was piloted and conducted in Tanzania and India. This project was launched in 2003 and the curriculum was developed initially focusing developing world. The main aim of this project was to create awareness on diabetic foot, to provide sustainable training on diabetic foot, to transfer knowledge to other colleagues and export ideas to other developing countries, to reduce the risk of lower limb complications and to empower people with diabetes regarding diabetic foot. Several successful projects were done in Tanzania targeting physicians and nurses [69–74]. It was always aimed to train a team from each centre. It all started in Tanzania, developing world exported to other developing countries, later to the second world and finally the first world in Europe [69–74]. Step by step has already touched about 110 countries in the world. In 2009 it was decided to bring surgeons on board. It felt that surgeons should be trained for salvaging diabetic foot. So those centres where physician and nurses were already trained surgeon were asked to join to complete the team. First course of its kind for surgeons was held in Tanzania [69–74]. Several other groups of surgeons were later formed in Europe and Asia. Step by step foot project showed us that ulceration, infection and amputation all are prevented through organised diabetic foot care programmes. Regular education of the staffs and patients, regular follow of the patients and multidiscipline approach to manage diabetic foot ulcers. Step by step reported that above strategic plan there was greater than 50% reduction rates in amputation rate [5, 6, 69–74].

2.4.2 Train the Foot Trainer (*TtFT*) Project

In December 2012, a decision was made to introduce Train the foot Trainer project (*TtFT*). It is almost similar to the original step by step foot project, but here health care workers from different countries in that region are asked to come under one roof. Once health care workers go back to their own countries, they need to disseminate the knowledges by conducting step by step foot projects. The first successful *TtFT* course was conducted in Brazil in 2012 [75].

2.5 Conclusion

Africa is in epidemiological transition with a massive projected increase in diabetes and diabetes-related lower limb complications including peripheral neuropathy, peripheral arterial disease, DFUs and amputations. Unless urgent action is taken to tackle these by developing cost-effective and evidence-based strategies, a situation that is already challenging will become substantially worse. DFUs and amputations rates in patients with diabetes can be reduced by >50% by better education of patients. Education on diabetic foot is the only tool we have in Africa that should be part of the curriculum. It should be targeted at both health care workers and patients.

Acknowledgments I would like to acknowledge all our colleagues for their constructive discussion during the genesis of this manuscript. We usually highly appreciate Shabneez Gangji and other staff in diabetes centre's in Dar es Salaam for their assistance.

References

1. Abbas ZG (2013) The global burden of diabetic foot. In: Pendsey S (ed) Contemporary management of diabetic foot, 1st edn. JP Medical Ltd, London, pp 24–30
2. Atun R, Davies JI, Gale EAM et al (2017) Diabetes in sub-Saharan Africa: from clinical care to health policy. Lancet Diabetes Endocrinol 5:622–667
3. National Geography Encyclopaedic entry. Available from: https://www.nationalgeographic.org/encyclopedia/antarctica/. Accessed 24 June 2020
4. International Diabetes Federation, Diabetes Atlas, 9th edition (2019). Available from: https://www.diabetesatlas.org/en/resources/. Accessed 24 June 2020
5. Naemi R, Chockalingam N, Lutale JK, Abbas ZG (2020) Predicting the risk of future diabetic foot ulcer occurrence. A prospective cohort study of patients with diabetes in Tanzania. BMJ Open Diabetes Res Care 8(1) pii: e001122. https://doi.org/10.1136/bmjdrc-2019-001122
6. Abbas ZG (2013) Preventing foot care and reducing amputation: a step in right direction for diabetes care. Diab Manag 3:427–435
7. Abbas ZG (2017) Managing the diabetic foot in resource-poor settings: challenges and solutions. Chronic Wound Care Manag Res 4:135–142
8. Abbas ZG, Archibald LK (2006) Recent international development: Africa. In: AJM B, Cavanagh P, Rayman G (eds) The foot in diabetes, 4th edn. John Wiley & Sons Ltd, Hoboken, NJ, pp 379–385
9. Abbas ZG, Archibald LK (2007) Challenges for management of the diabetic foot in Africa: doing more with less. Int Wound J 4:305–313
10. Abbas ZG, Archibald LK (2005) Epidemiology of the diabetic foot in Africa. Med Sci Monit 11:RA262–RRA70
11. Abbas ZG, Viswanathan V (2007) The diabetic foot in Africa and India. Int Diab Monitor 19:8–12
12. Abbas ZG, Gill GV, Archibald LK (2002) The epidemiology of diabetic limb sepsis: an African perspective. Diabet Med 19:895–899
13. Abbas ZG, Archibald LK (2007) The diabetic foot in Sub-Saharan Africa: a new management paradigm. Diab Foot J 10:128–136

14. Abbas ZG, Lutale JK, Morbach S, Archibald LK (2002) Clinical outcome of diabetic patients hospitalized with foot ulcers, Dar es Salaam, Tanzania. Diabet Med 19:575–579
15. Tesfaye S, Gill G (2011) Chronic diabetic complications in Africa. Afr J Diabetes Med 19(1):4–8
16. Abbas ZG, Archibald LK (2000) Foot complications in diabetic patients with symptomatic peripheral neuropathy in Dar es Salaam. Tanzania Diabetes Int 10:52–56
17. Abbas ZG, Lutale JK, Archibald LK (2009) Diabetic foot ulcers and ethinicity in Tanzania: a contrast between African and Asian populations. Int Wound J 6:124–131
18. Morbach S, Lutale JK, Viswanathan V, Mollenberg J, Ochs HR, Rajashekart S, Ramachandran A, Abbas ZG (2004) Regional difference in risk factors and clinical presentation of diabetic foot lesions. Diabet Med 21:91–95
19. Zulfiqarali G. Abbas, Janet K. Lutale, Lennox K. Archibald, William J. Jeffcoate (2020) Rat bite as a cause of diabetic foot ulcer in sub-Saharan Africa. International Wound Journal 17(4):897–899
20. Abbas ZG, Lutale JK, Archibald LK (2005) Rodent bites on the feet of diabetic patients in Tanzania. Diabetes Med 22:631–633
21. Abbas ZG, Bal A (eds) (2019) Pocket guideline of diabetic foot 2019, 2nd edn. Jaypee Brothers Medical Publishers (P) Ltd, New Delhi
22. International Working group on the Diabetic Foot (IWGDF). The development of global consensus guidelines on the management and prevention of the Diabetic Foot 2019, www.iwgdf.org. https://iwgdfguidelines.org/guidelines/guidelines/. Accessed 24 June 2020
23. Lipsky BA, Senneville É, Abbas ZG, Aragón-Sánchez J, Diggle M, Embil JM, Kono S, Lavery LA, Malone M, van Asten SA, Urbančič-Rovan V, EJG P, International Working Group on the Diabetic Foot (IWGDF) (2020) Guidelines on the diagnosis and treatment of foot infection in persons with diabetes (IWGDF 2019 update). Diabetes Metab Res Rev 36(Suppl 1):e3280. https://doi.org/10.1002/dmrr.3280
24. Peters EJG, Lipsky BA, Senneville É, Abbas ZG, Aragón-Sánchez J, Diggle M, Embil JM, Kono S, Lavery LA, Malone M, Urbančič-Rovan V, Van Asten SA (2020) Interventions in the management of infection in the foot in diabetes: a systematic review. Diabetes Metab Res Rev 36(Suppl 1):e3282. https://doi.org/10.1002/dmrr.3282
25. Senneville É, Lipsky BA, Abbas ZG, Aragón-Sánchez J, Diggle M, Embil JM, Kono S, Lavery LA, Malone M, van Asten SA, Urbančič-Rovan V, Peters EJG (2020) Diagnosis of infection in the foot in diabetes: a systematic review. Diabetes Metab Res Rev 36(Suppl 1):e3281. https://doi.org/10.1002/dmrr.3281
26. Cavanagh P, Attinger C, Abbas ZG et al (2012) Cost of treating diabetic foot ulcers in five different countries. Diabetes Metab Res Rev 28:107–111
27. Edmonds M, Boulton A, Buckenham T, Every N, Foster A, Freeman D, Gadsby R, Gibby O, Knowles A, Pooke M, Tovey F, Unwin N, Wolfe J (1996) Report of the diabetic foot and amputation group. Diabet Med 13:S27–S42
28. Jeffcoat WJ, Harding KG (2003) Diabetic foot ulcers. Lancet 361:1545–1551
29. Garoushi S, Johnson MI, Tashani OA (2019) A cross-sectional study to estimate the point prevalence of painful diabetic neuropathy in Eastern Libya. BMC Public Health 19(1):78
30. Khalil SA, Megallaa MH, Rohoma KH, Guindy MA, Zaki A, Hassanein M, Malaty AH, Ismael HM, Kharboush IF, El Kafash DN, Sallam HN, Desouky IA (2019) Prevalence of chronic diabetic complications in newly diagnosed versus known type 2 diabetic subjects in a sample of Alexandria population, Egypt. Curr Diabetes Rev 15(1):74–83
31. Chahbi Z, Lahmar B, Hadri SE, Abainou L, Kaddouri S, Qacif H, Baizri H, Zyani M (2018) The prevalence of painful diabetic neuropathy in 300 Moroccan diabetics. Pan Afr Med J 31:158
32. Khalifa WA (2018) Risk factors for diabetic foot ulcer recurrence: a prospective 2-year follow-up study in Egypt. Foot (Edinb) 35:11–15. https://doi.org/10.1016/j.foot.2017.12.004
33. Kisozi T, Mutebi E, Kisekka M, Lhatoo S, Sajatovic M, Kaddumukasa M, Nakwagala FN, Katabira E (2017) Prevalence, severity and factors associated with peripheral neuropathy

among newly diagnosed diabetic patients attending Mulago hospital: a cross-sectional study. Afr Health Sci 17(2):463–473
34. Awadalla H, Noor SK, Elmadhoun WM, Almobarak AO, Elmak NE, Abdelaziz SI, Sulaiman AA, Ahmed MH (2017) Diabetes complications in Sudanese individuals with type 2 diabetes: overlooked problems in sub-Saharan Africa? Diabetes Metab Syndr 11(Suppl 2):S1047–S1051
35. Assaad-Khalil SH, Zaki A, Abdel Rehim A, Megallaa MH, Gaber N, Gamal H, Rohoma KH (2015) Prevalence of diabetic foot disorders and related risk factors among Egyptian subjects with diabetes. Prim Care Diabetes 9(4):297–303
36. Olamoyegun M, Ibraheem W, Iwuala S, Audu M, Kolawole B (2015) Burden and pattern of micro vascular complications in type 2 diabetes in a tertiary health institution in Nigeria. Afr Health Sci 15(4):1136–1141
37. Ogbera AO, Adeleye O, Solagberu B et al (2015) Screening for peripheral neuropathy and peripheral arterial disease in persons with diabetes mellitus in a Nigerian University Teaching Hospital. BMC Res Notes 8:533
38. Kuate-Tegueu C, Temfack E, Ngankou S et al (2015) Prevalence and determinants of diabetic polyneuropathy in a Sub-Saharan African referral hospital. J Neurol Sci 355:108–112
39. Owolabi MO, Ipadeola A (2012) Total vascular risk as a strong correlate of severity of diabetic peripheral neuropathy in Nigerian Africans. Ethn Dis 22:106–112
40. Jarso G, Ahmed A, Feleke Y (2011) The prevalence, clinical features and management of peripheral neuropathy among diabetic patients in Tikur Anbessa and St. Paul's Specialized University Hospitals, Addis Ababa, Ethiopia. Ethiop Med J 49:299–311
41. Oguejiofor OC, Oli JM, Ajaero CN, Odenigbo CU, Odike MA (2009) Are the symptoms of diabetic peripheral neuropathy in Nigerian patients objective? An evaluation using the United Kingdom Screening Test (UKST) and Bio-Thesiometry. Niger J Clin Pract 12(2):113–119
42. Mugambi-Nturibi E, Otieno CF, Kwasa TO et al (2009) Stratification of persons with diabetes into risk categories for foot ulceration. East Afr Med J 86:233–239
43. Gill G, Gebrekidan A, English P, Wile D, Tesfaye S (2008) Diabetic complications and glycaemic control in remote North Africa. QJM Int J Med 101(10):793–798
44. Ndip EA, Tchakonte B, Mbanya JC (2006) A study of the prevalence and risk factors of foot problems in a population of diabetic patients in Cameroon. Int J Low Extrem Wounds 5:83–88
45. Ugoya SO, Echejoh GO, Ugoya TA, Agaba EI, Puepet FH, Ogunniyi A (2006) Clinically diagnosed diabetic neuropathy: frequency, types and severity. J Natl Med Assoc 98(11):1763–1766
46. Moulik PK, Mtonga R, Gill GV (2003) Amputation and mortality in new-onset diabetic foot ulcer stratified by etiology. Diabetes Care 26:491–494
47. Benotmane A, Mohammedi F, Ayad F, Kadi K, Azzouz A (2000) Service d'Endocrinologie-Diabetologie, Centre Hospitalo-Universitaire, Oran, Algerie. Diabetic foot lesions: etiologic and prognostic factors. Diabetes Metab 26(2):113–117
48. Kadiki OA, Roaed RB (1999) Epidemiological and clinical patterns of diabetes mellitus in Benghazi, Libyan Arab Jamahiriya. Benghazi Diabetic Clinic, Benghazi, Libyan Arab Jamahiriya. East Mediterr Health J 5:6–13
49. Codjo HL, Adoukonou TA, Wanvoegbe A et al (2016) Prevalence of peripheral artery disease among diabetics in Parakou in 2013. Ann Cardiol Angeiol 65:260–264
50. Konin C, Essam N'loo AS, Adoubi A et al (2014) Peripheral arterial disease of the lower limbs in African diabetic patients: ultrasonography and determining factors. J Mal Vasc 39:373–381
51. Mwebaze RM, Kibirige D (2014) Peripheral arterial disease among adult diabetic patients attending a large outpatient diabetic clinic at a national referral hospital in Uganda: a descriptive cross sectional study. PLoS One 9(8):e105211
52. Okello S, Millard A, Owori R, Asiimwe SB, Siedner MJ, Rwebembera J, Wilson LA, Moore CC, Annex BH (2014) Prevalence of lower extremity peripheral artery disease among adult diabetes patients in south-western Uganda. BMC Cardiovasc Disord 14:75
53. Oyelade BO, Olaolorun AD, Odeigah LO, Amole IO, Aderibigbe SA (2014) The relationship between obesity and peripheral arterial disease in adult Nigerian diabetics. Niger Postgrad Med J. 21(1):57-60.

54. Umuerri EM, Obasohan AO (2013) Lower extremity peripheral artery disease: prevalence and risk factors among adult Nigerians with diabetes mellitus. West Afr J Med 32:200–205
55. Kumar A, Mash B, Rupesinghe G (2007) Peripheral arterial disease—high prevalence in rural black South Africans. S Afr Med J 97:285–288
56. Levitt NS, Bradshaw D, Zwarenstein MF et al (1997) Audit of public sector primary diabetes care in Cape Town, South Africa: high prevalence of complications, uncontrolled hyperglycaemia, and hypertension. Diabet Med 14:1073–1077
57. Mamo T, Yifter H, Lemessa T (2015) Risk factors assessment of diabetic foot ulcer using the sixty seconds screening tool: a hospital based cross sectional study at Tikur Anbessa specialized hospital. Ethiop Med J (Suppl 2):45–49
58. Kengne AP, Djouogo CF, Dehayem MY et al (2009) Admission trends over 8 years for diabetic foot ulceration in a specialized diabetes unit in Cameroon. Int J Low Extrem Wounds 8:180–186
59. Muthuuri JM (2007) Characteristics of patients with diabetic foot in Mombasa, Kenya. East Afr Med J 84(6):251–258
60. Nouedoui C, Teyang A, Djoumessi S (2003) Epidemiologic profile and treatment of diabetic foot at the National Diabetic Center of Yaounde-Cameroon. Tunis Med 81(1):20–25
61. Sano D, Tieno H, Drabo Y, Sanou A (1998) Service de Chirurgie Generale et Digestive, CHU de Ouagadougou. Management of the diabetic foot, apropos of 42 cases at the Ougadougou University Hospital Center. Dakar Med 43(1):109–113
62. Isiguzo CM, Jac-Okereke C (2015) Diabetic foot ulcer—12 months prospective review of pattern of presentation at Enugu State University of Technology Teaching Hospital, Parklane, Enugu: a basis for diabetic foot clinic? Niger J Med 24:125–130
63. Ngim NE, Ndifon WO, Udosen AM et al (2012) Lower limb amputation in diabetic foot disease: experience in a tertiary hospital in southern Nigeria. Afr J Diabetes Med 1:13–15
64. Chalya PL, Mabula JB, Dass RM, Ngayomela IH, Chandika AB, Mbelenge N, Gilyoma JM (2012) Major limb amputations: a tertiary hospital experience in north-western Tanzania. J Orthop Surg Res 7:18
65. Enweluzo GO, Giwa SO, Adekoya-Cole TO et al (2010) Profile of amputations in Lagos University Teaching Hospital, Lagos, Nigeria. Nig Q J Hosp Med 20:205–208
66. Sié Essoh JB, Kodo M, Djè Bi Djè V et al (2009) Limb amputations in adults in an Ivorian teaching hospital. Niger J Clin Pract 12:245–247
67. Muyembe VM, Muhinga MN (1999) Department of Surgery, Central Provincial Hospital, Nyeri, Kenya. Major limb amputation at a provincial general hospital in Kenya. East Afr Med J 76(3):163–166
68. Abbas ZG, Lutale JK, Ilondo MM, Archibald LK (2012) The utility of Gram stains and culture in the management of limb ulcers in persons with diabetes. Int Wound J 9(6):677–682
69. Abbas Z, Morbach S (2005) Diabetes foot damage in developing countries: the urgent need for education. Diabetes Voice 50:15–17
70. Abbas ZG, Lutale JK, Bakker K, Baker N, Archibald LK (2011) The 'Step by Step' Diabetic Foot Project in Tanzania: a model for improving patient outcomes in less-developed countries. Int Wound J 8:169–175
71. Bakker K, Abbas ZG, Pendsey S (2006) Step by step, improving diabetic foot care in the developing world. A pilot study for India, Bangladesh, The "*Step by Step*" Diabetic Foot Project in Tanzania, 2004–2010 Sri Lanka and Tanzania. Pract Diab Intern 23:365–369
72. Pendsey S, Abbas ZG (2007) The *Step-by-Step* program for reducing diabetic foot problems: a model for the developing world. Curr Diab Rep 7(6):425–428
73. Abbas ZG (2015) Reducing diabetic limb amputations in developing countries. Expert Rev Endocrinol Metab 10(4):425–434
74. Abbas ZG (2014) Chapter 39: Preventive foot care programs. In: Hinchliffe RJ, Schaper NC, Thompson MM, Tripathi RK, Timaran CH (eds) The diabetic foot, 1st edn. JP Medical Ltd, London., www.jpeedigital.com, pp 24–30
75. Baker N, Van Acker K, Urbancic-Rovan V, Abbas ZG, Morbach S (2017) The worldwide implementation of the '*Train the Foot Trainer*' programme. Diabet Foot J 20(2):71–76

Diabetic-Foot Complications in American and Australian Continents

3

Kanakamani Jeyaraman

3.1 Introduction

Diabetic foot problems are a challenging health issue with clinical, social, and economic implications and are set to increase in the future, with the world facing the epidemic of type 2 DM. Though developing countries in Africa, Asia, and South America are likely to see the greatest rise, developed countries also are facing similar uptrends. Foot problems consume about 10–12% of the health-care resources available for diabetes and potentially up to 40% in developing countries [1]. It is estimated that every 30 seconds in some parts of the world, a limb is lost due to diabetes and the average annual cost is $8659 per patient. The cost of treating a diabetic patient with foot problems is 5.4 times higher than treating a patient without foot problems in the year of the first episode and eight times higher for higher grade ulcers than lower grade ulcers [2].

Worldwide, about 9.1–26.1 million people with diabetes develop foot ulcers every year [3]. Understanding the epidemiology of the diabetic foot problems is important for the appropriate allocation of health-care resources and budget planning. Knowing the region-specific risk factors can help to develop prevention and treatment strategies relevant to that region. More information is available on the epidemiology of diabetes-related lower extremity amputations (LEA) than the epidemiology of the diabetic foot problem, itself. The incidence and prevalence of diabetic foot problems and diabetes-related LEA vary significantly between different countries and between different regions within countries. The point prevalence of diabetic foot ulcer (DFU) in developed countries range from 1.5–10%. The incidence of DFU in community-based studies in Europe is between 0.5–2.2% and is high at 3–6% in clinic-based studies from developing countries. The incidence rate

K. Jeyaraman (✉)
Royal Darwin Hospital, Darwin, NT, Australia

Northern Territory Medical Program, Flinders University, Darwin, NT, Australia

M. Zubair et al. (eds.), *Diabetic Foot Ulcer*,
https://doi.org/10.1007/978-981-15-7639-3_3

could be even higher in high-risk select population, e.g., 30–50% in a diabetic population with previously healed ulcer [1]. Therefore, it is difficult to compare the incidence and prevalence rates from different studies. Factors like the methodology, the study setting, population studied, the definition of the DFU, and the denominator used to calculate the incidence/prevalence rates should be carefully considered for proper interpretation of the data.

3.2 Epidemiology of Diabetic Foot Complications

The International Diabetes Federation (IDF) has organized the countries in American continent into two regions—North America and Caribbean (NAC) and South and Central America (SACA). The NAC region consists of the USA, Mexico, Canada, and 21 Caribbean countries and territories. An estimated 357.1 million adults aged 20–79 years have diabetes in this region, with a regional prevalence of 13.3%, the highest of all IDF regions. The SACA region with 20 countries and territories has a regional prevalence of 9.4% with 335.1 million diabetic population living in this region. The Australian continent with three countries Australia, New Zealand, and Papua New Guinea comes under the Western Pacific IDF region. The 2019 IDF data shows that the annual incidence of foot ulceration is 2% and of amputation is 1% in patients with diabetes in high-income countries [4]. This is expected to be even higher in low- and middle-income countries.

Globally, North America has the highest prevalence of diabetic foot problems, about 13.0% (10–15.9%) and Oceania has the least, about 3.0% (0.9–5.0%). Within North America, Canada had a higher prevalence of 14.8% compared to the USA prevalence of 13.0% [5]. Differences in age, duration of diabetes, BMI, presence of hypertension, smoking, and diabetic retinopathy might explain the high prevalence in American countries. There are very few studies from South America regarding the epidemiology of diabetic foot problems.

3.2.1 North America and Caribbean

Globally, North America has the highest health-care and economic burden due to diabetic foot problems. Every 30 seconds, about, one million dollars is spent on the inpatient and outpatient care of the diabetic foot, in the USA alone. The estimate of the annual US burden of DFUs is at least $15 billion. The 1999–2000 NHANES data showed a prevalence of 7.7% foot ulcers in patients with diabetes [6]. Data analysis of a subpopulation of Medicare beneficiaries with diabetes in the USA in 2008 showed a point prevalence of 8.0% for white, 8.7% for African-Americans, 4.2% for Asian, 8.6% for Hispanic, 9.6% for American Indian/Alaska Natives, and 5.5% for others [7]. Another analysis of a 5% random sample of Medicare and Private insurance beneficiaries for the period between 2007 and 2011 showed an incidence of 12.8% in Medicare and 4.8% in privately insured patients with diabetes [8].

The Center for Disease Control and Prevention reported that the age-adjusted prevalence of a history of DFU in adults with diabetes in the USA in 2000–2002 was 12.7%. The highest prevalence was in the states of California, Indiana, and Nevada with a prevalence of about 16%. DFU prevalence was lowest in the states of Colorado, North Carolina, North Dakota, Ohio, West Virginia, and Wisconsin at about 10%. In a multivariate analysis, the significant risk factors identified were younger age, longer duration of diabetes, white race, Hispanic ethnicity, obesity, insulin use, and smoking [9].

The Seattle diabetic foot study is one of the few longest and largest prospective studies on the epidemiology of DFU. The study reported an incidence of 5.0 per 100 person-years [10]. Another prospective observational study, the TRIAD study in Michigan conducted between 1999 and 2003 showed that 3% of diabetic patients in managed care had DFU and 2% had amputations [11]. A study from Texas in 2003, reported an incidence of ulceration, infection, and amputation in patients with diabetes was 68.4, 36.5, and 5.9 per 1000 patients with diabetes per year, respectively [12]. Veterans Health administration and Medicare claims data for a cohort of 255,234 patients with diabetes was analyzed for the period from 2000–2004. This data showed that 54.8% had a documented foot condition in 1999 and 26.9 per 1000 had an LEA over the period of 2000–2004 [13].

The prevalence of DFU in Canada is estimated to be around 14.8% (9.4–20.1%) [5]. A nation-wide study in Canada using four linked databases showed a prevalence of 75 per 100,000 and an incidence rate of 42.4 per 100,000 of the general population. The highest prevalence was in Manitoba at 106.2 per 100,000 and the lowest was in Ontario 64.7 per 100,000 population. The average cost per prevalent case was $21,371 [14]. In the ABCD study conducted in the Alberta province of Canada where 2040 diabetic patients self-reported, 18% of the respondents reported peripheral neuropathy, 28% had peripheral vasculopathy, 6% had foot ulcer or infection and 1.4% has had gangrene or amputation [15]. In a recent report, 27.4% of the ABCD cohort in Alberta, reported having diabetic foot problems [16]. Another prevalence study in a remote Northern Canadian Aboriginal community in Manitoba showed that amongst 169 diabetic patients 82% were at high risk of developing ulcers in the future [17].

There is no nation-wide prevalence or incidence data available on diabetic foot problems from Mexico. A small clinic-based study from Tijuana, Mexico showed that 44% of the 205 patients studied were at high risk of developing diabetic foot problems [18]. Diabetic foot problems are very common in the Caribbean region. Foot infections are the leading cause of hospital admissions to the surgical floors in Caribbean public hospitals. In 2001, Walrond reported that on average, 75% of the beds in the surgical wards of a public hospital in Barbados were occupied by patients with diabetic foot problems [19]. A 1-year prospective study in an Eastern Caribbean population showed 13.7% of hospitalized patients had major and 30.0% had minor amputations [20]. A study from a specialist diabetes clinic in Jamaica showed that amongst 188 diabetic patients, the prevalence of amputations was 8.5%, current ulcers were 4.3%, and current foot infections were 3.7% [21]. Amongst 2106 patients with diabetes attending primary care in Trinidad, the prevalence of neuropathy was 49%, previous foot ulceration was 12% and amputation was 4% [22]. Annually, the government of Trinidad and Tobago spends about US $85 million, solely for the inpatient care of patients with diabetic foot infections [23].

3.2.2 South and Central America

A cross-sectional study of 11,357 inpatients across 135 health centres in 9 Latin American countries showed a diabetic foot prevalence of 14.8% in hospitalized patients. The prevalence was highest in Chile at 13% and lowest in Bolivia at 3.8% [24]. An epidemiological survey conducted in six health districts in Brazil showed that among 1374 diabetic patients, the diabetic foot was observed in 9%. The prevalence of lower limb amputations was 2.3% of the total sample and 25.6% among individuals with foot complications [25]. A large multicentre cross-sectional study BRAZUPA conducted across 19 centres in Brazil showed a prevalence of active ulcer in 18.6% and amputation in 13.7% of the 1455 patients with high-risk feet [26]. The BRAZUPA study found that younger age at presentation and neuropathy as a significant risk factor for DFU than ischaemic foot, whereas ischemia was more associated with poor outcomes and amputation. In 2014, Brazil spent about Int$ 361 million for the treatment of patients with diabetic foot complications, which is about 0.31% of public health expenses for this period [27]. In a rural community in Ecuador, the prevalence of active diabetic foot disease was 7% in patients with diabetes [28]. A cross-sectional study on 307 diabetic patients from Colombia showed that 13.0% had a history of previous ulcers and 1.6% had amputations [29]. In 2015, a study from Peru reported that US$ 74.5million was attributable to the prevention and management of high-risk diabetic foot [30].

3.2.3 Oceania

The Diabetic Foot Australia (DFA) is a national body established in 2005 with the primary goal to end avoidable amputations within a generation, i.e., by 2040. The DFA has recently established a national diabetes-related foot disease strategy for 2018–2022 [31]. The DFA has estimated that in any given day in Australia:

- Thousand people will be hospitalized with diabetic foot problem
- Twelve will undergo diabetes-related amputation
- Four will die due to diabetic foot disease
- Four million dollars will be spent treating diabetic foot disease

The Australian Diabetes Obesity and lifestyle study (AusDiab) is a population-based study in Australia which included 11,247 people aged ≥25 years from 42 randomly selected areas of Australia. This study showed that 19.6% were at risk for foot ulceration [32]. The Fremantle Diabetes study showed a DFU prevalence of 1.2% in patients with diabetes in Phase I (1993–1996) and 1.5% in Phase II (2008–2011) [33].

There are no population-based studies from New Zealand on the epidemiology of diabetic foot problems. In a study from the Waikato region of New Zealand, out of the 2192 diabetic patients who attended for retinopathy screening, 13% were at high risk of developing diabetic foot disease [34]. Two Maori primary health organizations in Northcote in 2012 reported that 8% of diabetic patients had active foot ulcer [35]. The prevalence of abnormal foot sensations in 459 diabetic patients was 30% in Nauru, 23% in Solomon Islands, and 19% in Vanuatu [36].

3.3 Geographic Variations in the Characteristics, Risk Factors, and Outcomes of DFU

The type, site, and etiology of ulcer can vary from country to country depending on the climate, use of footwear, access to health care, physical activity, and culture. In general, diabetic foot problems are predominantly ischemic in developed countries and neuropathic/neuro-ischemic in developing countries [3]. It is believed that due to resource-poor settings, diabetic patients in developing countries have long-term suboptimal glycemic control and are more prone to develop neuropathy. However, the scenario is now changing, and the occurrence of peripheral vascular disease is increasing in developing nations [37]. Similarly, the outcome of the DFU is dependant not only on the biological factors of the individual but also on the management decisions of the health-care professional and the availability of health-care resources.

3.3.1 Characteristics of DFU

In the Seattle diabetic foot study, out of 1483 limbs prospectively followed up, 162 ulcers developed over a mean follow-up period of 3.7 years. About half of the limbs with ulcers (49.1%) had clinicians diagnosed with peripheral vascular disease (PVD) and 67.9% had absent monofilament sensations [38]. A study from Ontario on 87 patients showed that 54.4% of DFUs were non-planar, 60.8% were small <1 cm^2, 14.4% had gangrene, and 2.4% had osteomyelitis. Preexisting DFUs, multiple DFUs at first presentation, ulcer size >3 cm^2 and PVD were associated with delayed healing [39]. In another single center hospital-based study in Ontario, 279 DFU patients were studied over 5 years. Majority of the ulcers (82.5%) were in the forefoot. Palpable pedal pulse and use of total contact cast were associated with better wound healing [40].

A longitudinal study in a tertiary care hospital in Mexico from 2012–2015 on 100 patients with DFU showed that inappropriate shoes and formation of blisters were the two main causes for foot lesions. The size of ulcer ranged from 1.5–8 cm^2.

Majority (75%) were plantar; 48% were forefoot ulcers; and 29% were in hindfoot. During the study period, 15% had major and 30% had minor amputations. Wagner Grade 3 and 4 accounted for 73% of the ulcers [41]. In the BRAZUPA study, 14.2% were ischemic, 39.3% were neuro-ischemic, and 45.1% were neuropathic ulcers. Male gender, ischemic foot, hypertension, South/Southeast region of origin, previous history of ulcer, and altered vibration sensations were associated with amputation [26].

A study from a tertiary care hospital at the Northern Territory of Australia reported ulcers in the plantar surface of forefoot (74.9%) were common. More than half (54.8%) had Wagner grade 2 and above [42]. A clinic-based study at the Foot wound clinic in Western Sydney described a median ulcer area of 1.5 cm^2 and 45.1% on the plantar aspect of the foot, 16.6% had ischaemic ulcers, and 25.6% had osteomyelitis [43].

Cultural barriers and access to health care also affect the clinical presentation and outcomes of DFU. In Trinidad and Tribago, out of the 446 patients admitted with DFU, about 36.6% were walking barefoot, 42.4% had footwear-related injuries, and 1.6% were due to burns. More than half of them identified the foot injury early but there was a median delay of about 6 days before presentation to the medical practitioner. About one third had tried some home remedies before presenting to the health-care providers [44]. Of note, most of the Caribbean patients with diabetes routinely wear "flip-flops" and the Caribbean health care has successfully used the "slipping slipper" sign in public education campaigns to identify patients with high-risk feet [20]. In Colombia, 76.2% of diabetic patients did not have foot examination over a period of 1 year and many were not asked about dysesthesia and claudication, despite >85% having such symptoms [29].

3.3.2 Risk Factors for DFU

Various studies from many different parts of the world have reported the risk factors associated with DFU. Many of these studies analyzed retrospective data. Various demographic and clinical risk factors have been studied and shown to be associated with increased risk of DFU. Age, male gender, height, weight, BMI, ethnicity, poor socioeconomic status, smoking, and alcohol use are the demographic factors that have demonstrated a relationship with DFU. Indigenous populations have long been known to have poor health outcomes and are expected to be at higher risk of diabetes-related foot disease and amputations. The data on the association of ethnicity and the occurrence of DFU is scarce. A study done in 200 patients in Mexico showed that there was no relationship between sociodemographic variables and risk of DFU. Rather, poor knowledge and poor foot care practices have a significant correlation with the development of DFU [45].

A systematic review of 67 studies from 33 countries showed that the patients with diabetic foot were older, had a lower body mass index, longer diabetic duration, and had more hypertension, diabetic retinopathy, and smoking history than patients without diabetic foot [5]. A systematic review and meta-analysis done by

Crawford et al. collated 16,385 individual patient data from ten cohort studies conducted worldwide. Age, sex, height, BMI, smoking, alcohol use, duration of diabetes, HbA1c, Insulin treatment, vision problems, retinopathy, kidney problems, inability to feel 10 g monofilament, absent pedal pulses, absent ankle reflex, reduced vibration perception threshold (VPT), abnormal ankle-brachial index (ABI), foot deformities, history of ulcer, and history of amputation have all been reported to be associated with DFU. However, the meta-analysis found that three factors—history of foot ulceration, inability to feel 10 g monofilament, and absence of any pedal pulse—were consistently and independently predictive of DFU. A combination of these three factors is comparable to other complex approaches to predict the occurrence of DFU and is very simple for clinical use [46].

The Seattle diabetic foot study prospectively looked at the independent effects of multiple potential risk factors. Participants were recruited in 1990 at a single Veteran Affairs Medical clinic in Seattle and followed up until 2012. Significant predictors of foot ulcer were glycosylated hemoglobin (HbA1c), impaired vision, prior foot ulcer, monofilament insensitivity, tinea pedis, and onychomycosis. They concluded that this readily available clinical information can predict the development of DFU and hence help to target the patients who are at high risk of DFU [10]. Another multicenter prospective follow-up study from Massachusetts showed that clinical examination and monofilament tests are the most sensitive to identify feet at risk, whereas foot pressures are very specific and can be used for providing advice on footwear [47]. A cross-sectional study of 117 patients in the Federal district of Brazil identified similar risk factors for DFU—peripheral arterial disease, painful peripheral polyneuropathy, foot deformities, loss of protective sensations, and dry skin [48]. Risk factors identified for DFU in an Australian study were diabetes duration, height, age, and uric acid levels [32].

3.3.3 Outcomes of DFU

The natural history of DFU is sobering. About 50–60% die within 5 years. About 50% of DFUs get infected and about 20% end up in amputation. The outcome of the DFU varies widely between and within countries [1]. A pooled analysis of 5 randomized controlled trials (RCTs) in the USA showed that 23.9% ulcers healed within 12 weeks and another 32.8% healed within 20 weeks of receiving good standard care [49]. In Canada, after a 52 weeks follow-up, 86.6% ulcers healed and the mean time to healing was 10.2 ± 10.2 weeks. At 52 weeks, 7.1% have had amputation and 8.9% had died [15]. A prospective cohort study in Brazil showed that 61.8% healed after 1 year [48].

The story does not end with healing and the DFUs that have healed have a high chance to recur. The recurrence rate is 17% per person-year in North America and was not significant in Canada and Cuba [50]. A prospective study from Maryland, the USA between 2012 and 2016 showed a recurrence rate of 30.6% at 1 year and 64.4% at 3 years, in a multidisciplinary setting [51]. Another study from multiple centers including one from Australia showed a similar recurrence rate of 31% at

1 year. The median ulcer-free survival in the healed group was 233 days [52]. A meta-analysis of risk factors for recurrence reported that male gender, smoking, duration of DM, duration of past DFUs, plantar ulcers, PAD, and peripheral neuropathy are associated with recurrence [53].

3.4 Epidemiology of Lower Limb Amputation

Lower extremity amputation (LEA) remains the major and most serious outcome of DFU. Globally, 50–70% of all nontraumatic amputations are due to diabetes. Persons with diabetes are 15–40 times more likely to lose a limb than someone without diabetes. About 1.3–7% of the world population has already undergone diabetes-related amputation and, in a year, about 0.9–2.4% will lose their limbs to diabetes [1]. Data on diabetes-related LEAs are abundant. However, comparing the results from the epidemiological studies on LEA is beset by major differences in the study population (general vs. at risk), setting (community vs hospital-based), and the definition of major and minor amputations, to mention a few. Some studies report the rates in the general population and others to report the rates in population at risk, e.g., in patients with DM.

3.4.1 Incidence and Prevalence of Diabetes-Related LEA

Great geographic variations exist in the rates of diabetes-related LEA and regional variations within a country are also common. In some countries, amputation rates have declined as a result of foot care initiative programs and projects. In others, either no reduction or an increase in LEA rate has been reported. A nation-wide cross-sectional data from the USA, between 2000 and 2015, has shown a resurgence of LEA after a two-decade long decline. This increase in LEA was more pronounced in men and in the younger age group [54]. Another interesting observation from the US data is the wide variation in the LEA rates between different states. It has been shown using Medicare beneficiaries data that in contiguous portions of southeast Texas, southern Oklahoma, Louisiana, Arkansas, and Mississippi have disproportionately high LEA rates. Low rates of LEA were found through contiguous portions of southern Florida, New Mexico, Arizona, and eastern Michigan [55]. This geographical clustering remained after adjusting for known confounders like age, race, socioeconomic status, access to health care, and frequency of microvascular and macrovascular complications. It is unclear as to the cause of such high variation. It is plausible that this could be due to the biological differences in the disease process itself or due to variations in the implementation of guidelines, availability of health-care resources, health-care provider training, and/or therapeutic preference or patient preference.

Data from the Canadian Institute for health information's discharge abstract database for the period between 2006–2011 shows that the average age-adjusted incidence rate of LEA among people with diabetes was 280.5 per 100,000, whereas for people without diabetes it was 9.7 per 100,000. Quebec and British Columbia had the lowest and New Foundland and Labrador had the highest incidence rates [56]. A cross-sectional study from the Mexican social security Institute compared the diabetes-related LEA incidence between 2004 and 2013. Sadly, the amputation rates in Mexico increased from 2004 to 2013 [57]. Diabetes-related LEA rates are among the world's highest in Barbados. A prospective study conducted in 1999 for 1 year showed an incidence rate of 936 per 10^5 patients with DM [58].

There is not much-published data from South America on the epidemiology of lower limb amputations. From 2011 to 2016, 102,056 amputation surgeries were performed in the Brazilian Unified National Health System (SUS), of which 70% occurred in individuals with diabetes mellitus [59]. Another study using the discharge data from 32 hospitals in Brazil for the period between 1985 and 2008 showed an average annual incidence rate of 30 per 100,000 inhabitants of nontraumatic amputations out of which 95% were due to DM [60]. A narrative review by Seguel, from the University of Chile, has reported that the diabetes-related LEA rates have increased by 28% from 2002 to 2006 [61]. A study from Costa Rica between 2001–2007 showed a diabetes-related incidence of amputation was 6.02 per 1000 person-years (8.65 in men and 4.50 in women) (Table 3.1) [62].

The Diabetic foot Australia reports that 12 in 100,000 general population will have diabetes-related LEA every 20 days. Regional variations do exist within Australia. Northern Territory has the highest rates of lower limb amputations, both traumatic and nontraumatic [31]. This disparity in the incidence is thought to be due to the high proportion of Indigenous population in this part of Australia, a population well known to have high incidence of type 2 DM. A clinic-based study in a tertiary care hospital in the Northern Territory showed a high amputation rate of 51.3% after a median follow-up of 5.8 years [63]. A nation-wide study in New Zealand using the Virtual Diabetes Register and the hospitalization data for the period between 2011–2014, showed an annual incidence rate of 98 per 10^5 diabetic population of major and 152 per 10^5 of minor. The amputation rates varied fourfold across New

Table 3.1 Summary of the incidence data from various countries in the NAC, SACA, and Oceania regions

Country	Year	Incidence (per 10^5)	Population
USA [54]	2000, 2009, 2015	538, 307, 462	People with DM
Canada [56]	2006–2011	280.5	People with DM
Mexico [57]	2004, 2013	Major—100.9, 111.1 Minor—168.8, 162.5	People with DM
Barbados [58]	2000	936 (557 minor and 379 major)	People with DM
Brazil [60]	1985–2008	30	General population
Costa Rica [62]	2001–2007	920 (360 major and 560 minor)	People with DM
Chile [61]	2002, 2006	602	People with DM
Australia [31]	2012–2013	219	General population
New Zealand [63]	2010–2013	250 (98 major and 152 minor)	People with DM

Some of the incidence rates shown in this table are derived from the original study to get a number equivalent to per 10^5 population per year

Zealand the lowest observed in Waitemata (53.3 per 10^5 major amputations) and the highest rate of 190 per 10^5 in the Tairawhiti district health board. Ethnicity could explain a part of the variation with Tairawhiti having a higher proportion of Maoris than the national average. However, this variation is only marginally affected by other known comorbidities, which indicates that more work is needed to find out the causes of this variation, and more efforts are needed to close this gap [64].

3.4.2 Risk Factors for Diabetes-Related LEA

The demographic factors well known to be associated with diabetes-related LEA are age, gender, ethnicity, and socioeconomic status. Marked ethnic differences exist in the incidence of amputation. American studies suggest that LEAs are more likely to occur in African-Americans than in Caucasians. This difference cannot just be explained by differences in access to health care. Studies in Veterans with equal access to health care confirms than Native and African-Americans are at higher risk for diabetes-related LEA when compared to Caucasians, whereas Asian-Americans are at lower risk than Caucasians [65]. Similarly, in Australia Indigenous ethnicity is shown to be a risk factor for amputation [63]. Other person-specific risk factors described in literature are smoking, alcohol use, poor glycemic control, longer duration of DM, presence of other diabetes-related micro and macrovascular complications, insulin treatment, previous DFU, previous amputation, and foot deformities. The Seattle prospective diabetic foot study showed arterial disease and sensory neuropathy are the only limb specific risk factors associated with amputation [66].

3.5 Diabetic Foot Infections

Infections of the feet in diabetic patients can develop through DFUs, trauma, skin cracks, fissures, or other defects in the nail bed such as paronychia. The infection can either be a localized superficial skin involvement or can involve deeper skin structures beyond the site of local trauma. The different types of diabetic foot infections (DFI) include cellulitis, abscess, tendinitis, necrotizing fasciitis, septic arthritis, and osteomyelitis. The most common predisposing factor for DFI in a diabetic foot with loss of sensations is DFU. It is estimated that about 59% of DFUs are infected at presentation and infections result in multiple hospitalizations and multiple antibiotic courses, poor wound healing and increased risk of amputations, frequently systemic compromise, and increase in mortality. DFI in combination with PAD significantly increases the risk of amputations [67].

3.5.1 Microbial Epidemiology of Infection in Diabetic Foot Patients

The microbiology of the DFI is well studied. With various bacterial culture and molecular approaches, diverse microbiota have been reported in the DFUs/DFIs. Geographic features, patient metadata (e.g., Smoking), duration and location of infection, and previous antibiotic use will influence the bacterial distribution in an individual patient. For example, in Western countries Gram-positive aerobic bacteria are commonly reported. In warmer climates particularly in Asia and Africa, Gram-negative bacteria are more prevalent. DFUs of shorter duration tend to have simpler microbiota mainly Gram-positive cocci (GPC) and chronic DFUs are usually polymicrobial. Aerobic bacteria are localized in the upper surfaces where the oxygen content is high and anaerobic bacteria are found in deeper infections. Globally, the most common GPC isolated form DFU is Staphylococcus and the most frequent Gram-negative rods (GNB) are from the Enterobacteriaceae family (*E. coli*, Klebsiella, Proteus, etc.). The anerobic bacteria isolated from up to 95% of deep diabetic infections are *Peptostreptococcus* spp., *Bacteroides* spp., and *Prevotella* spp. [68]. Some of the studies from the American and Australian continents are summarized in Table 3.2.

Table 3.2 Summary of a few studies on the microbial pattern of diabetic foot infections in the American and Australian continents

Author, year	Country, period of study	Specimen	Bacteria	Most efficient antibiotic	Antibiotic resistance
Henig et al. [69]	USA, 2018	77% tissue and 22% swab	72% Polymicrobial; 57% of monomicrobial was SA	Not reported	MRSA 31.4%; 56.2% had at least 1 MDRO
Citron et al. [70]	USA, 2001–2004	Tissue culture	83% polymicrobial; SA in 76.6% and GNB in 19.7% in all cultures	Ertapenem, piperacillin-tazobactam	MRSA 11.8%
Sánchez-Sánchez et al. [71]	Mexico, 2011–2016	Tissue sample	87.3% SA in all cultures	Levofloxacin, cefalotin, and amikacin	MRSA 42%
Víquez-Molina et al. [72]	Costa Rica, 2014–2016	Tissue sample	26.6% Staphylococcus in monomicrobial cultures	Not reported	MRSA 9.2%
Islam et al. [73]	Trinidad and Tribago, 2011–2012	Not available	56.8% polymicrobial; 64.7% GNB	Ciprofloxacin and ceftazidime	MDRO 25.9%; ESBL producing 11.3% MRSA 4.5%
Perim et al. [74]	Brazil, 2013	Tissue sample	70% polymicrobial 40% GPC in all cultures	Imipenem and gentamicin for GNB	59% MRSA, 26% of SA were vancomycin resistant
Carro et al. [75]	Argentina, 2018	Soft tissue samples	53.8% polymicrobial; 47.1% of monomicrobial were GNB	GNB-ciprofloxacin	Not reported

(continued)

Table 3.2 (continued)

Author, year	Country, period of study	Specimen	Bacteria	Most efficient antibiotic	Antibiotic resistance
Kurup et al. [76]	Guyana, 2019	Not available	42.1% polymicrobial; 63% of all culturesweréGNB-Pseudomonas was common among GNB; SA 20% of all GPC	Not reported	MRSA 12.1% of all GPC cultures
Valenzuela et al. [77]	Chile, 2013–2018	Bone culture	26% polymicrobial; GP 68.4% of all Entercoccus faecalis is the most common GPC	Carbapenems	44.5% of SA resistant to cefoxitin and 59% of COL SA oxacillin resistant. No vancomycin resistance. 87% of Klebsieallaand 63% of *E. coli* were ESBL producing
Commons et al. [78]	Australia, 2012–2013	67.3% were non-sterile superficial and deep swabs	30.5% of all were SA and 20.9% were Pseudomonas	NR	MRSA 11.9% of sterile specimens

Few studies report the proportion in all positive cultures and others report the proportion only in monomicrobial cultures. *GPC* Gram-positive cocci, *GNB* Gram-negative bacteria, *MDRO* multi-drug resistant organism, *SA Staphylococcus aureus*, *MRSA* methicillin resistant *Staphylococcus aureus*, *ESBL* extended spectrum beta-lactamase, *COL SA* coagulase negative *Staphylococcus aureus*

3.5.2 Diagnosis and Assessing Severity of DFI

According to existing literature, many of the noninfected DFUs receive antibiotics leading to antibiotic resistance. It is critical to diagnose an infected diabetic foot for the appropriate use of antibiotics. The diagnosis of infection should be based on the presence of at least two of the following signs: induration, perilesional erythema, hyperesthesia, tenderness, warmth, and purulent exudate. These local signs especially warmth and erythema may not manifest in severe ischemia. Other nonspecific signs are non-purulent discharge, undermining of edges, and friable discolored granulation tissue [79]. Cutaneous bulla, discolored skin, soft tissue crepitus, and fetid odor indicate necrotizing infections. The following findings support the presence of osteomyelitis which can further be confirmed by imaging [80]

- Grossly visible bone or positive probe test
- Larger Ulcers >2 cm^2

- Ulcers present for >1–2 weeks
- ESR >70 mm per hour

Several wound classification systems exist to assess the severity of DFI, but none are universally accepted. Meggit-Wagner, ANM-SEGAL, University of Texas, SAD, SSS, GIBBONS, PEDIS, SEWSS, WIFI classification systems combine scores for various elements of diabetic foot characteristics, such as infection, neuropathy, location, ischemia, edema, and the degree of tissue involvement. The International Working Group on the Diabetic Foot (IWGDF) recommends not to use these classification systems to decide management or to assess prognosis in an individual patient with DFU. The only classification systems which would guide to decide treatment in an individual patient are IWGDF/IDSA (Infectious Diseases Society of America) and the WIfI (Wound/Infection/Ischemia) classification in patients with PAD. The IWGDF/ISDA has four grades of severity and will assist with decisions on hospitalization for parenteral antibiotics. Where the appropriate setting is available, WiFi should be used to assess the perfusion and the likelihood of benefit from revascularisation [81]. The SINBAD system is recommended for communications between health-care professionals and for conducting regional/national/international audits to allow comparisons on the outcomes of DFU.

3.5.3 Antibiotic Treatment of DFI

The microbiology of DFI is diverse and multidrug-resistant organisms (MDRO) are rapidly emerging all around the world, mostly due to the inappropriate use of antibiotics. The selection of empirical antibiotic therapy is a clinical challenge and should consider MRSA, Pseudomonas, and anaerobes. A metanalysis of 16 RCTs (8 from the USA and 1 multinational study involving the USA, Canada, Latin America, and Australia) including 4158 patients concluded that (a) Piperacillin/Tazobactam was superior to Ertapenem in severe infections but similar for moderate infections; (b) Ertapenem was more effective than tigecycline for moderate to severe infections; (c) the adjuvant use of topical agents such as topical pexiganan and topical gentamycin collagen sponge with systemic antibiotics improved the outcomes, compared with systemic antibiotics alone; (d) the rate of recurrence was significantly lower with the amino-penicillin regimen, compared with those using oral/intravenous ofloxacin, and (5) lower rates of complications with the imipenem/cilastatin regimen, compared with the piperacillin/tazobactam regimen [82]. A Cochrane review in 2015 had some key results on the adverse events and could not conclude the most efficient antibiotics—(a) carbapenems combined with anti-pseudomonal agents had fewer side effects than anti-pseudomonal penicillins, (b) Tigecycline produced more adverse effects than Ertapenem ± Vancomycin, (c) Linezolid caused more harm than ampicillin-sulbactam, and (d) Daptomycin had less adverse effects than vancomycin and other semisynthetic penicillins [83].

3.6 Conclusion

Given the devastating effects of the diabetic foot disease on the individual and the nation, many countries have established foot care programs nationally and/or in collaboration with other countries. The EVA project involving five Andean countries—Bolivia, Ecuador, Peru, Columbia, and Venezuela, focuses on education, treatment, and care of diabetes with the primary goal to reduce and prevent diabetes-related amputations. The action plan was to educate both patients with diabetes and healthcare professionals. The Brazilian "Save the diabetic foot Project" was started in 1992 and in the first decade of its activities was successful increasing the awareness on diabetic foot screening and improving management, by setting up foot care teams throughout the country. There are unresolved problems that the project is now confronting, particularly financial barriers. The Guyana Diabetes and Foot Care Project (GDFP) was created in 2008–2013. In phase 1 Interprofessional Diabetes foot center was established at the national referral hospital, and in Phase 2 this expanded to 6 administrative regions covering 90% of the population. This intervention resulted in a 68% reduction in the rate of major amputations and this reduction sustained over 5 years. The Diabetic Foot Canada and Diabetic foot Australia are similar initiatives aiming to reduce the burden of diabetic foot complications. Even with all these initiatives and efforts, diabetic foot problems will continue to rise in pandemic proportions and we should all be well prepared to face this significant public health issue.

References

1. Piaggesi A, Apelqvist J (eds) (2018) The diabetic foot syndrome. Front diabetes, vol 26. Karger, Basel, pp 1–18. https://doi.org/10.1159/000480040
2. Driver VR, Fabbi M, Lavery LA, Gibbons G (2010) The costs of diabetic foot: the economic case for the limb salvage team. J Am Podiatr Med Assoc 100(5):335–341
3. Armstrong DG, Boulton AJM, Bus SA (2017) Diabetic foot ulcers and their recurrence. N Engl J Med 376(24):2367–2375. https://doi.org/10.1056/NEJMra1615439. Review
4. https://diabetesatlas.org/upload/resources/2019/IDF_Atlas_9th_Edition_2019.pdf. Accessed 27 Nov 2019
5. Zhang P, Lu J, Jing Y, Tang S, Zhu D, Bi Y (2017) Global epidemiology of diabetic foot ulceration: a systematic review and meta-analysis. Ann Med 49(2):106–116. https://doi.org/10.1080/07853890.2016.1231932. Review
6. Gregg EW, Sorlie P, Paulose-Ram R, Gu Q, Eberhardt MS, Wolz M, Burt V, Curtin L, Engelgau M, Geiss L, 1999–2000 national health and nutrition examination survey (2004) Prevalence of lower-extremity disease in the US adult population >=40years of age with and without diabetes: 1999–2000 national health and nutrition examination survey. Diabetes Care 27(7):1591–1597
7. Margolis DJ, Malay DS, Hoffstad OJ et al (2011) Prevalence of diabetes, diabetic foot ulcer, and lower extremity amputation among Medicare beneficiaries, 2006 to 2008: Data Points #1. 2011 Feb 17. In: Data points publication series. Agency for Healthcare Research and Quality (US), Rockville, MD. Available from: https://www.ncbi.nlm.nih.gov/books/NBK63602/
8. Rice JB, Desai U, Cummings AK et al (2014) Burden of DFUs for medicare and private insurers. Diabetes Care 37:651–658

9. Centers for Disease Control and Prevention (CDC) (2003) History of foot ulcer among persons with diabetes—United States, 2000–2002. MMWR Morb Mortal Wkly Rep 52(45):1098–1102
10. Boyko EJ, Ahroni JH, Cohen V, Nelson KM, Heagerty PJ (2006) Prediction of diabetic foot ulcer occurrence using commonly available clinical information: the Seattle Diabetic Foot Study. Diabetes Care 29(6):1202–1207
11. McEwen LN, Ylitalo KR, Munson M, Herman WH, Wrobel JS (2016) Foot complications and mortality: results from translating research into action for diabetes (TRIAD). J Am Podiatr Med Assoc 106(1):7–14
12. Lavery LA, Armstrong DG, Wunderlich RP, Tredwell J, Boulton AJ (2003) Diabetic foot syndrome: evaluating the prevalence and incidence of foot pathology in Mexican Americans and non-Hispanic whites from a diabetes disease management cohort. Diabetes Care 26(5):1435–1438
13. Helmer D, Tseng CL, Wrobel J, Tiwari A, Rajan M, Pogach L, Sambamoorthi U, Feinglass J (2011) Assessing the risk of lower extremity amputations using an administrative data-based foot risk index in elderly patients with diabetes. J Diabetes 3(3):248–255
14. Hopkins RB, Burke N, Harlock J, Jegathisawaran J, Goeree R (2015) Economic burden of illness associated with diabetic foot ulcers in Canada. BMC Health Serv Res 15:13
15. Al Sayah F, Soprovich A, Qiu W, Edwards AL, Johnson JA (2015) Diabetic foot disease, self-care and clinical monitoring in adults with type 2 diabetes: the Alberta's caring for diabetes (ABCD) cohort study. Can J Diabetes 39(Suppl 3):S120–S126. https://doi.org/10.1016/j.jcjd.2015.05.006
16. Zhao H, McClure NS, Johnson JA, Soprovich A, Al Sayah F, Eurich DT (2019. pii: S1499-2671(19)30612-4) A longitudinal study on the association between diabetic foot disease and health-related quality of life in adults with type 2 diabetes. Can J Diabetes. https://doi.org/10.1016/j.jcjd.2019.08.008
17. Reid KS, Martin BD, Duerksen F, Nicolle LE, Garrett M, Simonsen JN, Trepman E, Embil JM (2006) Diabetic foot complications in a northern Canadian Aboriginal community. Foot Ankle Int 27(12):1065–1073
18. Márquez-Godínez SA, Zonana-Nacach A, Anzaldo-Campos MC, Muñoz-Martínez JA (2014) Diabetic foot risk in patients with type II diabetes mellitus in a family medicine unit. SEMERGEN 40(4):183–188. https://doi.org/10.1016/j.semerg.2013.10.004. Spanish
19. Walrond ER (2001) The Caribbean experience with the diabetic foot management of the diabetic foot. West Indian Med J 50(Suppl 1):24–26
20. Islam S, Harnarayan P, Cawich SO, Budhooram S, Bheem V, Mahabir V, Ramsewak S, Aziz I, Naraynsingh V (2013) Epidemiology of diabetic foot infections in an eastern Caribbean population: a prospective study. Perm J 17(2):37–40. https://doi.org/10.7812/TPP/12-126. PubMed PMID: 23704841; PubMed Central PMCID: PMC3662275
21. Ferguson TS, Tulloch-Reid MK, Younger NO, Wright-Pascoe RA, Boyne MS, McFarlane SR, Francis DK, Wilks RJ (2013) Diabetic foot complications among patients attending a specialist diabetes clinic in Jamaica: prevalence and associated factors. West Indian Med J 62(3):216–223
22. Gulliford MC, Mahabir D (2002) Diabetic foot disease and foot care in a Caribbean community. Diabetes Res Clin Pract 56(1):35–40
23. Cawich SO, Islam S, Hariharan S, Harnarayan P, Budhooram S, Ramsewak S, Naraynsingh V (2014) The economic impact of hospitalization for diabetic foot infections in a Caribbean nation. Perm J 18(1):e101–e104. https://doi.org/10.7812/TPP/13-096. PubMed PMID: 24626079; PubMed Central PMCID: PMC3951038
24. Carro GV, Saurral R, Sagüez FS, Witman EL (2018) Diabetic foot among hospitalized patients in Latin America. Medicina (B Aires) 78(4):243–251. Spanish
25. Vieira-Santos IC, Souza WV, Carvalho EF, Medeiros MC, Nóbrega MG, Lima PM (2008) Prevalence of diabetic foot and associated factors in the family health units of the city of Recife, Pernambuco State, Brazil, in 2005. Cad Saude Publica 24(12):2861–2870. Portuguese
26. Parisi MC, Moura Neto A, Menezes FH, Gomes MB, Teixeira RM, de Oliveira JE, Pereira JR, Fonseca RM, Guedes LB, Costa E Forti A, de Oliveira AM, de Medeiros Nóbrega MB, Colares

VN, Schmid H, Nienov OH, Nery M, Fernandes TD, Pedrosa HC, Schreiber de Oliveira Cda S, Ronsoni M, Rezende KF, Quilici MT, Vieira AE, de Macedo GM, Stuchi-Perez EG, Dinhane KG, Pace AE, de Freitas MC, Calsolari MR, Saad MJ (2016) Baseline characteristics and risk factors for ulcer, amputation and severe neuropathy in diabetic foot at risk: the BRAZUPA study. Diabetol Metab Syndr 8:25

27. Del Brutto OH, Mera RM, King NR, Zambrano M, Sullivan LJ (2016) The burden of diabetes-related foot disorders in community-dwellers living in rural Ecuador: Results of the Atahualpa Project. Foot (Edinb) 28:26–29. https://doi.org/10.1016/j.foot.2016.05.003
28. Toscano CM, Sugita TH, Rosa MQM, Pedrosa HC, Rosa RDS, Bahia LR (2018) Annual direct medical costs of diabetic foot disease in Brazil: a cost of illness study. Int J Environ Res Public Health 15(1) pii: E89
29. Pinilla AE, Sánchez AL, Mejía A, Barrera MP (2011) Primary-care prevention activities in outpatients suffering from diabetic foot care. Rev Salud Publica (Bogota) 13(2):262–273. Spanish
30. Cárdenas MK, Mirelman AJ, Galvin CJ, Lazo-Porras M, Pinto M, Miranda JJ, Gilman RH (2015) The cost of illness attributable to diabetic foot and cost-effectiveness of secondary prevention in Peru. BMC Health Serv Res 15:483
31. Van Netten JJ, Lazzarini PA, Fitridge R, Kinnear E, Griffiths I, Malone M, Perrin BM, Prentice J, Sethi S, Wraight PR (2017) Australian diabetes-related foot disease strategy 2018–2022: the first step towards ending avoidable amputations within a generation. Diabetic Foot Australia, Wound Management CRC, Brisbane
32. Tapp RJ, Shaw JE, de Courten MP, Dunstan DW, Welborn TA, Zimmet PZ, AusDiab Study Group (2003) Foot complications in Type 2 diabetes: an Australian population-based study. Diabet Med 20(2):105–113
33. Baba M, Davis WA, Norman PE, Davis TM (2015) Temporal changes in the prevalence and associates of foot ulceration in type 2 diabetes: the Fremantle Diabetes Study. J Diabetes Complicat 29(3):356–361
34. O'Shea C, McClintock J, Lawrenson R (2017) The prevalence of diabetic foot disease in the Waikato region. Diabetes Res Clin Pract 129:79–85. https://doi.org/10.1016/j.diabres.2017.04.020
35. Ihaka B, Bayley A, Rome K (2012) Foot problems in Maori with diabetes. N Z Med J 125(1360):48–56
36. Win Tin ST, Kenilorea G, Gadabu E, Tasserei J, Colagiuri R (2014) The prevalence of diabetes complications and associated risk factors in Pacific Islands countries. Diabetes Res Clin Pract 103(1):114–118
37. Abbas Z (2017) Managing the diabetic foot in resource-poor settings: challenges and solutions. Chronic Wound Care Manag Res 4:135–142. https://doi.org/10.2147/CWCMR.S98762
38. Boyko EJ, Ahroni JH, Stensel V, Forsberg RC, Davignon DR, Smith DG (1999) A prospective study of risk factors for diabetic foot ulcer. The Seattle Diabetic Foot Study. Diabetes Care 22(7):1036–1042
39. Roth-Albin I, Mai SHC, Ahmed Z, Cheng J, Choong K, Mayer PV (2017) Outcomes following advanced wound care for diabetic foot ulcers: a Canadian study. Can J Diabetes 41(1):26–32. https://doi.org/10.1016/j.jcjd.2016.06.007
40. Lu SH, McLaren AM (2017) Wound healing outcomes in a diabetic foot ulcer outpatient clinic at an acute care hospital: a retrospective study. J Wound Care 26(Suppl 10):S4–S11
41. Cervantes-García E, Salazar-Schettino PM (2017) Clinical and surgical characteristics of infected diabetic foot ulcers in a tertiary hospital of Mexico. Diabet Foot Ankle 8(1):1367210
42. Jeyaraman K, Berhane T, Hamilton M, Chandra AP, Falhammar H (2019) Mortality in patients with diabetic foot ulcer: a retrospective study of 513 cases from a single Centre in the Northern Territory of Australia. BMC Endocr Disord 19(1):1. https://doi.org/10.1186/s12902-018-0327-2. PubMed PMID: 30606164; PubMed Central PMCID: PMC6318899
43. Haji Zaine N, Burns J, Vicaretti M, Fletcher JP, Begg L, Hitos K (2014) Characteristics of diabetic foot ulcers in Western Sydney, Australia. J Foot Ankle Res 7(1):39. https://doi.org/10.1186/s13047-014-0039-4. eCollection 2014. PubMed PMID: 25279002; PubMed Central PMCID: PMC4182857

44. Islam S, Harnarayan P, Cawich S, Mahabir V, Budhooram S, Bheem V, Ramsewak S, Naraynsingh V (2013) Secondary prevention of diabetic foot infections in a Caribbean nation: a call for improved patient education. Int J Low Extrem Wounds 12(3):234–238. https://doi.org/10.1177/1534734613486151
45. Robles R, Compeán Ortiz L, Quirarte N, Berry D, Pérez P, Martínez S (2017) Knowledge and practices of diabetes foot care and risk of developing foot ulcers in México may have implications for patients of Méxican heritage living in the United States. Diabetes Educ 43:297–303. https://doi.org/10.1177/0145721717706417
46. Crawford F, Cezard G, Chappell FM, Murray GD, Price JF, Sheikh A, Simpson CR, Stansby GP, Young MJ (2015) A systematic review and individual patient data meta-analysis of prognostic factors for foot ulceration in people with diabetes: the international research collaboration for the prediction of diabetic foot ulcerations (PODUS). Health Technol Assess 19(57):1–210. https://doi.org/10.3310/hta19570. Review. PubMed PMID: 26211920; PubMed Central PMCID:PMC4781379
47. Pham H, Armstrong DG, Harvey C, Harkless LB, Giurini JM, Veves A (2000) Screening techniques to identify people at high risk for diabetic foot ulceration: a prospective multicenter trial. Diabetes Care 23(5):606–611
48. Dutra LMA, Melo MC, Moura MC, Leme LAP, De Carvalho MR, Mascarenhas AN, Novaes MRCG (2019) Prognosis of the outcome of severe diabetic foot ulcers with multidisciplinary care. J Multidiscip Healthc 12:349–359. https://doi.org/10.2147/JMDH.S194969. eCollection 2019. PubMed PMID: 31118658; PubMed Central PMCID: PMC6506632.5:483
49. Margolis DJ, Kantor J, Santanna J, Strom BL, Berlin JA (2000) Risk factors for delayed healing of neuropathic diabetic foot ulcers: a pooled analysis. Arch Dermatol 136(12):1531–1535
50. Fu XL, Ding H, Miao WW, Mao CX, Zhan MQ, Chen HL (2019) Global recurrence rates in diabetic foot ulcers: a systematic review and meta-analysis. Diabetes Metab Res Rev 35(6):e3160. https://doi.org/10.1002/dmrr.3160. Review
51. Hicks CW, Canner JK, Mathioudakis N, Lippincott C, Sherman RL, Abularrage CJ (2020) Incidence and Risk Factors Associated With Ulcer Recurrence Among Patients With Diabetic Foot Ulcers Treated in a Multidisciplinary Setting. J Surg Res 246:243–250
52. Akturk A, van Netten JJ, Scheer R, Vermeer M, van Baal JG (2019) Ulcer-free survival days and ulcer healing in patients with diabetic foot ulcers: a prospective cohort study. Int Wound J 16:1365. https://doi.org/10.1111/iwj.13199
53. Huang ZH, Li SQ, Kou Y, Huang L, Yu T, Hu A (2019) Risk factors for the recurrence of diabetic foot ulcers among diabetic patients: a meta-analysis. Int Wound J 16(6):1373–1382. https://doi.org/10.1111/iwj.13200
54. Geiss LS, Li Y, Hora I, Albright A, Rolka D, Gregg EW (2019) Resurgence of diabetes-related nontraumatic lower-extremity amputation in the young and middle-aged adult U.S. population. Diabetes Care 42(1):50–54
55. Margolis DJ, Hoffstad O, Nafash J, Leonard CE, Freeman CP, Hennessy S, Wiebe DJ (2011) Location, location, location: geographic clustering of lower-extremity amputation among Medicare beneficiaries with diabetes. Diabetes Care 34(11):2363–2367. https://doi.org/10.2337/dc11-0807. PubMed PMID: 21933906; PubMed Central PMCID: PMC3198303
56. Imam B, Miller WC, Finlayson HC, Eng JJ, Jarus T (2017) Incidence of lower limb amputation in Canada. Can J Public Health 108(4):e374–e380
57. Cisneros-González N, Ascencio-Montiel IJ, Libreros-Bango VN, Rodríguez-Vázquez H, Campos-Hernández Á, Dávila-Torres J, Kumate-Rodríguez J, Borja-Aburto VH (2016) Lower extremity amputation rates in diabetic patients. Rev Med Inst Mex Seguro Soc 54(4):472–479
58. Hennis AJ, Fraser HS, Jonnalagadda R, Fuller J, Chaturvedi N (2004) Explanations for the high risk of diabetes-related amputation in a Caribbean population of black African descent and potential for prevention. Diabetes Care 27(11):2636–2641
59. Santos KPBD, Luz SCTD, Mochizuki L, d'Orsi E (2018) Burden of disease from lower limb amputations attributable to diabetes mellitus in Santa Catarina State, Brazil, 2008–2013. Cad Saude Publica 34(1):e00013116

60. Barbosa BM, Monteiro RA, Sparano LF, Bareiro RF, Passos AD, Engel EE (2016) Incidence and causes of lower-limb amputations in the city of Ribeirão Preto from 1985 to 2008: evaluation of the medical records from 3,274 cases. Rev Bras Epidemiol 19(2):317–325. https://doi.org/10.1590/1980-5497201600020009
61. Seguel G (2013) An update on diabetic foot. Rev Med Chil 141(11):1464–1469. https://doi.org/10.4067/S0034-98872013001100014
62. Laclé A, Valero-Juan LF (2012) Diabetes-related lower-extremity amputation incidence and risk factors: a prospective seven-year study in Costa Rica. Rev Panam Salud Publica 32(3):192–198
63. Jeyaraman K, Berhane T, Hamilton M, Chandra AP, Falhammar H (2019) Amputations in patients with diabetic foot ulcer: a retrospective study from a single centre in the Northern Territory of Australia. ANZ J Surg 89(7–8):874–879. https://doi.org/10.1111/ans.15351
64. Gurney JK, Stanley J, York S, Sarfati D (2019) Regional variation in the risk of lower-limb amputation among patients with diabetes in New Zealand. ANZ J Surg 89(7–8):868–873. https://doi.org/10.1111/ans.15079
65. Young BA, Maynard C, Reiber G, Boyko EJ (2003) Effects of ethnicity and nephropathy on lower-extremity amputation risk among diabetic veterans. Diabetes Care 26(2):495–501
66. Boyko EJ, Seelig AD, Ahroni JH (2018) Limb- and person-level risk factors for lower-limb amputation in the prospective Seattle diabetic foot study. Diabetes Care 41(4):891–898. https://doi.org/10.2337/dc17-2210
67. Kwon KT, Armstrong DG (2018) Microbiology and antimicrobial therapy for diabetic foot infections. Infect Chemother 50(1):11–20. https://doi.org/10.3947/ic.2018.50.1.11. Review. PubMed PMID: 29637748; PubMed Central PMCID: PMC5895826
68. Ramirez-Acuña JM, Cardenas-Cadena SA, Marquez-Salas PA, Garza-Veloz I, Perez-Favila A, Cid-Baez MA, Flores-Morales V, Martinez-Fierro ML (2019) Diabetic foot ulcers: current advances in antimicrobial therapies and emerging treatments. Antibiotics (Basel) 8(4) pii: E193. Review. https://doi.org/10.3390/antibiotics8040193
69. Henig O, Pogue JM, Cha R, Kilgore PE, Hayat U, Ja'ara M, Ali RM, Mahboob S, Pansare R, Deeds K, Joarder B, Kandala H, Dhar S, Kaye KS (2018) Epidemiology of diabetic foot infection in the metro-detroit area with a focus on independent predictors for pathogens resistant to recommended empiric antimicrobial therapy. Open Forum Infect Dis 5(11):ofy245. https://doi.org/10.1093/ofid/ofy245. eCollection 2018 Nov. PubMed PMID: 30402532; PubMed Central PMCID: PMC6215454
70. Citron DM, Goldstein EJ, Merriam CV, Lipsky BA, Abramson MA (2007) Bacteriology of moderate-to-severe diabetic foot infections and in vitro activity of antimicrobial agents. J Clin Microbiol 45(9):2819–2828. PubMed PMID: 17609322; PubMed Central PMCID: PMC2045270
71. Sánchez-Sánchez M, Cruz-Pulido WL, Bladinieres-Cámara E, Alcalá-Durán R, Rivera-Sánchez G, Bocanegra-García V (2017) Bacterial prevalence and antibiotic resistance in clinical isolates of diabetic foot ulcers in the northeast of Tamaulipas, Mexico. Int J Low Extrem Wounds 16(2):129–134. https://doi.org/10.1177/1534734617705254
72. Víquez-Molina G, Aragón-Sánchez J, Pérez-Corrales C, Murillo-Vargas C, López-Valverde ME, Lipsky BA (2018) Virulence factor genes in *Staphylococcus aureus* isolated from diabetic foot soft tissue and bone infections. Int J Low Extrem Wounds 17(1):36–41. https://doi.org/10.1177/1534734618764237
73. Islam S, Cawich SO, Budhooram S, Harnarayan P, Mahabir V, Ramsewak S, Naraynsingh V (2013) Microbial profile of diabetic foot infections in Trinidad and Tobago. Prim Care Diabetes 7(4):303–308. https://doi.org/10.1016/j.pcd.2013.05.001
74. Perim MC, Borges Jda C, Celeste SR, Orsolin Ede F, Mendes RR, Mendes GO, Ferreira RL, Carreiro SC, Pranchevicius MC (2015) Aerobic bacterial profile and antibiotic resistance in patients with diabetic foot infections. Rev Soc Bras Med Trop 48(5):546–554. https://doi.org/10.1590/0037-8682-0146-2015

75. Carro GV, Carlucci E, Priore G, Gette F, Llanos MLA, Dicatarina Losada MV, Noli ML, Amato PS (2019) Infections in diabetic foot. Choice of empirical antibiotic regimen. Medicina (B Aires) 79(3):167–173. Spanish
76. Kurup R, Ansari AA (2019) A study to identify bacteriological profile and other risk factors among diabetic and non-diabetic foot ulcer patients in a Guyanese hospital setting. Diabetes Metab Syndr 13(3):1871–1876. https://doi.org/10.1016/j.dsx.2019.04.024
77. Valenzuela PT, Mühlhauser ME, Palma S, Escobar C, Marin M (2019) 1421. Microbiology and resistance of diabetic foot osteomyelitis in a teaching hospital in Santiago, Chile. Open Forum Infect Dis 6(Suppl 2):S517–S518. https://doi.org/10.1093/ofid/ofz360.1285
78. Commons RJ, Robinson CH, Gawler D, Davis JS, Price RN (2015) High burden of diabetic foot infections in the top end of Australia: an emerging health crisis (DEFINE study). Diabetes Res Clin Pract 110(2):147–157. https://doi.org/10.1016/j.diabres.2015.09.016. PubMed PMID: 26453263; PubMed Central PMCID: PMC4684095
79. Lipsky BA, Berendt AR, Cornia PB, Pile JC, Peters EJ, Armstrong DG, Deery HG, Embil JM, Joseph WS, Karchmer AW, Pinzur MS, Senneville E, Infectious Diseases Society of America (2012) 2012 Infectious Diseases Society of America clinical practice guideline for the diagnosis and treatment of diabetic foot infections. Clin Infect Dis 54(12):e132–e173. https://doi.org/10.1093/cid/cis346
80. Butalia S, Palda VA, Sargeant RJ, Detsky AS, Mourad O (2008) Does this patient with diabetes have osteomyelitis of the lower extremity? JAMA 299(7):806–813. https://doi.org/10.1001/jama.299.7.806. Review
81. https://iwgdfguidelines.org/wp-content/uploads/2019/05/IWGDF-Guidelines-2019.pdf. Accessed 29 Nov 2019
82. Tchero H, Kangambega P, Noubou L, Becsangele B, Fluieraru S, Teot L (2018) Antibiotic therapy of diabetic foot infections: a systematic review of randomized controlled trials. Wound Repair Regen 26(5):381–391. https://doi.org/10.1111/wrr.12649
83. Selva Olid A, Solà I, Barajas-Nava LA, Gianneo OD, Bonfill Cosp X, Lipsky BA (2015) Systemic antibiotics for treating diabetic foot infections. Cochrane Database Syst Rev (9):CD009061. https://doi.org/10.1002/14651858.CD009061.pub2. Review

Part II

Complications and Treatments Updates

Acute and Chronic Wound Healing Physiology

4

Ayman Fisal Ahmed Foad

4.1 Introduction

Diabetic patients are prone to develop wounds in the lower limbs. The predisposing factors include neuropathy, which is a common chronic complication of persistent hyperglycemia, affecting the autonomic nervous system render their skin dry, with a loss of the accommodating sweating reflex, furthermore, the sensory loss for touch and minor injuries let them a prey for repetitive injuries without adopting protective measures. The microvascular and macrovascular complications ultimately result in hemodynamics disturbances and peripheral ischemia. Immunological responses are dampened by diabetes, further enhancing the chance for deteriorating and delaying the healing of the wounds.

Wounds are defined as injury in the skin, mucus membranes, or connective tissues resulting in defects in the structure and/or the function of the organs. Skin ulcers are commonly encountered in diabetics, and they are defined as loss of the continuity of the lining epithelium, which is a stratified squamous epithelium of the dry variety, which reveals the raw surface of the underlying tissue. Ulcers cause a breach in the skin by the loss of the protective keratin, keratinocytes, and a defect in the anchoring basement membrane.

The body response and attempt to repair is dictated by the type of tissue inflicted and by local and systemic factors. The capacity of the cell in the different tissue holds different aptitudes to replicate, divide, and differentiate. The cleanest of the wounds, without foreign bodies contamination facilitating the production of biofilms of potential pathogens has the potential to heal utmost compared to dirty and contaminated wound sites. The cultivation of pathogens at the site of the wound in diabetics is augmented and fostered by hyperglycemia, and low immunity. Wound

A. F. A. Foad (✉)
Faculty of Medicine, University of Tabuk, Tabuk, Kingdom of Saudi Arabia

Orotta College of Medicine & Health Sciences, Asmara, Eritrea

M. Zubair et al. (eds.), *Diabetic Foot Ulcer*,
https://doi.org/10.1007/978-981-15-7639-3_4

healing is notably slower in the lower limbs compared to the scalp or upper limbs. And the closure of the wound or advised timing of removal of the surgical suture is often delayed in the lower limb wounds, this mostly attributed to density of blood supply per surface area. Personal factors have a profound impact on healing. As healing a pone fide anabolic process, the availability of nutritional components essential for building and restoration influences the tempo and the structure of the healing process. Proteins are the building blocks for repairing the damaged structure of tissue and acts as chemical messengers among other substances, governing and orchestrating the healing process, the influx of inflammatory cells, and the differentiation of stromal, endothelial, and epithelial cells. Vitamin C has a pivotal role in cross-linking of collagen fibers and fostering their tensile strength.

4.2 Tissue Repair

In the attempt of repair, tissue may undertake tow routes, either healing by regeneration or healing by connective tissue and scar formation. The former route constitutes the complete restitution of the morphology and the function of the injured tissue, and this encompasses a myriad of barrier and secretary functions of the skin. In healing by connective tissue, the gap is filled by the lay down of collagen by fibroblasts and a nonspecialized cell, sealing the gap and resulting in a deranged morphology and function of the skin.

The main factors dictating which repair route execution prevail are:

1. *The Capacity of the Indigenous Cells to Divide*: Epithelial tissues constituting cells are considered as labile cell, and they are constantly dividing and replicating because they are shed on the surfaces, they are in a constant state of renewal, and stem cells often found in a specific niche are capable of divergent asymmetrical replications yielding two daughter cells, one aimed for further division, replication, and differentiation and the other to preserve the stem cell line. The stem cell reserve loses its merit of replication with the advancing age of the subject due to cumulative oxidative cell membrane, organelles, and DNA damage and telomere shortening. Visceral epithelial cells (Liver) assume a dormant behavior notwithstanding they have the capacity to replicate vividly if they summoned. They stay on the side track of the cell cycle and after stimulation enter the cycle and adopt a rapid dividing profile to renovate missing cells or part of organs in a brief time has been noticed after hepatic live donor lobe donation. On the other hand, permanent cells, are terminally differentiating cells incapable of replication, once lost by the injury they are replaced by scar formation. Injury endured on labile cells in case all the other confounding factors are optimized results in a rapid and cosmetically appealing scar.
2. *The Maintenance of the Scaffolding Connective Tissue Frame*: This constitutes the blueprint of the tissue and forms the track through which the new cells can pave and arrange to replace missing or injured cells. Without these blueprints,

there is no trace of the repair system to follow, and this results in haphazard attempts, culminating in healing by collagen deposition and scar formation.

3. *The Resolution of Inflammation at the Site of Injury*: *Mikhail Bakunin* once said "The urge to destroy is also a creative urge." Repetitive injuries create a milieu of chronic inflammation. By definition chronic inflammation constitutes three processes going simultaneously hand-by-hand; inflammation, tissue injury and loss, and a unremitting attempts of repair. The halt of this vicious cycle compels cessation of the injurious process and its resultant inflammatory process.

4.3 Extracellular Matrix

These are structural proteins or proteins complexed with carbohydrates.

They maintain the tensile strength of the tissues, which is mainly attained by collagen, which is imposed by cross-linking of collagen fibers resulting in bundles arranged and aligned toward lines of stress. They give the elasticity of the tissues, which is mainly mediated by elastin. Glycoproteins and mucopolysaccharides can hold water in their cervices and provide the turgor of our organs and tissues. Many growth factors are quenched within their matrices and released after tissue injury to exert their actions. Basement membrane is composed of organized fibrillar collagen anchoring the surface epithelium on one side and attached to subepithelial connective tissue framework on the other side, it provides the sense of polarity to the surface epithelium cells and prevents *anoikis*, a type of programmed cell death occurring upon detachment of the epithelial cell from its basement membrane. Fibronectin, which acts as an adhesive protein anchoring other structural proteins and quenching growth factors.

4.4 Cytokines [1]

The cross-talk between the cells in our body is mediated by chemical compounds. These substances mediate and orchestrate highly complexed and tightly controlled processes including housekeeping, tissue maintenance, and repair. Cytokines, growth factors, and mediators ordinarily have *hierarchical* properties; in which one factor can activate many downstream factors. They are also promiscuous in a sense that many factors can activate or culminate in activating a singular downstream effectors or pathways. Many cytokines are promiscuous, in regard they can stimulate many effectors, and they are not faithful for one downstream effector. The cytokines are either secreted in a steady level and their actions determined by tipping of the scale between pro and anti-mediators, or they been secreted only on demand and disappear after achieving their purpose. Cytokines are labile chemical compounds with a finite lifespan, and their secretion start by their release from ready-made stored vesicles with a brief and limited storage, and a subsequent induced prompt synthesis and secretion with a potentially prolonged action.

The action of cytokines can be exerted by four means:

(a) *A paracrine* mode of action when the cell secretes the chemical mediator, which exert its function in neighboring cells in its vicinity.
(b) *Autocrine* stimulation when cell secretes the chemical substance that is released one it is surface to bound to a surface receptor, culminating in a self-stimulation loop.
(c) *An endocrine* method in which an endocrine gland or cell secretes a chemical mediator to the bloodstream to circulate and activate distant cells, tissues, or organs.
(d) Lastly, some neurotransmitters are secreted through *synapses* to activate post-synaptic cell.

The first three aforementioned modes of stimulation act in a cascade fashion with downstream amplification and feedback mechanism, the latter, synaptic stimulation often fades and weakens with increased distance.

Cytokines and chemical mediators are classified as cell derived or plasma (liver) derived.

Plasma-derived mediators are synthesized mainly in the liver and secreted and circulate in the plasma as inactive precursors forms, which upon activation enter a cascade loop of activation and amplification. Complement component system and Hageman factor system are examples of liver-derived mediators having intricate relations with the coagulation system and with other loops of amplifications and control proteins. Cell-derived mediators are secreted from inflammatory cells in areas of injury and from quenched reserve within the connective tissue matrix. The ultimate goal of these factors is the fine-tuning of the healing process, otherwise unchecked trophic stimuli might get strayed and result in suboptimal healing or emergence of neoplastic growth.

4.5 Healing by Regeneration [2]

It signifies the complete restitution of the original structure and function of the injured tissue with minimum or no scarring. The healing process must endure optimal conditions to secure this option; local factors must be permissible including small wound with approximated clean edges, noninfected wound, and the absence of detritus tissue or foreign bodies. The scaffolding connective tissue framework must be maintained, as the loss of the blueprint yield chaotic infidel restoration. Cell or tissue factors also can influence this option by the regenerative capacity of the injured cells; as labile tissues fare better than stable and permanent cells. Systemic factors also influence this option, including the well-being of the patient, the control of his diabetes, and nutritional status. The healing attempt under these conditions referred by clinicians as the first intension. Optimal conditions may present de novo in the wound or optimized after medical intervention.

4.6 Repair with Scar Formation

This type of healing often referred to as second intention healing, and it results in a prolonged healing process, weak scar, and ugly scar (Fig. 4.1). All the aforementioned optimal conditions are not met in this case, or further appropriate interventions were not applied. Local factors controlling wound healing are many, one of the most important factors is the extend of the injury or tissue loss, considering the remaining of scaffolding structure of the tissue made by the basement membrane and tissue framework.

4.7 Predisposing Factors for Injuries in Diabetics (Fig. 4.2)

Glucose as a fuel providing molecules is often abundant, due to the relative insulin lacking or resistance, its surplus becomes a bacterial growth-enhancing factor rather than a tissue source of energy. The evidence supporting this notion is not conclusive yet and further researches in this matter are warranted, but some researchers found an increased incidence of surgical wound infection related to hyperglycemia [3, 4]. As the majority of diabetics presenting with DSF complications are elderly, and often share a myriad of diabetic associated macrovascular and microvascular

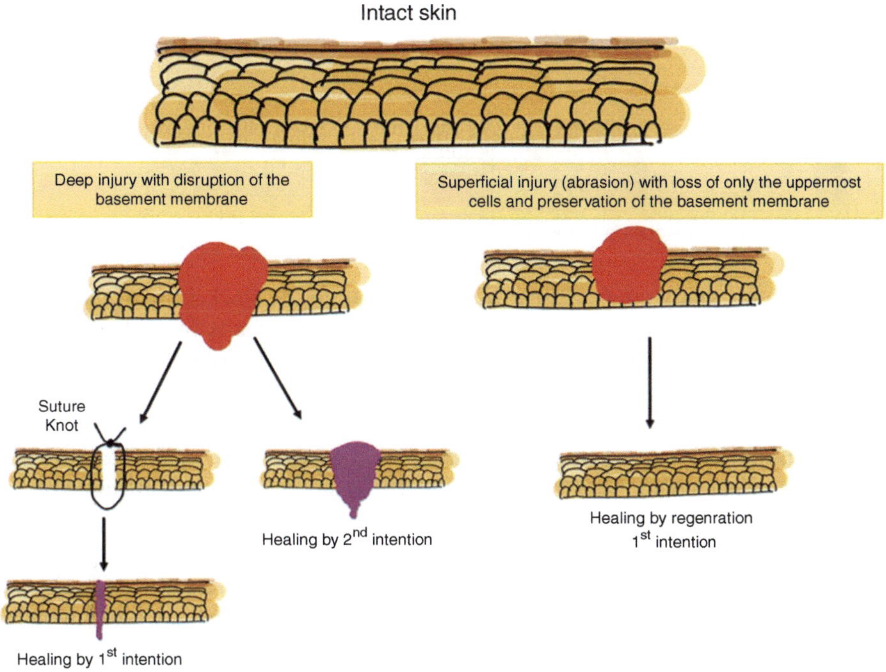

Fig. 4.1 Healing by regeneration, the first and the second intention

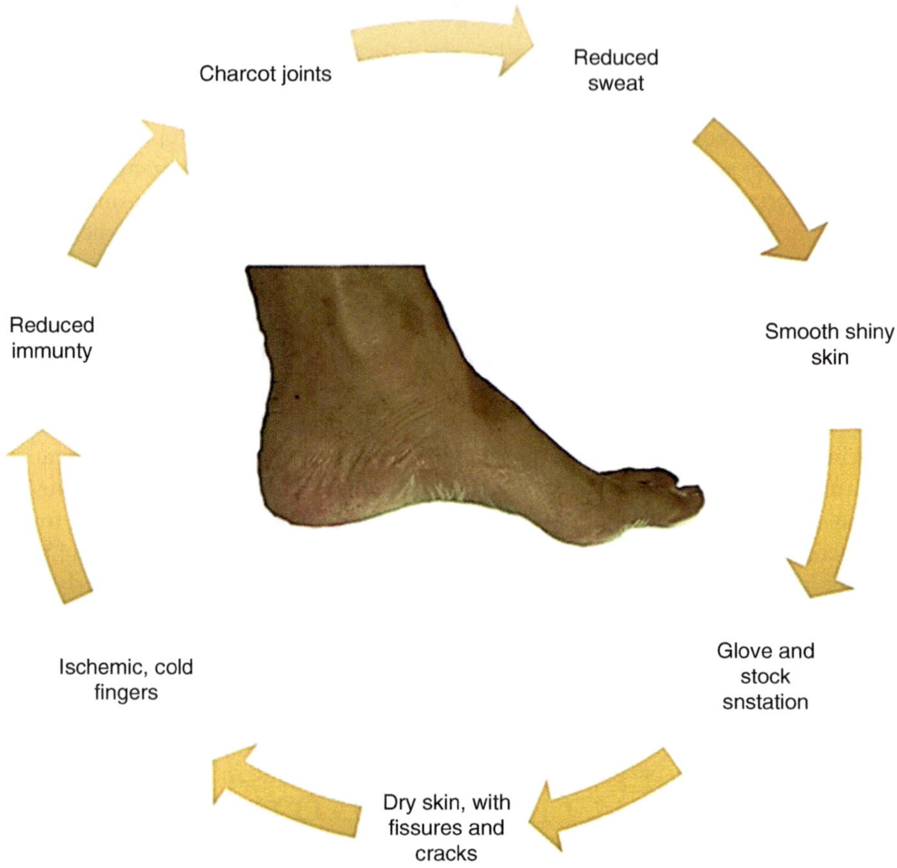

Fig. 4.2 Factors predisposing to foot injury in diabetics

complications, many confounding factors attribute to the slackening of the healing including cell senescence of fibroblasts and the limited capacity of epithelial cells to cover tissue defects. Diabetic patients often have reduced immunity toward infections. Such infections may cause death in about 5% of diabetics. The pathogenesis beyond this is attributed to the reduced chemotactic, phagocytic, and secretory function of inflammatory cells. Macrovascular and microvascular complications also adversely affect small blood vessels, and capillary culminating in less optimal inflammatory vascular events, vasodilatation, and enhanced permeability. Diabetic retinopathy and cataract affect visual fields and acuity. This may result in repeated and inadvertent traumatic pumping of the lower limbs in furniture within the house hold. Diabetic patients with DSF may show comorbidities of the cardiovascular and renal system resulting in reflective hemodynamic changes in the systemic and local circulation, and a buildup of toxic levels of metabolites adversely affecting hematopoiesis and the immune system. The loss of sensory feedback imposes the lower limb to repeated trauma, and subsequent gradual injuries and tear of ligaments culminating in subluxation of small joints, malposition of bones, and loss of the normal arches of the feet. This might result in repeated frictions and pressure ischemia of soft tissue due to unfitting shoes. These deformities lead to a condition known as Charcot joint and compel a special attention by chiropodist or at least a caring household personnel. Diabetic autonomic nervous system dysfunction may cause loss of the skin turgor, with shiny brittle dermis, loss of skin adnexa, and dryness due to lack of sweating.

4.8 Phases of Wound Healing [5]

1. *Inflammation Phase*: This is the response of vascularized living tissue to injury and trauma. Ischemic limb may show minimal inflammatory response and necrotic gangrenous tissue only show inflammation at the interface with viable tissue margins. The attempt of the inflammation is to remove and debride the injured areas form offending agents and to scavenge dead cells. The main effectors of inflammation are to display a cellular response with an influx of a myriad of inflammatory cells through the blood vessel portal, which also facilitates edema formation.
2. *Proliferative Phase: and This Is Comprised*:
   (a) *Angiogenesis*: In acute inflammation, the vascular response comprises dilatation and hyperemia at the arterial end and increased permeability at the venular end of the vascular bed. In persistent and chronic inflammation, the continuous injury, inflammation, and attempt to repair go hand-by-hand simultaneously. This necessitates the formation and sprouting of new blood vessels to provide fuel and nutrients and building blocks for the repair process (Fig. 4.3).

   The process of angiogenesis in diabetics is dampened and not optimal, due to microvascular and microvacuolar complications usually encountered in long-standing diabetes and metabolic syndrome. After the injury, the defect of lost or crushed tissue will be filled by inflammatory cells and protein-rich exudation. Proteins dry on the surface and form a scab, which is a coagulated serum on the surface of the wound, and usually overlies a raw granular oozy surface. If the injured epidermis is overlined by a necrotic layer of tissue, an eschar is formed, which can be pearly white and pale in case of ischemia necrosis, or black/black brown in case of vascularized tissue. Circumferential eschar can some time act as napkin-ring or as a plaster which can induce compartment syndrome and impede blood flow to the distal part of the limb, causing Volkmann contracture or necrosis; escharotomy may resolve this issue [6].

   (b) *Collagen Formation*: As the wound mature granulation tissue is formed, which is composed of immature leaky blood vessels within edematous stroma rich in proteins and newly formed extracellular matrix with a plethora of inflammatory cells.

   (c) *Epithelization*: Epithelial cells from the base of the epidermis of flanking skin edges start to form a monolayer from the edges to cover the gap, and as they reach the mid-line and seal the gap they activate a contact inhibition

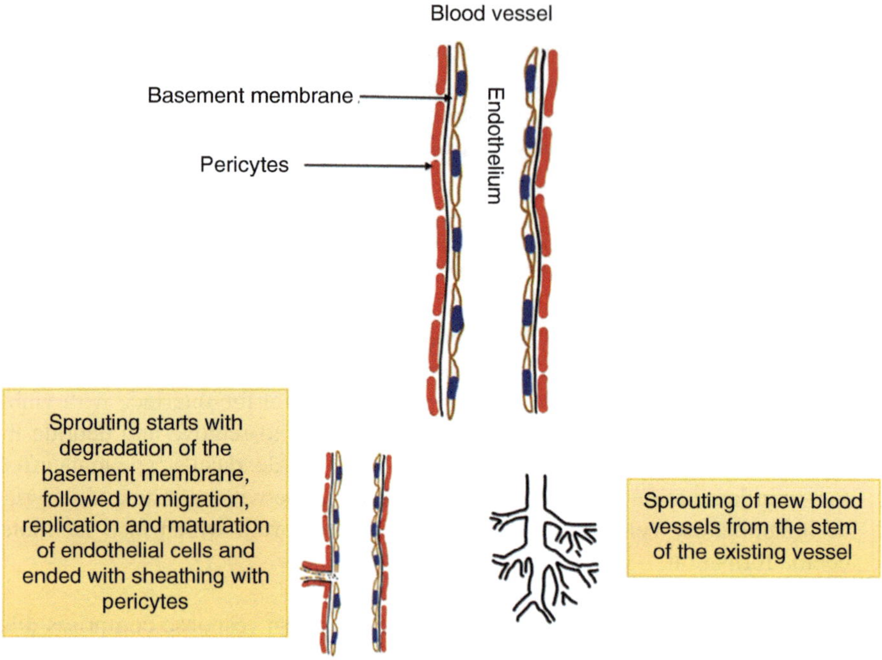

Fig. 4.3 Angiogenesis is a step of paramount importance in healing

program, a merit of normal non-neoplastic cells, they stop dividing and start a vertical maturation step. This is mediated by the APC β-catenin pathway, in which β-catenin is located in sub-membranous location associated with E-cadherin, a transmembrane protein which functions as an adhesive structure linked in homodimer fashion with adjacent cell proteins. Some times in case of repetitive trauma an exuberant granulation tissue is formed protruding as a hill above the horizontal level of the wound plane, which impedes the union of the epithelial cells coming from the edges of the wound, the term proud flesh is applied to this condition, mimicking the lordotic posture of a proud person. In this case, the epithelial cell should climb up the protuberance of the granulation tissue to meat at the summit.

3. *Maturation Phase*: This is a continuous process. The color of the scar fades from cherry red to pale pink to white as it matures and ages with a more organized matrix and more mature blood vessel surrounded by a dual layer of endothelial and pericyte.

4.9 Timing Sequences of Skin Wound Healing

1. *Blood clot (scab)*: its purpose is to stanch the bleeding and provides a matrix rich in growth factors and chemokines. It is formed within 24 h, and neutrophils are noticed crouching from the margins.
2. *Granulation tissue*: starts to develop 1–2 days (peaking at 5–7 days), and is composed of proliferating fibroblasts and endothelium (vascularized loose CT). The

vessels are leaky leading to extravasation of proteins and fluids and creating edema. It provides a framework for subsequent scar formation and continues remodeling.

3. *Cell proliferation and collagen deposition*: primes within 2–4 days after wounding, and neutrophils are largely replaced by macrophages. The granulation tissue scaffolding is converted into a scar (fibroblasts and collagen).
4. *Scar formation*: *starts* 2 weeks with sequential collagen deposition and gradual fading of the vasculature. The red granulation tissue is converted into a relatively avascular scar with a reduction of the inflammatory cells and marching of the epithelial cells to seal the gap.
5. *Wound contraction*: of larger wounds, proceed with the dominance of myofibroblasts having combined features of fibroblasts with laying downing of collagen, and smooth muscle contractile features causing wound contracture culminating in reduction the surface of the wound.
6. *Tensile strength*: within 1 week is 10% of the initial strength of the healthy tissue, and increases gradually with advanced bundling and alignment of the collagen fibers towards the line of stress reaching about 70–80% of the initial strength within 3–4 months.

4.10 Complications of Wounds in Diabetics

1. *Venous leg ulcers (congested)*: occur in elderly people with chronic venous hypertension (severe varicose veins or congestive heart failure). It fails to heal because of the poor delivery of oxygen to the site of the ulcer.
2. *Arterial ulcers (pale)*: atherosclerosis, Ischemia → atrophy, and necrosis of the skin and underlying tissues (painful).
3. *Neurotrophic ulcers*: found at sites under mechanical pressure, and characteristically appear as friable punched out ulcers surrounded with dry scaly skin [7].
4. *Pressure sores (Decubitus ulcer)*: mechanical pressure and local ischemia pose a dramatic impact in wound healing; this leads to a vicious circle of partial healing and repeated injuries. Protection and guarding against it is more attenable than healing.
5. *Atrophic scar* this leads to a very scant and weak connective tissue lay down, rendering the injured tissue a prey for repeated trauma and dehiscence, which can be brought upon by trivial trauma.
6. *Hypertrophic scar*: this results from excessive scar tissue confined to the edges of the wound. Adversely this may cause ugly big protruding scar and contracture of the skin.
7. *Keloid formation*: this occurs with racial predisposition noticed in black ethnicity. The healing is characterized by exuberant scar formation which is not confined to the edges of the wound.
8. *Wound contracture* occurs if a large area of fibrotic tissue is crossing a joint, this might restrict the full range of joint movement. This is usually anticipated if the wound left to heal under low tension on the relaxed flexed position of the joint.

4.11 Factors Influencing Wound Healing [8]

1. *Site of the wound*, it is noticeable that skin injuries in head and neck heals faster than torso, abdomen, and lower limb injury in a descendant order. This is credited to the density of blood supply per surface area in the corresponding tissues.
2. *Type of the tissue*: determine the outcome of the healing process. Labile continuously dividing cells are capable of continuous division and can replace the lost and injured tissues as long as other confounding factors are controlled. Stable tissues have a lesser potential for division. On the other hand, permanent cells or tissue are incapable of division, and cell death is only replaced by fibrosis.
3. *Amount of lost tissue*: small superficial tissue with minimal loss of cells has the potential to heal optimally compared to big wounds with large gaps. With a proper surgical intervention, healing can be augmented.
4. *General condition of the patient*: the presence comorbidities, such as critical atherosclerosis, ischemic heart disease, and heart failure among others, which are frequently encountered in long-lasting and poorly controlled diabetes may adversely interfere or delay healing.
5. *Nutritional status*: well-fed subjects replenished with nutrients, essential minerals and vitamin fare better than starved or deficient subjects. Vitamin D is required for the optimization of almost all steps of cutaneous wound healing [9], nonetheless, vitamin C is also required for the cross-linking of collagen bundles the building blocks of scar tissue. Diabetic patients often are deficient in micronutrient and this may interfere with proper wound healing process [10].
6. *Steroid use* retards the process of wound healing, the administration of dexamethasone in postoperatively increase morbidity and delay wound healing [11]. Glucocorticoids slow the healing and dampen the strength and the abundance of collagen fibers. Researchers found the excess glucocorticoids in patients with *Cushing* syndrome reduces the level of heat shock proteins in wounds, this results in a consequent reduction in angiogenesis and resultant delayed healing [12].
7. *Direction of the wound*: if injuries run parallel to the *Langer* lines, they heal with an esthetically minimal scar compared with injuries running perpendicular to these lines.
8. *Age*: wounds in young individuals or patients with short-lasting diabetes, characteristically have a good and prompt wound healing compared with elderly, long-lasting diabetes, and poorly controlled diabetes [13]. Some researchers argue that the healing in elderlies is merely delayed but the end results are almost the same [14]. There are both undisputable evidence supporting that skin of the geriatric population has both morphological features of skin atrophy and reduction of physiological qualities with advanced aging [15].
9. *Racial factor* also may influence the healing of wounds, as an example, patients with the black ethnic background may have a higher tendency to develop keloids, exuberant scar tissue often exceeds the limit of the wound lead to disfiguring ugly scars [16].

10. *Infection*: can adversely sluggish wound healing as clean wound fares better than, contaminated, dirty, and infected wounds.
11. *Foreign body*: debridement of wounds and removal of contaminants and foreign bodies foster the speed of wound healing.
12. *Genetics*: polymorphism in genes controlling inflammatory response have a slightly deranged healing process. Mutations of structural proteins present with the noticeably delayed healing process.

4.12 Muscle, Tendon and Bone Healing

1. *Skeletal muscular tissues* are incapable of dividing and is usually replaced by connective tissues. If severe infection spread and induce a systemic inflammatory response syndrome, skeletal muscles (not necessary at the site of injury) may undergo a waxy coagulative necrosis pattern known as *Zenker's* degeneration.
2. *Tendons* have a capacity of healing and should be optimally kept under tension to reduce contracture and restriction of joint movement.
3. *Bone* has a virtuous capacity to heal, and if infected this capacity is noticeably hindered. Treatment of infection and removal of dead sequestrum hasten healing, on the other hand, the persistence of infection with resurging draining sinuses may be almost sturdy to healing. Diabetic patients may suffer from stubborn bone injuries and delayed union of bone fragments, there are noticeable reduced osteoblastic activity and increased apoptosis especially with accompanied infections. The growth factors controlling the healing process are scarce in the milieu of diabetic ulcers including bone morphogenetic protein and tumor necrosis factor (BMP, TNF) [17, 18].

4.13 Gangrene

Diabetic patient develops as a consequence of progressive macroangiopathy and microangiopathy a broad spectrum of potential complications. Gangrene is an atrocious known concern of poorly controlled diabetics. It is a consequence of vascular, neural, and immunological dysfunctions often encountered in diabetic patients. The term originates from the Latin root *gangraena*, which literally means "an eating or gnawing sore." This a special type of cell death is due to peripheral ischemia owed to vascular comprise [7].

1. *Dry gangrene* is a type of gangrene characterized by changes in skin color from shades of redness and blackness with a subsequent tissue breakdown and putrefaction of protein contents resulting in a foul odor [19]. Inflammation only occurs at the margin of the living tissue, manifesting the cardinal signs of inflammation; redness, swelling, hotness, pain (which may be dampened as a result of peripheral neuropathy), and loss of function. Systemic manifestations develop as a response of the body to injury manifesting as fever, anorexia, nau-

sea, and fatigue. Dead tissue falls off spontaneously, with unnoticeable minor trauma, or by surgical debridement [20]. There are no signs of infections at the site of the injury.

2. *Wet gangrene* ensues with secondary bacterial infections, noticeable with pockets of pus and weeping wounds. This poses a more serious impact on the health of the subject and warrants an urgent surgical and medical intervention. Septicemia and septic shock are a frightful complication.
3. *Gas gangrene* on the other hand results from infection with *Clostridium perfringens*, a gram-positive spore-forming bacilli, with a resultant myonecrosis, the spread of infection through tissue plains and liberation of toxins into the bloodstream. Grossly the wound is crepitus upon palpation and shows bubbles and air-filled bullae.

4.14 Classification of Diabetic Wounds [21]

Classification systems help to triage patients for suitable clinical care and follow-up. A score also services as a fast-universal way to describe the wound, and alarms for deterioration or assures in case of improvement.

There are multiple widely used classification systems for diabetic wounds, nevertheless, the widely used systems in clinical practice are *Wagner* (Fig. 4.4) and of the *University of Texas* systems.

1. *Wagner system*: in this system, there are 5 grades, grade-0 indicates an intact skin in a diabetic patient, grade-1 signifies the presence of a superficial wound involving the epidermis, dermis, or down to the subcutaneous tissues, grade-2 designates deep extension of the wound to the tendons, underlying bone or a joint

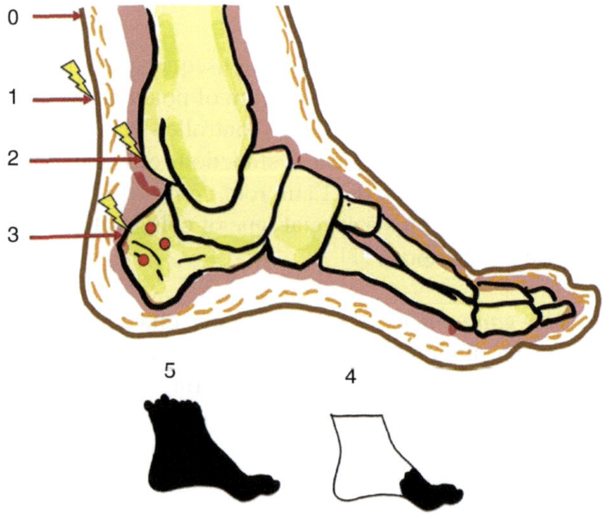

Fig. 4.4 Wagner classification of diabetic wounds, 0 = intact skin, 1 = epidermal, dermal and subcutaneous tissues, 2 = extension to tendons, muscle, capsule, and bone, 3 = 2+ infection (abscess or osteomyelitis), 4 = partial gangrene, 5 = extensive gangrene

capsule, grade-3 indicates grade-2 lesions with a superimposed infection of the bone or a localized suppurative inflammation, while grade-4 and 5 reserved for partial or extensive gangrene of the foot [22].

2. *University of Texas system*: is a combined system in which stages and grades the wound. Grading of the wound starts with grad-0 for intact skin or a healed remote wound in diabetic patients, grade-1 indicates a superficial cutaneous wound, grade-2 describes a deep wound affecting muscle, tendons, or a joint capsule, grade-3 denotes an extensive wound penetrating the underlying bone or reaching a joint cavity. The staging system of wounds classifies them according to ischemia and infection as follows; stage-A for clean wounds, stage-B for infected wound without peripheral ischemia, stage-C for ischemic clean noninfected wound, and stage-D for infected wounds with ischemia [22].

References

1. Werner S, Grose R (2003) Regulation of wound healing by growth factors and cytokines. Physiol Rev 83(3):835–870
2. Gantwerker EA, Hom DB (2011) Skin: histology and physiology of wound healing. Facial Plast Surg Clin North Am 19(3):441–453
3. Ramos M, Khalpey Z, Lipsitz S, Steinberg J, Panizales MT, Zinner M et al (2008) Relationship of perioperative hyperglycemia and postoperative infections in patients who undergo general and vascular surgery. Ann Surg 248(4):585–591
4. Showen A, Russell TA, Young S, Gupta S, Gibbons MM (2017) Hyperglycemia is associated with surgical site infections among general and vascular surgery patients. Am Surg 83(10):1108–1111
5. Velnar T, Bailey T, Smrkolj V (2009) The wound healing process: an overview of the cellular and molecular mechanisms. J Int Med Res 37(5):1528–1542
6. Martin P, Nunan R (2015) Cellular and molecular mechanisms of repair in acute and chronic wound healing. Br J Dermatol 173(2):370–378
7. Leg and foot ulcers. https://my.clevelandclinic.org/health/diseases/17169-leg-and-foot-ulcers
8. Guo S, Dipietro LA (2010) Factors affecting wound healing. J Dent Res 89(3):219–229
9. Oda Y, Hu L, Nguyen T, Fong C, Zhang J, Guo P et al (2018) Vitamin D receptor is required for proliferation, migration, and differentiation of epidermal stem cells and progeny during cutaneous wound repair. J Invest Dermatol 138(11):2423–2431
10. Pena G, Kuang B, Cowled P, Howell S, Dawson J, Philpot R et al (2020) Micronutrient status in diabetic patients with foot ulcers. Adv Wound Care 9(1):9–15
11. Polderman JA, Farhang-Razi V, Van Dieren S, Kranke P, DeVries JH, Hollmann MW et al (2018) Adverse side effects of dexamethasone in surgical patients. Cochrane Database Syst Rev 11:CD011940
12. Gordon CB, Li DG, Stagg CA, Manson P, Udelsman R (1994) Impaired wound healing in Cushing's syndrome: the role of heat shock proteins. Surgery 116(6):1082–1087
13. Wang P-H, Huang B-S, Horng H-C, Yeh C-C, Chen Y-J (2018) Wound healing. J Chin Med Assoc 81(2):94–101
14. Gosain A, DiPietro LA (2004) Aging and wound healing. World J Surg 28(3):321–326
15. Sgonc R, Gruber J (2013) Age-related aspects of cutaneous wound healing: a mini-review. Gerontology 59(2):159–164
16. Chike-Obi CJ, Cole PD, Brissett AE (2009) Keloids: pathogenesis, clinical features, and management. Semin Plast Surg 23(3):178–184

17. Sun M, Yang J, Wang J, Hao T, Jiang D, Bao G et al (2016) TNF-alpha is upregulated in T2DM patients with fracture and promotes the apoptosis of osteoblast cells in vitro in the presence of high glucose. Cytokine 80:35–42
18. Jiao H, Xiao E, Graves DT (2015) Diabetes and its effect on bone and fracture healing. Curr Osteoporos Rep 13(5):327–335
19. Rettger LF (1908) Further studies on putrefaction. J Biol Chem 4:45–55
20. Biehl C, Eckhard M, Szalay G, Heiss C (2016) Minor foot amputations in diabetic foot syndrome. Oper Orthop Traumatol 28(5):365–372
21. Shatnawi NJ, Al-Zoubi NA, Hawamdeh H, Khader YS, Omari AE-K, Khammash MR (2018) Redefined clinical spectra of diabetic foot syndrome. Vasc Health Risk Manag 14:291–298
22. Game F (2016) Classification of diabetic foot ulcers. Diabetes Metab Res Rev 32(Suppl 1):186–194

Screening of Foot Inflammation in Diabetic Patients by Noninvasive Imaging Modalities

5

Hyder O. Mirghani

5.1 Introduction

Diabetic foot problems (DFP) are common disabling syndromes. DFP is on the rise due to increasing age and high body mass index. DFP is costly, and with a tendency for recurrence. Diabetic foot syndrome which is characterized by high morbidity and mortality is defined as an ulcer of the foot of diabetic patients distal to the malleoli associated with diabetes-related complications. There are several classifications of DFS with some integrating infections [1, 2]. The diabetic septic foot is a component of DFP where infections are categorized as mild, moderate, and severe [3]. Foot inflammation includes osteomyelitis, joint infections, rheumatological diseases, and tenosynovitis. The diagnosis of foot inflammation remains a great challenge particularly in diabetic septic foot and when degenerative diseases are present, mainly due to the overlap between different components (neuropathy, and neuropathic arthropathy). The role of clinical and conventional imaging in the diagnosis of the diabetic septic foot may be limited due to accuracy. The musculoskeletal manifestation of diabetes mellitus including diabetic septic foot become an important focus of diagnostic and therapeutic procedures. Many imaging modalities are in use including plain radiography and to some extent ultrasonography (U/S), computed tomography (CT), and magnetic resonance imaging (MRI). Being a large issue in radiologic units serving other medical departments, musculoskeletal imaging influences further management of patients with diabetes in many aspects. However, it is not always possible to draw a fully reliable unequivocal interpretation in particular for diabetic septic foot [4, 5]. Differentiating soft tissue infections from osseous infection is vital to determine the appropriate therapeutic course. Radiographs are the initially recommended methods of evaluation that can provide

H. O. Mirghani (✉)
Department of Internal Medicine, Faculty of Medicine, University of Tabuk, Tabuk, Kingdom of Saudi Arabia
e-mail: h.mirghani@ut.edu.sa

M. Zubair et al. (eds.), *Diabetic Foot Ulcer*,
https://doi.org/10.1007/978-981-15-7639-3_5

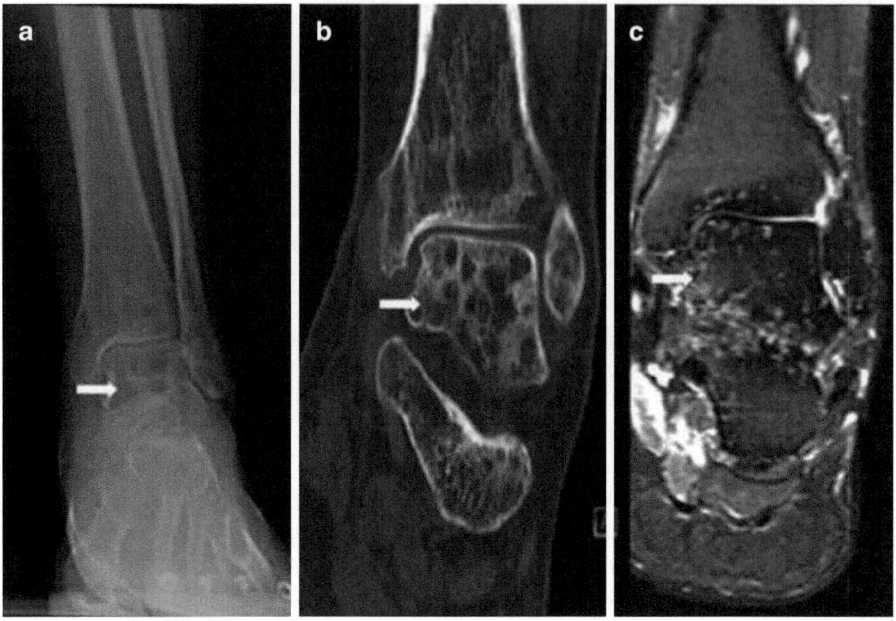

Fig. 5.1 Plain radiograph, CT, and MRI: A 53-year-old diabetic presenting with pain in the left ankle: AP radiograph (**a**) and the corresponding coronal reformatted CT image (**b**) showing patchy lucencies predominantly in the talus (arrow), also in the distal tibia and fibula. MR image (STIR coronal) (**c**) also demonstrates patchy juxta articular heterogenous signal intensities (arrow) in the talus. This was diagnosed as reflex sympathetic dystrophy. *AP* anteroposterior, *STIR* short tau inversion-recovery [26]

anatomic features and guiding the subsequent mode of imaging, however, they are not often diagnostic of osteomyelitis [6]. A great qualitative leap had been achieved since the introduction of morphologic magnetic resonance (MRI) imaging. MRI can differentiate between soft tissue and bone marrow edema. However, the application may be difficult due to the co-existence of infection and neuropathy [7]. A very interesting and promising is the introduction of electromagnetic simulation (EMS) as a noninvasive diagnostic approach. EMS can predict and diagnose peripheral vascular disease with great accuracy than Doppler studies and ankle-brachial index in terms of the extent and site of vessel involvement [8]. In the current chapter, non-invasive imaging of inflammation (mainly thermography, radiography, U/S, CT, MRI, and nuclear studies) regarding diabetic septic foot was discussed (Fig. 5.1).

5.2 Skin Temperature and Thermography

5.2.1 Skin Temperature Recording

Temperature monitoring of the foot has been used in the prevention of diabetic foot ulcers because abnormal skin temperature distribution can indicate ulcer risk. Skin temperature had been shown to correlate with peripheral neuropathy.

Randomized controlled trials with low risk of bias concluded the effectiveness of daily measurement of feet skin temperature in the prevention of foot ulcers [9]. Many devices are used to measure skin temperature including wearable temperature sensors at certain areas of the sole with alarm signals provided to the user. The temperature data collected can be displayed to the user, sent to other devices, or stored for future use [10]. It is interesting to note that wireless socks are found to be effective, reliable, and accurate in the contiguous measurement of foot skin temperature, the patients found them not different from standard socks [11]. Infrared cameras are a quick, fast, inexpensive, and noncontact tool for assessing skin temperature [12]. A cohort study conducted among patients with diabetic neuropathy and followed for foot ulcers after assessing the difference in temperature between the feet. The temperature was measured by an infrared thermometer, the authors found >2·2 °C difference in feet temperature for impending ulceration is not valid as single measurement, however, validity improves when confirmed the following day and further improves with individual correction [13]. Skin temperature measurement was found to be feasible when combined with the educational component and counseling of patients with foot ulcers [14].

5.2.2 Thermography (Thermal Imaging)

Thermographic (thermal imaging) patterns showed various variations between patients with diabetes mellitus and their counterparts without the diseases and can be used for assessing the circulatory status [15]. Furthermore, thermography could be useful for screening of foot ulcers with osteomyelitis [16], A relatively recent cohort with three arms (neuroischemic foot with ulcer, neuroischemic without ulcer, and controls without neuroischemia or ulcers) found that skin temperature was higher among patients with neuroischemia with or without ulceration, no statistically significant difference was observed between neuroischemic feet indicating that the ono-ulcerated feet are of risk of ulcers that can be predicted by thermography [17].

5.2.3 Plain Radiographs of the Feet

Due to the presence of deep fascia in the feet, the absence of pain due to neuropathy, and minimal inflammation rubor, it is not easy to assess diabetic septic on the clinical ground especially puncture wounds. Plain X-rays could be of great help. A radiograph is usually ordered first, an excellent overview of structural damage, previous surgery, and neuropathic arthropathy [18, 19]. However, the role of X-ray may be limited due to inaccuracy [5]. Imaging that answered specific questions including ultrasonography and computed tomography will be discussed in the following section (Fig. 5.2).

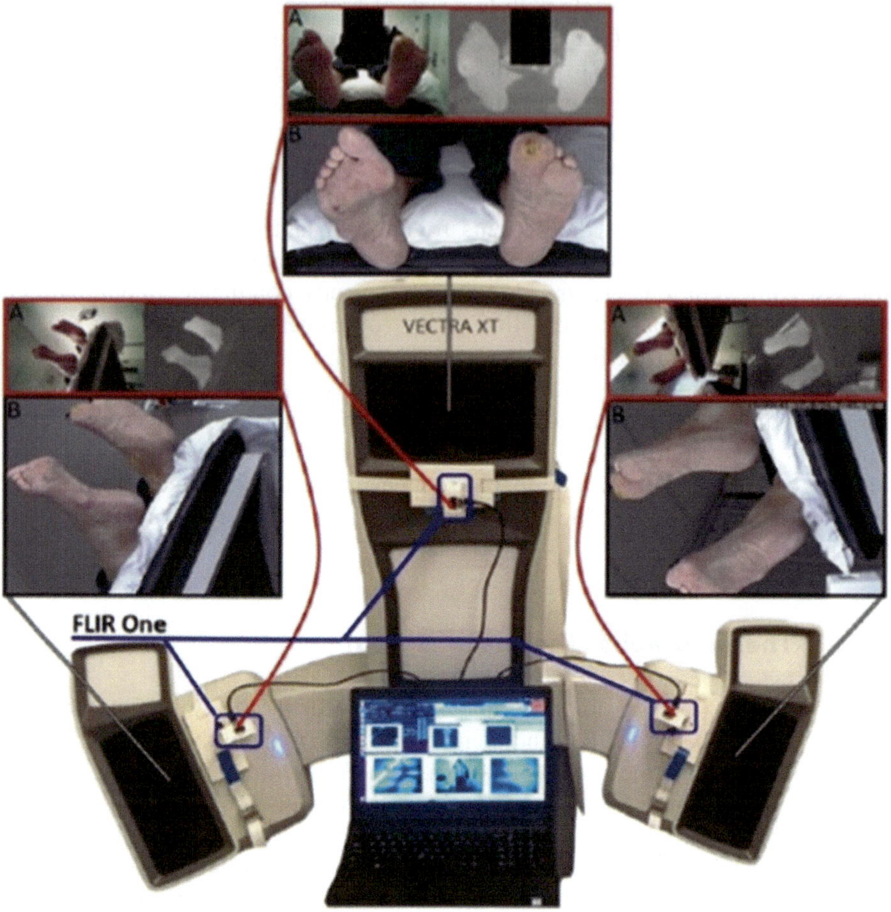

Fig. 5.2 Imaging setup. In the middle the Vectra XT, 3D imaging system can be seen (white). On the inner side of every viewpoint of the 3D imaging system, a FLIR One IR camera was attached (blue indicator), and connected to the laptop in front of the 3D imaging system. (A) Above each viewpoint the resulting 2D images are provided. On top, framed in red, the two images from the IR camera are shown (left: color image; right: thermal IR image in grayscale). (B) Bottom image, framed in black, is the texture map from the 3D image system [33]

5.2.4 Ultrasonography of the Feet

Ultrasonography is easily accessible and helpful for an accurate diagnosis. U/S is helpful in infectious diseases including cellulitis, pyomyositis, tenosynovitis, septic arthritis, and necrotizing fasciitis. The sonographic features include cobblestoning, air collection, abscesses, hyper, or hypoechoic changes. Color Doppler scans help to differentiate infectious from noninfectious causes. U/S is not good in osteomyelitis discrimination and neuropathic osteodystrophy, however, it can guide fluid aspiration for further evaluation. Imaging findings that showed ulcers, sinuses, abscesses,

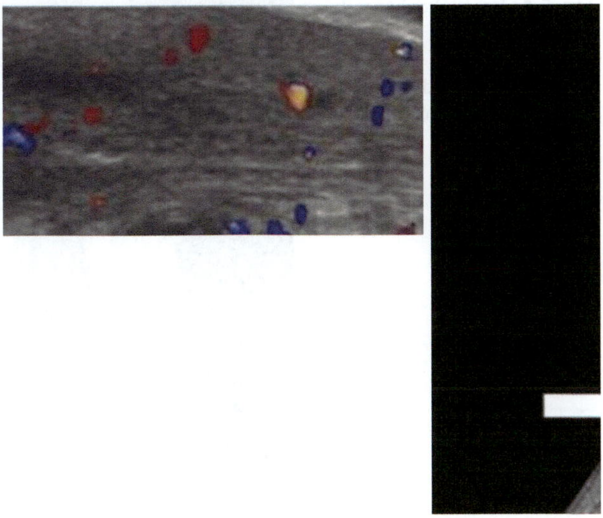

Fig. 5.3 Transverse color Doppler sonography. *MRI*: The imaging of choice (90% and 83% sensitivity and specificity, respectively) for diabetic septic foot including osteomyelitis and soft tissue infections

or cellulitis favor septic foot rather than osteodystrophy. X-Ray and MRI are other complementary tools [20] (Fig. 5.3).

The sensitivity and specificity are shown as follows [21]:

- Bone marrow edema (100% sensitivity and 90% specificity when occurred with tenosynovitis)
- Soft tissue swelling (85.7% sensitivity), soft tissue destruction sensitivity, and specificity (57.1% and 42.9%, respectively)
- Bone destruction (sensitivity of 14.3% and a specificity of 10%)
- Tenosynovitis (55% sensitivity and 50%specificity)

Short tau inversion-recovery (STIR) T2 weighted is the most sensitive modality, MRI can differentiate between osteomyelitis and neuropathic joints. Diabetic Charcot neuroarthropathy (DCN) is a great challenge to both radiologists and the treating physicians, especially in its early stages. In early DCN, the plaint radiographs may not detect osseous fragmentation or dislocation [21, 22], diffusion-weighted MR imaging (with short imaging time and not requiring contrast) are also helpful in differentiation of diabetic osteoarthropathy from osteomyelitis. Recent advances in MR imaging can provide functional quantitative information in addition to structural information, dynamic contrast imaging may detect differences in between the vascularization patterns of neuropathic arthropathy and osteomyelitis. MR angiography and MR neuropathy are discussed elsewhere in this book [23–25]. Also, periarticular and subchondral predilection, multiple bone and joint involvement, the absence of ulcers and sinus tracts, and intact overlying skin, favor the diagnosis of Charcot's neuropathic joint rather than osteomyelitis. Intraarticular loose bodies are also less in neuropathic joints. MR studies help differentiate viable

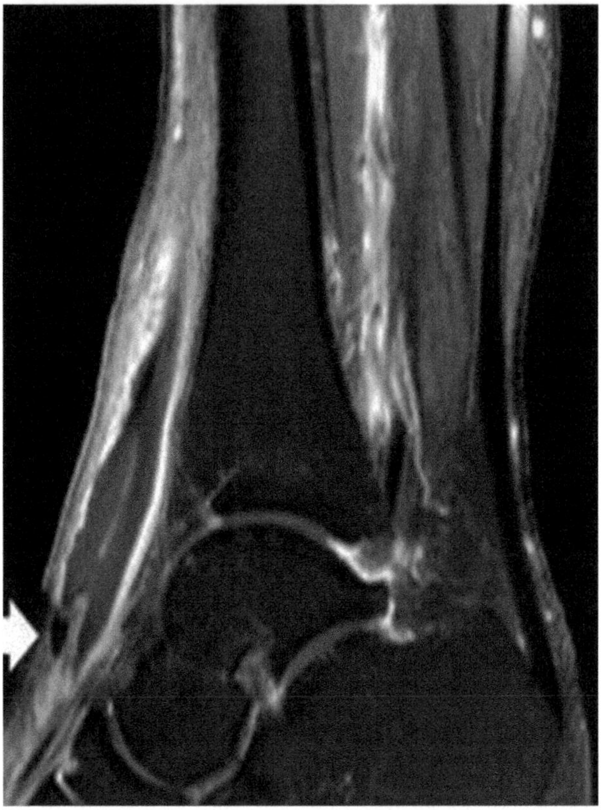

Fig. 5.4 Sagittal enhanced T1-weighted fat-suppressed image shows subcutaneous fluid collection with rim-like enhancement

from non-viable tissue directing surgery. Furthermore, it helps detect loculated infections after the failure of joint aspiration and for post-surgery follow-up. Pitfalls of MRI include noninfectious inflammatory conditions including gout, fracture, and neoplasm [19]. Radiographs are insensitive and take 7–15 days to show periostitis and cortical destruction [26].

NB: Sixty-one percent of patients with diabetic foot who initially showed T2 marrow signal abnormality (osteitis) are eventually diagnosed as osteomyelitis and deserve aggressive therapy [27] (Fig. 5.4).

5.2.5 Computed Tomography (CT)

CT scan is helpful in the diagnosis of soft tissue infections and osteomyelitis (together with sulfur colloid and leucocyte scan) in particular if an MRI scan is contraindicated or extensive artifact from metal is present [6]. Newer hybrid imaging techniques (SPECT/CT, PET/CT, and positron emission tomography/magnetic resonance imaging) are useful techniques [28]. PET/CT with fluorine-18-fluorodeoxyglucose-labeled autologous leukocytes was shown to sensitive (83.3%)

and specific (100%) for the diagnosis of diabetic foot infection complicated by Charcot's neuroarthropathy compared to CEMRI (83.3% and 63.6% respectively) [29].

5.3 Radionuclide Procedures

The radiolabeled leukocytes with either ^{99m}Tc-HMPAO or ^{111}In-oxine are the standard when osteomyelitis is suspected, it gives 95% accuracy and allowed the differentiation of soft infection. SPECT/CT is mandatory in addition to plantar images to determine the exact location and extent of infection. Radiolabeled non-colloid and white blood cells of bone marrow may differentiate osteomyelitis from Charcot neuroarthropathy and osteomyelitis [30].

5.4 Infections of the Feet

Foot infection among patients with diabetes is even more challenging, a reliable and unequivocal answer is not always possible [3]. A multidisciplinary approach is the art of the task to diagnose and follow infection. Infection is defined as the presence of two signs of inflammation or purulence as is classified as follows [31]:

- Superficial: limited in size and depth
- Moderate: deeper or more extensive
- Severe: accompanied by systemic signs or metabolic perturbations

Imaging plays a major role, plain radiographs are the usual initial approach. MRI is the imaging of choice, computed tomography, positron emission tomography, and single-photon emission (SPECT)/CT are increasingly used with different radiotracers [32].

5.5 Conclusion

Diabetic foot inflammation can be challenging in terms of diagnosis and thus management, in particular when Charcot osteoarthropathy, infections, fracture, other noninfectious inflammatory disorders including gouty arthritis, and neoplasm. Early diagnosis is vital for the early introduction of a specific therapy. MRI, especially STIR, diffusion-weighted, and dynamic contrast imaging are the modalities of choice for both inflammation and infections. Plain radiographs are the initial investigation providing anatomic and structural features. Computed tomography and ultrasonography are used for special purposes and when magnetic resonance imaging is contraindicated or not sensitive and specific (bone marrow or soft tissue destruction). Radionuclide scans are not in common use due to cost and they are not readily available. Thermography is quick, cheap, and sensitive when available.

References

1. Shatnawi NJ, Al-Zoubi NA, Hawamdeh H, Khader YS, Omari AE, Khammash MR (2018) Redefined clinical spectra of diabetic foot syndrome. Vasc Health Risk Manag 14:291–298. https://doi.org/10.2147/VHRM.S169502
2. Jeffcoate WJ, Macfarlane RM, Fletcher EM (1993) The description and classification of diabetic foot lesions. Diabet Med 10(7):676–679
3. Brtková J (2015) The imaging of musculoskeletal manifestations and complications in diabetes mellitus. Vnitr Lek 61(6):552–558
4. Sprengel SD, Klaan B, Kintzele L (2018) Inflammatory changes of the foot. Radiologe 58(5):433–441. https://doi.org/10.1007/s00117-018-0364-x
5. Lipsky BA, Berendt AR, Cornia PB et al (2012) Infectious Diseases Society of America 2012 Infectious Diseases Society of America clinical practice guideline for the diagnosis and treatment of diabetic foot infections. Clin Infect Dis 54(12):e132–e173
6. Beaman FD, von Herrmann PF, Kransdorf MJ, Adler RS, Amini B, Appel M et al (2017) ACR appropriateness criteria suspected osteomyelitis, septic arthritis, or soft tissue infection (excluding spine and diabetic foot). J Am Coll Radiol 14(5S):S326–S337. https://doi.org/10.1016/j.jacr.2017.02.008
7. Martín Noguerol T, Luna Alcalá A, Beltrán LS, Gómez Cabrera M, BroncanoCabrero J, Vilanova JC (2017) Advanced MR imaging techniques for differentiation of neuropathic arthropathy and osteomyelitis in the diabetic foot. Radiographics 37(4):1161–1180. https://doi.org/10.1148/rg.2017160101
8. Borkar R, Rizkalla J, Kwon Y, Salama P, Rizkalla M (2018) Electromagnetic simulation of non-invasive approach for the diagnosis of diabetic foot ulcers. J Orthop 15(2):514–521. https://doi.org/10.1016/j.jor.2018.03.024
9. van Netten JJ, Price PE, Lavery LA, Monteiro-Soares M, Rasmussen A, Jubiz Y et al (2016) Prevention of foot ulcers in the at-risk patient with diabetes: a systematic review. Diabetes Metab Res Rev 32(Suppl 1):84–98. https://doi.org/10.1002/dmrr.2701
10. Martín-Vaquero J, Hernández Encinas A, Queiruga-Dios A, José Bullón J, Martínez-Nova A, Torreblanca González J et al (2019) Review on wearables to monitor foot temperature in diabetic patients. Sensors (Basel) 19(4) pii: E776. https://doi.org/10.3390/s19040776
11. Reyzelman AM, Koelewyn K, Murphy M, Shen X, Yu E, Pillai R et al (2018) Continuous temperature-monitoring socks for home use in patients with diabetes: observational study. J Med Internet Res 20(12):e12460. https://doi.org/10.2196/12460
12. Keenan E, Gethin G, Flynn L, Watterson D, O'Connor GM (2017) Enhanced thermal imaging of wound tissue for better clinical decision making. Physiol Meas 38(6):1104–1115. https://doi.org/10.1088/1361-6579/aa6ea0
13. Wijlens AM, Holloway S, Bus SA, van Netten JJ (2017) An explorative study on the validity of various definitions of a 2·2°C temperature threshold as warning signal for impending diabetic foot ulceration. Int Wound J 14(6):1346–1351. https://doi.org/10.1111/iwj.12811
14. Skafjeld A, Iversen MM, Holme I, Ribu L, Hvaal K, Kilhovd BK (2015) A pilot study testing the feasibility of skin temperature monitoring to reduce recurrent foot ulcers in patients with diabetes—a randomized controlled trial. BMC Endocr Disord 15:55. https://doi.org/10.1186/s12902-015-0054-x
15. Nagase T, Sanada H, Takehara K, Oe M, Iizaka S, Ohashi Y (2011) Variations of plantar thermographic patterns in normal controls and non-ulcer diabetic patients: novel classification using angiosome concept. J Plast Reconstr Aesthet Surg 64(7):860–866. https://doi.org/10.1016/j.bjps.2010.12.003
16. Oe M, Yotsu RR, Sanada H, Nagase T, Tamaki T (2012) Thermographic findings in a case of type 2 diabetes with foot ulcer and osteomyelitis. J Wound Care 21(6):274. 276-8
17. Gatt A, Falzon O, Cassar K, Camilleri KP, Gauci J, Ellul C et al (2018) The application of medical thermography to discriminate neuroischemic toe ulceration in the diabetic foot. Int J Low Extrem Wounds 17(2):102–105. https://doi.org/10.1177/1534734618783910

18. Naraynsingh V, Maharaj R, Dan D, Hariharan S (2011) Puncture wounds in the diabetic foot: importance of X-ray in diagnosis. Int J Low Extrem Wounds 10(2):98–100. https://doi.org/10.1177/1534734611411572
19. Tsang KW, Morrison WB (2016) Update: imaging of lower extremity infection. Semin Musculoskelet Radiol 20(2):175–191. https://doi.org/10.1055/s-0036-1581116
20. Park M, Park JS, Ahn SE, Ryu KN, Park SY, Jin W (2016) Sonographic findings of common musculoskeletal diseases in patients with diabetes mellitus. Korean J Radiol 17(2):245–254. https://doi.org/10.3348/kjr.2016.17.2.245
21. Zamyshevskaia MA, Zavadovskaia VD, Udodov VD, Zorkal'tsev MA, Grigor'ev EG (2014) Role of magnetic resonance imaging in the study of patients with diabetic foot syndrome. Vestn Rentgenol Radiol (4):31–37. (Article in Russian)
22. Short DJ, Zgonis T (2017) Medical imaging in differentiating the diabetic Charcot foot from osteomyelitis. Clin Podiatr Med Surg 34(1):9–14. https://doi.org/10.1016/j.cpm.2016.07.002
23. Eren MA, Karakaş E, Torun AN, Sabuncu T (2018) The clinical value of diffusion weighted magnetic resonance imaging in diabetic foot infection. J Am Podiatr Med Assoc 109:277. https://doi.org/10.7547/17-066
24. Abdel Razek AAK, Samir S (2017) Diagnostic performance of diffusion-weighted MR imaging in differentiation of diabetic osteoarthropathy and osteomyelitis in diabetic foot. Eur J Radiol 89:221–225. https://doi.org/10.1016/j.ejrad.2017.02.015
25. Liao D, Xie L, Han Y, Du S, Wang H, Zeng C et al (2018) Dynamic contrast-enhanced magnetic resonance imaging for differentiating osteomyelitis from acute neuropathic arthropathy in the complicated diabetic foot. Skeletal Radiol 47(10):1337–1347. https://doi.org/10.1007/s00256-018-2942-4
26. Rao A, Gandikota G (2018) Beyond ulcers and osteomyelitis: imaging of less common musculoskeletal complications in diabetes mellitus. Br J Radiol 91(1088):20170301. https://doi.org/10.1259/bjr.20170301
27. Duryea D, Bernard S, Flemming D, Walker E, French C (2017) Outcomes in diabetic foot ulcer patients with isolated T2 marrow signal abnormality in the underlying bone: should the diagnosis of "osteitis" be changed to "early osteomyelitis"? Skeletal Radiol 46(10):1327–1333. https://doi.org/10.1007/s00256-017-2666-x
28. Glaudemans AW, Uçkay I, Lipsky BA (2015) Challenges in diagnosing infection in the diabetic foot. Diabet Med 32(6):748–759. https://doi.org/10.1111/dme.12750
29. Rastogi A, Bhattacharya A, Prakash M, Sharma S, Mittal BR, Khandelwal N et al (2016) Utility of PET/CT with fluorine-18-fluorodeoxyglucose-labeled autologous leukocytes for diagnosing diabetic foot osteomyelitis in patients with Charcot's neuroarthropathy. Nucl Med Commun 37(12):1253–1259
30. Lipsky BA, Berendt AR, Cornia PB, Pile JC, Peters EJ, Armstrong DG et al (2012) 2012 Infectious Diseases Society of America clinical practice guideline for the diagnosis and treatment of diabetic foot infections. Clin Infect Dis 54(12):e132–e173. https://doi.org/10.1093/cid/cis346
31. Israel O, Sconfienza LM, Lipsky BA (2014) Diagnosing diabetic foot infection: the role of imaging and a proposed flow chart for assessment. Q J Nucl Med Mol Imaging 58(1):33–45
32. Mandell JC, Khurana B, Smith JT, Czuczman GJ, Ghazikhanian V, Smith SE. Osteomyelitis of the lower extremity: pathophysiology, imaging, and classification, with an emphasis on diabetic foot infection. Emerg Radiol. 2018;25(2):175–188. https://doi.org/10.1007/s10140-017-1564-9
33. van Doremalen RFM, van Netten JJ, van Baal JG, Vollenbroek-Hutten MMR, van der Heijden F. Infrared 3D Thermography for Inflammation Detection in Diabetic Foot Disease: A Proof of Concept. J Diabetes Sci Technol. 2020;14(1):46–54. https://doi.org/10.1177/1932296819854062

6 Molecular Mechanism and Biomechanics of the Diabetic Foot: The Road to Foot Ulceration and Healing

Mohammad Zubair and Farha Fatima

6.1 Introduction

Diabetes Mellitus (DM) is often the most complex disease that is almost vulnerable to all the body organs. Around 415 million individuals are usually affected through diabetes mellitus and most of them are due to the adverse effect of type 2 DM. it is further predicted that by the year 2040, a significant growth is about to take place, as almost 642 million people are detected at the high risks of the given disease is the near future [1]. Since the problem majorly affect the overall human body, there are greater chances among patients for increased impact in the form of diabetic foot ulcer (DFU). It was further regarded that among the overall patients suffering through DM, almost 15% of them are at high risks of DFU. Chronic diseases, recurrence, or the formation of various highly effective diseases are the most popular problems of DFU and are powerful enough to affect the patient's mind. The prevalence of the disease is often found among diabetic patients with ulcers. Researchers suggested that the majority of the amputations are often connected to diabetes mellitus (DM), since the disease weakens the overall body functions of the affected patient. However, the prevalence of the disease in its increased forms often results in morbidity and mortality of the human body.

Diabetic Foot Ulcer (DFC) is defined as the foot affected through the ulceration and is related to the diseases belonging to the neuropathy and peripheral arterial diseases commonly located in the lower limbs of the diabetic patients [2]. The problem is directly associated with neuropathy, infection, and ischemia. Patients who have poor control over diabetes mellitus are usually at the risk of foot ulceration leading toward unfavorable consequences including the poor metabolism of wound

M. Zubair (✉)
Department of Medical Microbiology, Faculty of Medicine, University of Tabuk, Tabuk, Kingdom of Saudi Arabia

F. Fatima
Department of Zoology, Faculty of Life Science, Aligarh Muslim University, Aligarh, India

M. Zubair et al. (eds.), *Diabetic Foot Ulcer*,
https://doi.org/10.1007/978-981-15-7639-3_6

healing along with the increasing risk of infection. The competitive metabolism of the associated patients is often integrated through the decreasing growth of body cells and angiogenesis. It is further associated with the low levels of peripheral blood flow leading toward the damage of the peripheral nerves followed by ulcerations, deformation, vascular diseases, and gangrene. DFU is often regarded as the disease that is connected to the increased financial load over patients who are willing to undergo quality treatment. Clinical experts suggested that the prevention of the disease is possible and is often manageable through early diagnosis, followed by preventive measures and quality treatment through a multidisciplinary professionals and clinical experts associated with the given disease [3]. Since diabetes is detected as one of the growing diseases, it is potentially able to affect other important organs of the human body. The growth of the disease often leads to the disruption and damage of important body parts leading toward severe results. In many cases, the foot is the major affected part of the human body that is specifically found among patients with uncontrolled diabetes.

Significant growth has been observed in the prevalence of disease under certain individuals. It was further regarded that the prevalence of foot ulcers is expected to occur among 9.1–26.1 million individuals suffering from diabetes. The approximation regarding the given disease is provided on an annual basis. Studies further suggested that the proportion of the diseases, i.e., diabetes and foot ulcerations have been high in the past, however, similar consistency has been observed regarding the development of the disease in present. The proportion of the individuals suffering from foot ulcerations due to diabetes has been high than those suffering from active ulcers. The development of this lifetime disease among diabetic individuals has been observed among 15–25% patients [4]. In Indonesia, the given problem has been documented among patients between 17–32%, along with the overall proportion of amputation which is up to 30%. The survival rate of such patients has been observed with an increased limit, i.e., up to 37% in the following years [5].

Another huge concern is often regarded as different complications associated with the problem, which serves as the greatest cause of posing different threats to the economy and public health. The development of diabetes is associated to obesity which in most severe conditions leads toward the formation of chronic DFU and impaired healing of foot wounds. Researchers suggested that the number of diabetic patients is likely to increase up to 366 million till 2030, followed by the diabetic epidemic diseases. Diabetic patients are often exposed to different diseases including the bony wound infections, loss of soft tissues, increased cardiovascular diseases, low levels of extreme amputations, and in most complex and severe cases it leads toward patient's death. The most common problem associated with the disease includes the lifetime probabilities of ulcerations, where almost 25% of diabetic individuals are likely to have neuropathic foot ulcerations leading toward amputations [6].

One of the famous physicians of diabetes suggested that diabetic foot ulcer is not a natural disease, rather it is formed due to external and internal body conditions. This suggests that foot ulceration is not the entire consequence of diabetes rather it serves as the consequence to the unfavorable contact of environmental risks and pathological developments of the lower limb [7].

6.2 Probability of Infections in Nonphysiological Inflammatory Responses

Most of the chronic foot ulcers are usually found in the inflammatory cycle that is often integrated through the development of the granulation tissues. However, the long-term inflammation in the inflammatory phase contributes to the increased defects found in the microcellular defects that ultimately reduce the probabilities of wound recovery [8]. Hyperglycemia usually contributes to decreasing the efficiency of the inflammatory responses, this is due to the altered functions in lymphocytes, neutrophils, and macrophages with reduced phagocytic and cytotoxic abilities [9, 10]. Majorly, the alterations in the cell activities are due to the reduced pressure of the local oxygen, as the impaired processes often contributes to the maximum consumption of oxygen. When considering the wound infections in foot, it has been developed that such incidence is most common and evident among patients with diabetic ulcers rather than those in chronic wounds. This imitates the reduced function of leukocytes. Also, the compression and physical stress leads toward the increase in the loading of local bacteria [11]. In cases where lies a narcotic tissue, there is a greater probability of the rapid increase in the formation of a wide number of microorganisms. It was further indicated that there lies a smooth relationship between the number of local bacteria found in the wounded part and the speed of wound healing. For instance, a single gram of tissue consists of the 105 bacteria then there is an increased probability of the minimum levels of tissue repairs. However, the decreased number of bacteria, i.e., up to 103, usually results in the development of β streptococci in hemolytic. Therefore, in order to cater the increased load of bacteria, it is expected to have an increase in the overall proportion of the lymphocytes mainly belonging to CD4-CD8 ratios. In specific cases, a significant decrease has been detected in this type of relationship, which is followed by the increased number of CD8 cells and a reduction in the total number of CD4 cells. This further suggests that CD8 plays an active role in reducing the healing process of wounds among diabetic individuals. Evidences found through various studies further indicated that the following cells are responsible for the changes in tissue repairs.

Another form of inflammatory response is usually integrated through the increased levels of the oxidative stress that shares a causal linkage between oxidative stress and hyperglycemia, leading toward the major health-related complications and cell damages among diabetic patients. This oxidative stress is generated through several mechanisms such as, Vitamin C, oxygen-free radicals, protein kinase C, and hexosamine pathways [8]. The transfer of the most powerful antioxidant or ascorbic acid is mostly held through the intervention of hyperglycemia. The overall process takes place in fibroblasts and the emplastic. The reachability of the hyperglycemia is often restricted through glycose, due to the similarity found in both the structures. The activation of nicotinamide adenine dinucleotide phosphate (NADPH), which is a type of enzyme that helps in increasing the activities in the oxidative stress followed by the increase in PKC, and the depletion of NADPH. The effects are significant in increasing the development of the radicals free from oxidation, with reduced synthesis of the glutathione and nitric acid. Moreover, the increased glucose concentrations result in the saturation of the hexokinase enzymes in the glycolytic routes. This results in ceasing the activity of utilizing the altered route of degradation. Finally, the formation of hyperglycemia is undertaken through the intervention of sorbitol and the use of NADPH, which apparently decreases the concentration of the last substance [12].

Diabetes is further characterized through the increased activity of the hexosamine biosynthetic routes, which refers to a qualitative alteration of NADH into NADPH, which is possible due to the obstruction of the glyceraldehyde 6 phosphate dehydrogenase. Concerning the cases where the identification of disease is still not understood, a significant increase is observed in different activities of xanthine oxidase, NADPH oxidase, and arachidonic acid cascade. Among the given elements, superoxide is the only element that is potentially strong in reacting with nitric oxide to form peroxynitrite, which may convert in nitrogen peroxide through the intervention of superoxide dismutase. In the given process, nitrogen peroxide is often used in the formation of the hydroxyl radicals that are integrated through the ferrous and cuprous ions. The biodiversity of vasodilators is often reduced or limited by the superoxide anion through its reaction of nitric oxide. Titanium peroxide then helps in the perpetuation of the premature apoptosis and inflammation of cells that produce matrix. In the final phase, the interaction of the hydroxyl radicals and lipids, proteins, and DNA help in promoting conditions that include, dementia, atherosclerosis, and the reperfusion of injury [13].

6.3 Amputation Impaired Response to Infection Diabetic Foot Ulceration

The impact of the growing diabetes problem is however evident through the development and growth in different problems including renal failure (final stage), blindness, minimum extremity amputations, and other permanent disabilities leading toward death. The problem has caused a significant increase in mortality and morbidity of diabetic patients. The most highlighted and outlined effect of the disease is in the form of diabetic foot ulcer, where every 10–25% of patients suffer through the given problem [14]. Foot ulcers are also characterized as the major cause of patient's hospitalization leading toward several financial, social, and health-related consequences [15, 16]. The uncontrolled glycemic control along with foot ulcers also serves as the fundamental factor for limb amputations and further serves as the major consequence of the patient's death [17] (Fig. 6.1).

A significant association has been found between rate of mortality and the amputation among patients with the hemoglobin level of <0.0001 [18]. Infections taking place among diabetic patients such as, peripheral arterial disease is one of the major causes of amputation that usually take place among the old age diabetic population.

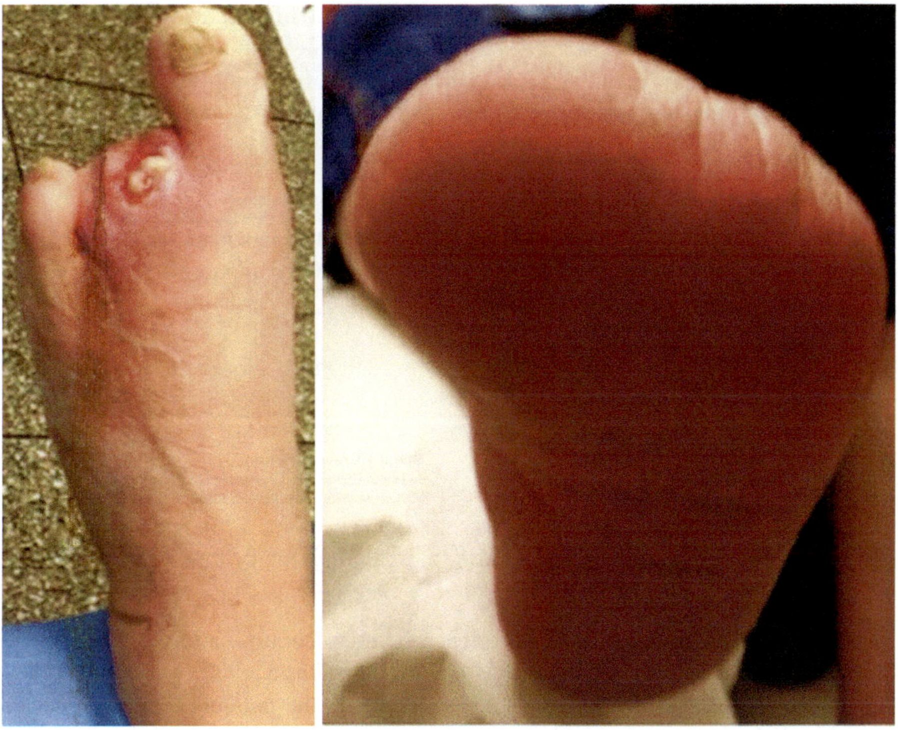

Fig. 6.1 Foot Amputation: Nonfunctional foot with underlying osteomyelitis successfully treated with transmetatarsal amputation and percutaneous tendon Achilles lengthening with 6-month follow-up (note lack of callus or recurrent ulceration). (Adapted from Ref. [86])

The problem has been studied by various scholars, as for instance; in Argentina. Sereday et al. [19] conducted a study by collecting data from 11 different hospitals. Findings of this study indicated that the amputation rate was common among diabetic patients. Besides, the infection was also identified as the fundamental cause of amputation along with the risks of peripheral arterial disease. The rate of amputation varies from country to country. As in Brazil only, Rezende et al. [20] found high rate of amputation, i.e., up to 47.7%. Similar, ratio was identified in Guiana, where before the development of structured national program for diabetes, the rate of amputation was approximately 42% which then decreased due to the increased awareness programs in the given region [18]. The amputation rate in Portugal was up to 5.8%. This was mostly found in the outpatient.

Since infections serve as the most common complication among diabetic patients and are highly associated with diseases such as; peripheral arterial disease and neuropathy, it is important for clinicians to have necessary knowledge regarding the severity of the infection. The idea is crucial as it may assist medical experts in providing the correct treatment to the affected patient. Figure 6.2 below provides important knowledge regarding the identification of infection in patients with diabetic foot ulcers at different stages.

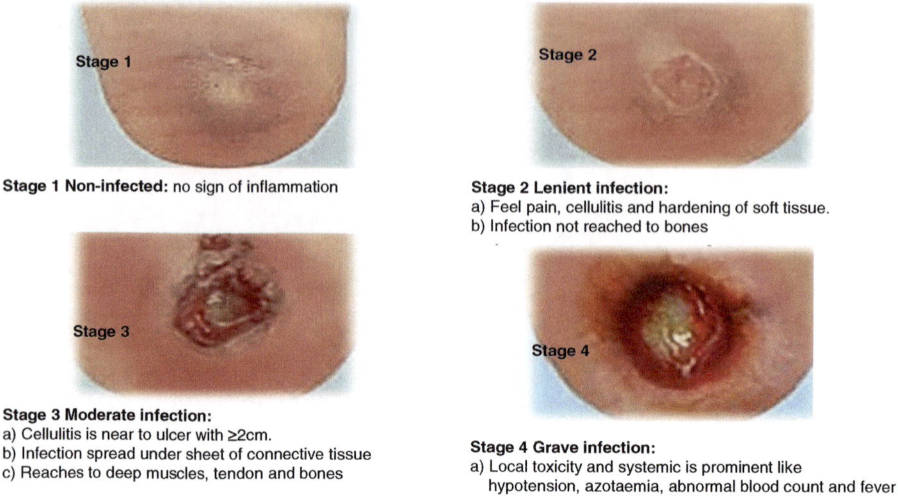

Fig. 6.2 Identification of different stages of infection. (Adapted and modified with license no. 4813661460709 from [88])

Most of the diabetic patients experience severe ulceration along with an active infection. The extent of the area that is being affected as a result of infection determines the type of disease management required by the patient. A necrotic lesion found in diabetic foot ulcers when acted by an infection lead toward the formation of wet gangrene. However, in most of cases where infections reach the final stages, the only option left for the treatment is amputation, which is also referred to as unsalvageable foot. Amputations occurring at any part of the foot increase the probability of infection and amputation in the remaining part of foot and thus require more critical care. Desormais et al. [21] in their study found that anemia is also highly associated to amputation resulting in patient's death. This usually happens due to the insufficient delivery of oxygen to the affected area, leading toward poor control of growing infection in diabetic patients [22].

6.4 Diabetic Foot Ulcerations and Risk Factors

Several risk factors have been associated with the prevalence of foot ulcers among diabetic patients leading toward the development and exposition of disease toward major threats.

6.4.1 Smoking

One of the most common risk factors associated with the given disease is smoking. According to the study conducted by Obaid and Eljedi [23], smoking is majorly associated with the diabetic foot ulcers. This is due to the toxic smoke that is inhaled during the process resulting in the hypoxia of body tissues that may cause several neuropathic and vascular disorders among patients with lower extremity of diabetes. Researchers suggested that cigarette smoking serves as one of the greatest causes that contributes to the worsening of diabetic neuropathy, which is a type of diabetic foot ulcerations. Oxidative stress produced by smoking creates adverse effects on diabetic individuals. It is further identified as an independent factor that is critical to the development of diabetic neuropathy [24]. The stimulation of the oxidative stress in various organs, including; the blood vessels and the nervous system results in severe damages in the cellular area. One important reason is the supplement of free radicals of oxygen in the human body, which is due to the presence of cigarette smoke [25].

The evidences gathered through in vivo and in vitro indicate the availability of the glycotoxins in the smoke released by the cigarette. These glycotoxins are considerably reactive in the formation of the advanced end products of the glycation (AGE). These end products are located outside the cell [26, 27]. In various smokers, the modification of lipids and proteins leads toward the incorporation of various receptors in order to develop the advanced end products glycation which ultimately results in the activation of the nicotinamide adenine dinucleotide phosphate oxidase (NADPO). The process further includes the induction of oxidative stress through the manifestation of the inflammatory chemokines and cytokines. The excessive development of the reactive oxygen species by the infusion of cigarette smoke leads toward the development of the nitric oxide synthase that increases the stress over glutamate leading toward the influx of Ca^{2+}. It further results in the dysfunction of mitochondria, inflammation, and the damage of the deoxyribonucleic acid [28, 29].

In addition, smoke caused by the cigarette develops a sense of resistance to insulin which apparently worsens neuropathy. Studies suggested that secretion of the insulin is at greater risks among smokers. The following conditions can only be catered through the development of maximum resistance to cigarette smoke resulting in the development of high insulin receptors such as the substrate-1ser^{636} phosphorylation.

The effects of cigarette smoking are not only limited to the formation of foot ulcerations among patients, rather it acts as one of the most prominent causes of delayed wound healing. The developments in the given area of knowledge suggested that smoking is mainly associated in producing the higher incidence of the postsurgical complexities. Whereas, ceasing smoking before 3 weeks of surgery reduces the probabilities of impaired wound healing and the rate of postsurgical morbidity is further decreased with a significance fall from 52% to 18%. This suggests that the cessation of smoking is effective in healing severe foot wounds among diabetics. Studies resulted in providing low-level evidences regarding the impact of smoking cessation in minimizing the risks of leg amputations and lesions among those with poor glycemic controls. However, studies suggested that quitting smoking before a certain duration of surgery helps in decreasing the chances of postoperative morbidity [30], which signifies the value of smoke cessation in increasing the chances of improvement in wound healing during the postoperative conditions.

Patients with controlled smoking contributes to reversing the consequences of the lack of oxygen and oxidative stress within human body.

Several clinical developments have been undertaken to develop smoke cessation with maximum probabilities of success among diabetic individuals. These therapies are in the form of bupropion, behavioral interventions, varenicline, and nicotine replacement therapy along with the induction of electronic cigarettes [31].

6.4.2 Obesity

Another common risk factor associated with the disease is obesity. Pham et al. [32] through detailed research suggested that diabetic foot ulcers are often related to obesity. While other researchers suggested that BMI ratios have no significant relationship with the prevalence of diabetic foot ulcer. Patients with diabetic foot ulcerations usually have low levels of BMI ranging from 25 kg to 30 kg/m^2. Since only few data is available regarding the significance of obesity in causing foot ulceration, therefore it may consider as one of the risks associated with the given problem. Another crucial information in similar cases indicated that the prevalence of the problem is more common among males in comparison to females. The reason includes the increased involvement of males toward the physical activities [33]. Obesity is further characterized as the cause of increasing the risks regarding the development of the peripheral neuropathy that does not depend on the level of glucose control. It also serves as an important source of affecting the small and large fibers in the human body, where large fibers are known to be highly impacted through hyperglycemia [34]. People suffering from both diabetes and obesity are more prone toward the risks of the peripheral developments of neuropathy. This indirectly exerts a greater significance over the idea of controlling both body weight and type 2 diabetes.

Individuals that lack the ability of undergoing through physical activities are more toward the development of obesity, leading toward other hazardous health risks. Contemporary developments in knowledge suggested that people that are least habitual of walking are at the minimal risks of undergoing through foot ulceration, in contrast to those who are more active and practice walking exercises. However, modern studies indicated that people that are not habitual of daily walking are at higher risks of foot ulceration [35]. The most amazing development in this regard initiated that people that undergo a variety of daily activities are at high risks regarding the development of foot ulceration. The idea is crucial here, as people that are not much habitual of undergoing through any such activity must be warned regarding the instant functionality of body in the form of increased variability in everyday activities. Since obesity is responsible for exerting the additional stress over the affected foot, controlled body weight may help in balancing the body forces that are exerted both at the ankle and foot of the affected individuals. The detailed analysis of the idea was developed through case-controlled study that was conducted. Ross et al. [36], according to which no significant association was detected between the increased BMI and the development of critical Charcot neuropathy among the diabetic patients.

6.4.3 Immunopathy

According to researchers, the immune system of diabetic patients is much weaker in comparison to those of healthy patients. Foot infection among diabetic patients contributes in weakening body functions that pose various threats on the appropriate functioning of limbs. Patients with uncontrolled diabetes generally cause the increased production of the pro-inflammatory cytokines leading toward inappropriate cell functions including phagocytosis, chemotaxis, intracellular, and phagocytosis killing. The immune system is further affected through the decreased functions of leukocytes, along with the destruction of cellular immunity [1]. Patients with poor glycemic controls usually have significantly low levels of leukocyte phagocytosis, while the development and increase in microbiocidal functions are directly related to the controlled hyperglycemia. Wound healing among individuals with normal glycemic controls is usually held through the low levels of chemotaxis and their impact on cytokines and growth factors followed by the expansion in metalloproteinases. In conditions where diabetic patients are affected through an open wound, a catabolic state is formed in the body of the affected person. The ineffective balance of nitrogen leads toward the lack of insulin. This is due to the breakdown of proteins also known as gluconeogenesis.

The dysfunctions in metabolisms are often followed by the impairment of different fibroblasts, collagens, and proteins that results in the lack of nutrition. Researches however suggested that the impairment of the diseases is mainly held in cases where the serum level of the glucose in the human body is usually decreased or is equal to the 150 ml/dl. High blood glucose serves as an immunity for the growth of bacteria including β-hemolytic streptococci, positive gram aerobic bacteria, etc. in human body. Other common organisms that are identified by the researchers include negative gram aerobes that are commonly found in the foot of the affected patients. Furthermore, it was developed that the soft tissues of foot, muscle sheaths, tendons, etc. are ineffective in resisting the development of the infection within foot. Since certain parts of foot are interconnected therefore the transfer of infection from one place to another is often impossible in most of the cases, leading toward the development of the osteitis. In most of the cases where necessary care is not provided toward the foot ulcers, the results are in the form of development of various complications including the gangrene.

6.4.4 Unbalance Between Metabolism and Nutrient Delivery

In most of the diabetic patients, the abnormal diabetic is mostly due to the low concentration levels of ATP (adenosine triphosphate) along with high concentration of lactate and glucose. Among diabetic, the low levels of wound healing are also due to the increased concentration of cellular metabolism, macrophages, fibroblasts along with other leukocytes. In other conditions, the insufficient concentration of the growth factors found in the diabetic ulcers promotes a significant decrease in growth factors including; PDGF, insulin-1 (IGF-), fibroblast growth factor (FGF),

Osteopontine, transforming factor-β1 in growth, TGF-β1, interleukin-8, and -10. It further contributes in the supra regulation of TNF-α, Il-1 and angiopoietin-21 [37]. The delay of angiogenesis is regulated with the low level of osteopontine along with the increased concentration of the angiopoietin-2, where the first contributes to the continuation of the process and latter restricts it.

A recent development suggested that micro RNA serves as an important contributor in the identification of the pathological developments of foot wounds among diabetic patients. In a physiological perspective, the precursor of the micro RNA, when evolved through the enzyme dicer is converted to the micro RNA, that functions in providing the translations of the RNA messengers [37]. A considerable change in the cellular gene expression has been observed with a significant decrease in the dicer enzymes among the diabetic group of rants. It was further observed that the biological mechanisms are highly impactful in decreasing the concentration of the keratinocyte proliferations among diabetic users. The expression of the micro RNA is integrated through the hypoxia-1α inducing factor, i.e., HIF-1 α, which serves as an important factor in promoting diabetes. This in turn provides the encoding of gene E2F3 transcription which helps in the provision of the keratinocytes. Finally, the increase in HIF-1α helps in the concentration of the proliferation of keratinocyte.

6.5 Altered Biomechanics in Diabetic Foot

Biomechanics serves as the basic art of implementing the rules and scientific laws that are associated with different fields of learning such as the architecture, engineering, physics, and mechanics that are usually applied to the living subjects. The committed practitioners of the present day, including those belonging to the Functional Lower Extremity Biomechanics (FLEB) have managed to conduct such interpersonal practices by implementing their abundant knowledge, professional experience followed by the use of technological devices that may contribute in providing the Evidence-based practice of Biomechanics [37, 38].

When discussing the biomechanics of the foot, it can be characterized into the functional segments following two fundamental ways. Following the first part, i.e., the Midtarsal joint it is divided into the forefoot and the rearfoot. While, latter divides the foot into second and the third rays reaching toward the medial and the lateral arch segments (as indicated in Fig. 6.3). The medial arch comprised talus, calcaneus, navicular, and talus along with the three cuneiforms and with three different metatarsals. Calcaneus, cuboids along with fourth and fifth metatarsals contributes to the development of the lateral arch. Both arches are further connected through transverse roof surface of the bone which is also known as the vault of the foot. The efficiency of vault in bearing heavyweights and related functioning is due to the support of healthy soft tissues that makes it compatible with the lifetime functioning [39]. Whereas, in cases where vault works in an off-centered position, it poses different challenges such as the excess in flexibility, arch, stiffness, or collapsing leading toward the excessive burden over postural

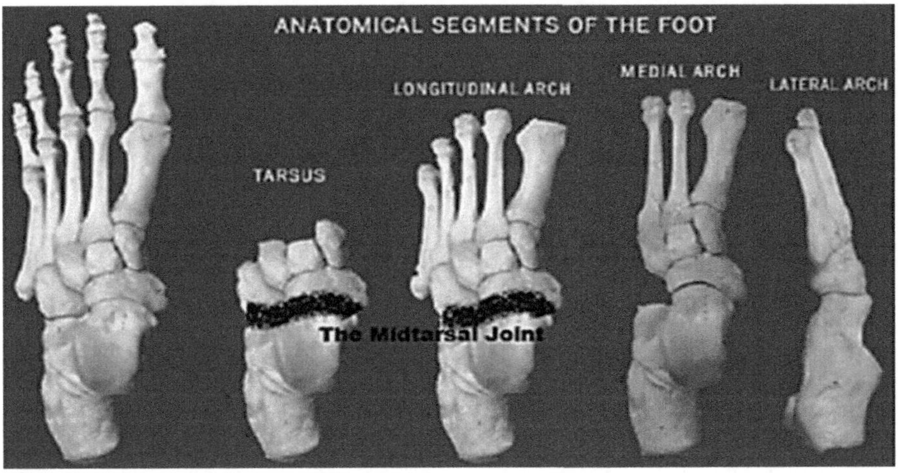

Fig. 6.3 Anatomical structure of the foot. (Adapted from Ref. [39])

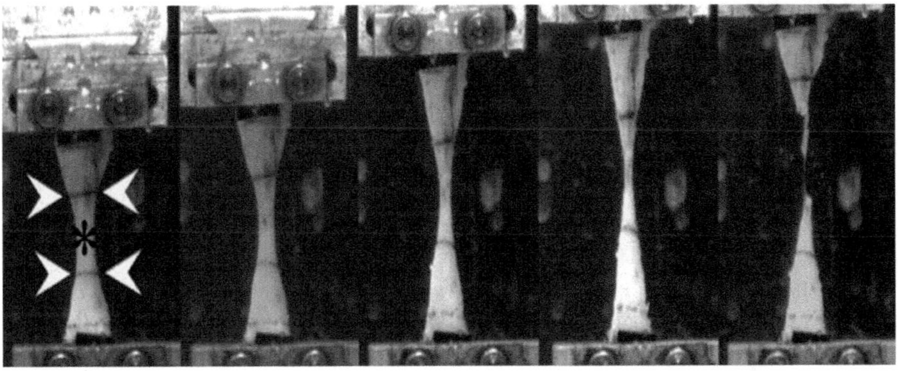

Fig. 6.4 Biomechanical testing of skin in Diabetic foot. (Adapted from Ref. [89])

and pedal bones, muscles, joints, tendons, integumentary organs, and ligaments. Among patients with diabetic foot ulcerations, several risks have been highlighted that are responsible toward altered biomechanics of the foot (Fig. 6.4). The overall situation is intervened through the loss of protective sensation (LOPS), peripheral arterial disease, and the loss of proprioception. The risk factors are however significant in maximizing the chances of the altered foot biomechanism and are highly connected in the form of the chained process leading toward the uncertain foot conditions. Certain important biomechanical risks have been outlined that are commonly found among diabetic patients. The factors include, ground reactive conditions and forces, stiff or hard shoes, the central elements of the biomechanical pathology, weight and mass of the diabetic individual, activity and the fitness level along with the state of health.

6.5.1 Contributing Factors to Altered Biomechanics in Diabetic Foot

Most of the deformities found in diabetic patients are held due to the altered foot biomechanics. Hyperglycemia causes the glycosylation of the connective tissues aggravates the hyper pronation of the foot, which ultimately increases the forefoot pressure over gait and stance [40]. Several causes have been identified that contributes to the development of the diabetic foot mechanism.

6.5.1.1 Diabetic Neuropathy

Neuropathy is often related to the loss of sensation that is majorly found among 20% of diabetic individuals. The problem is often encountered among patients suffering from type 2 diabetes and serve as the accommodating factor in developing a foot ulcer. Neuropathy or peripheral neuropathy serves as the loss of impairment of normal body functions related to the nervous system and is often related to the weakening of sensory, motor, and autonomic functions in diabetic patients. The prevalence of neuropathy among diabetic patients is comparatively high ranging from 16% to 66% [1].

The problem is mostly caused among diabetic patients resulting in the damage of various nerves found in the human body. However, in most of the patients, the problem is not visible through symptoms. While in others, signs such as chronic pain, numbness, tingling, loss of feeling at multiple body parts including, hands, legs, and feet are commonly associated with the presence of diabetic neuropathy. It has been estimated that approximately 60–70% of diabetic patients form neuropathy to a certain extent, where risks increase by the time with the gradual increase in the age of the affected patient. The most common signs of diabetic neuropathy are visible among those who had been suffering from diabetes for more than 25 years. Besides, it is also found among patients who have uncontrolled sugar and glucose level, and are overweighed [41].

6.5.1.2 Peripheral Neuropathy

Peripheral neuropathy acts as the fundamental causative factor for the altered biomechanics of the diabetic foot ulcer [32]. There lies a significant gap in the presence of normal protective and the proprioceptive abilities among patients with diabetic foot, and the given functions are almost absent by the time disease develops visible progress. Following this, peripheral neuropathy serves as the direct contributor for the inability of individuals in managing accommodation to the ground reactive forces and also acts as the fundamental source of joint subluxation. Since the diabetic foot works to make useful adjustments in the sensory feedback caused by gait. This feedback however is interrupted as a result of the development of peripheral neuropathy. For instance; in a standing position, the person managed to make minor adjustments by creating a balance through the body and the foot [42]. This helps in minimizing the prolonged pressure in any particular part of the body. Therefore, it can be inferred that peripheral neuropathy significantly contributes to increases the chances of problems during ambulation. Several causes have been identified that participate in the development of peripheral neuropathy. Some of them include, toxic exposures, excessive use of medicines, systemic disease, hereditary disorders, and other body infections. However, the most common causes that are easily controlled include; hypothyroidism, diabetes, and nutritional deficiency.

Peripheral neuropathy is also identified as one of the most common factors that contributes to the development of long-term complications specifically for diabetic neuropathy. It was further analyzed that almost 40% of patients suffering from type 2 diabetes show significant signs of neuropathy.

6.5.1.3 Peripheral Motor Neuropathy

Peripheral motor neuropathy is similar to that of the abnormality in the gait functions which will be discussed in the proceeding sections. Motor neuropathy is associated with developing the alterations in the anatomical structures of the foot and joint, which ultimately causes weakness and damage in the small intrinsic muscles. This leads toward the imbalance in movement causing muscle damage, followed by other significant characteristics including; plantar flexion taking place at the metatarsal head and clawing of toes.

6.5.1.4 Autonomic Neuropathy

Autonomic Neuropathy (AN) is commonly associated with the long-term occurrence of the diabetic mellitus. In most of the cases that are associated with lower probabilities of DM, AN result in the arteriovenous shunting leading toward the development of distension in the foot veins along with the dilation of the small arteries. Neuropathic edema is potentially strong enough to create different obstacles, hindering the treatment process of the diuretic therapy. Patients suffering through neuropathic experience swelling in feet, along with a sudden change in the body temperature.

Autonomic neuropathy further contributes to decreasing the autonomic nerve roots that are responsible for innervating the skin glands specifically responsible for sweating while involving the appendage tissue that ultimately causes dryness in the skin and low elasticity levels. This specifically takes place in the middle third region of the leg, where discoloration of the region takes place. The following conditions contributes to the formation of deep cracks on the downward region of the feet, resulting in the development of frequent injuries specifically among diabetic patients. The dryness occurring in the skin when forms a serious condition, develops the skin fissures that may ultimately cause infection proceeding toward the development of mild ulceration in diabetic feet.

6.5.2 Structural Foot Deformity

Restricted joint mobility, foot amputation, along with other structural foot deformities creates a significant impact on the diabetic patients who have problems associated with peripheral neuropathy, ranging from areas with increased pressure, ineffective weight bearing, along with abnormal obstruction of forces contributes in posing the maximum risks of ulcerations. Among diabetic patients, the structural deformity of the foot is highly associated with the decreased joint mobility. Nonenzymatic glycosylation that is found in the periarticular soft tissues exposes significant risk in the form of limited or reduced joint motion. The conditions are mainly common among diabetic patients with significant signs of neuropathy, resulting in the intrinsic musculature through atrophy that may cause hammering of different digits [43].

The reduction in motion then limits the ability of the foot in providing support to the ambulatory ground reactive forces which ultimately increases the plantar pressures. However, limited or reduced joint mobility is referred to as the hallux ability to bear the 50° of non-weight passive dorsiflexion [44]. In addition, glycosylation is potentially strong in affecting the resiliency factor in the Achilles tendon that pulls the foot toward the equinus, while potentially increasing the risk probabilities for foot ulcerations among diabetic patients. Therefore, to provide effective treatment, clinicians need to undertake the structural abnormalities among different patients. These structural abnormalities however include reduced joint mobility, claw toes, calluses, and bunions, along with flat feet that are significant in the identification of different pressure points on the foot that is susceptible to the future developments of the ulceration [45].

6.5.3 Gait Dysfunction

Gait refers to the way a person walks (Fig. 6.5). Whereas, abnormal gait or gait dysfunction refers to the type of abnormality that is specifically associated with the abnormality in walking and thus takes place when the human body is unable to

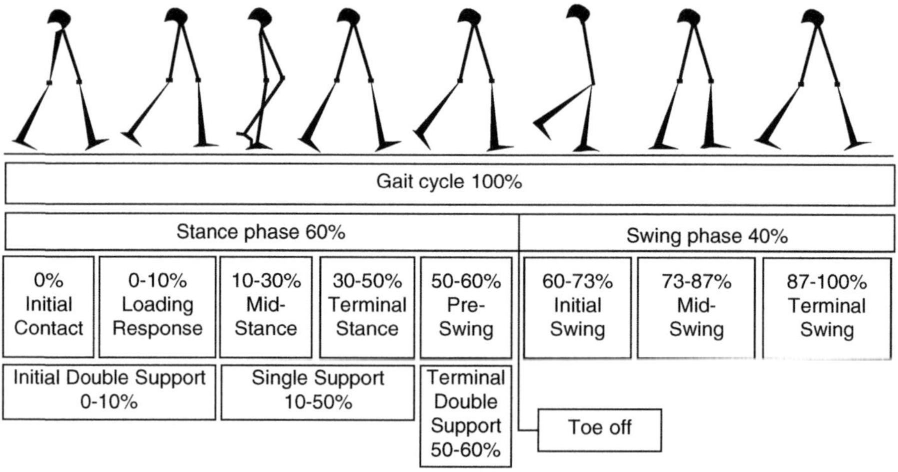

Fig. 6.5 Normal gait cycle source. (Adapted under license no. 4810900954855 from Ref. [90])

function in the usual manner. Factors such as; genetic characteristics, illness, injury, or any sort of abnormality associated with human leg or feet serve as the fundamental cause of gait abnormality. In certain cases, gait abnormalities are controlled by the time, while in other cases this acts as a permanent lifestyle.

The identification of the neurological disorders that are highly associated with developing changes in the human balance, posture, and gait functioning has been an important part of the clinical practice. The most foremost type of gait disability is significant in posing a substantial disability in completing the overall movement or the gait cycles. One of the most significant symptoms includes the occurrence of frequent falls creating prominent obstructions in walking smoothly. This is apparently connected to the development of injury, as a consequence where an individual fails to manage the recurrent falls. Another common issue associated with the gait includes the freeing of gait that acts as the fundamental cause of patient's fall that specifically takes place among those suffering from Parkinson disease (PD). In the given case, patient feels a sudden freeze of the leg while attempting to move forward [46, 47]. However, in most of the cases associated with gait disorders, the signs of the posture and balance are highly visible leading toward the early diagnosis of the disease.

Gait abnormality such as the asymmetrical reduced arm swing is the earliest symptom found among patients with PD [48, 49]. Foot injuries that commonly takes place among patients while walking are the consequences of gait occurrence during the normal walk. Diabetic patients tend to fall due to high risks of impaired vision, hypoglycemia along with the increased occurrence of the abnormal gait.

Normal gait functioning is interlinked to the individual ability of maintaining the safe gait, while acting effectively in the changing environments and in conditions that demand different gait functioning. The quality of an individual in maintaining the gait functioning is significantly associated with the person's ability of performing the everyday tasks in an independent manner while minimizing the risks of falling [50]. Diabetic patients due to internal weakness tend to take smaller steps while walking which actually demands an additional support [51]. Among various factors such as aging, psychological factors are also of fundamental importance in managing and influencing one's gait pattern. Patients suffering through peripheral neuropathy and diabetes mellitus are more toward gait instability [52].

Two common phases of gait, i.e., swing and stance serve as the essential components of ambulation. The swing phase is associated with the non-weight-bearing location where the foot is set free to move forward. Whereas, the stance phase takes place when the heel is in contact with the floor and ends with by lifting off the toes. Considering this, the stance phase takes place when limb bears the entire weight of the body. The foot is found to be more flexible during the stance phase of the gait, which allows it to absorb and bear the overall shock.

The extrinsic and intrinsic mobility plays an important role in managing the foot biomechanics among diabetic patients. Structural changes are further important that eventually takes place among diabetic patients. This is followed by the structural changes that take place within the capsule, ligament, and tendon of the diabetic patients followed by the disorganized patterns at the following places [53]. The changes are important as they lead toward reduced tensile strength and elasticity which ultimately result in the development of stiffness and subluxations in the foot. The overall changes occurring in the foot leads toward the altered biomechanics of foot [54].

In normal conditions, abnormal gait is characterized into different types depending upon the appearance and symptoms proposed by the individual walk. The first includes the spastic gait, which is in the form of dragging one's feet. This usually occurs when one is really stiff in managing the normal walk resulting in feet dragging.

Another type includes scissors gait, where the person tends to hit his/her legs during normal walking. This is due to the inward bending of one's leg which makes him/her unable to enjoy the normal work. Third type includes the steppage gait, this occurs in cases where an individual's toes are pointed toward the surface of the grounds. This type of movement usually takes while walking.

Waddling gait is another type of gait abnormality. A person suffering through this type of walking abnormality usually take each step from side to side. It is further held by undertaking short steps and involuntary body movement, i.e., body swinging. This type of problem is usually diagnosed through different imaging techniques to identify the type or the location of the injury, damages in body tissues, or broken or weaken bones of the affected person. Despite the treatment, the problem cannot be cured to the fullest.

6.5.4 Limited Joint Mobility

Limited Joint Mobility (also referred to as cheiroarthropathy) is a frequently inserted disease among ten diabetic patients. The disease is characterized based on its tendency to limit the mobility of the patients, particularly the joints. Other common characteristics associated with it include thickening of the skin as well as waxiness mostly for the fingers dorsal surface; however, the changes in the skin may also appear when the mobility is not restricted [55]. A proper definition of the limited joint mobility is difficult to gain consensus upon; however, the general idea is it causing finger joints nonpainful contracture. The most common and significant complication resulting from it is diabetic foot ulcer which is considered to be a major economic, social as well as medical burden globally. The occurrence of foot ulcers among diabetic patients accounts for almost 25% and is generally associated with limb amputation. Limited joint mobility is categorized as one of the major risk factors leading to the development of diabetic foot ulceration. Fernando et al. [56] showed that limited joint mobility leads to foot ulcers as it substantially damages tissue at the subtalar joint by exerting abnormal pressures at the susceptible sites.

The prevalence of limited joint mobility for diabetic patients is found to account for 8–58% [55]. The variation in this percentage is based on the population, and the way the mobility among the patients is measured. Studies have emphasized that substantial care must be practiced when the mobility of different parts is being examined to avoid any confusion resulting from other diabetic problems. The incidence of limited joint mobility is found for both type 1 diabetic patients as well as type 2 diabetic patients [55]. The risk of developing limited joint mobility is linked to the increase in the value of glycated hemoglobin (A1C) as well as the length of the prevalence of diabetics, though, it may emerge at the early stage. Smoking and age are categorized as other risk factors for the emergence of limited joint mobility among diabetic patients.

6.5.4.1 Classification

Over the years, the classification of the foot ulcer has emerged, though, none has been accepted at a universal level [57]. The classification of the foot ulcer as per Wagner-Meggitt is mainly based on the depth of the wound, which comprises of six grades of the wound [58]. These grades are intact skin, superficial ulcer, deep ulcer to the tendon, joint or bone, deep ulcer with osteomyelitis or abscess, forefoot gangrene, and last whole foot gangrene, ranging from 1 to 6, respectively. Similarly, the treatment method of limited joint mobility differs from the intensity of the disease. However, generally, strict diabetes control is recommended to any such patient.

6.6 Causal Pathways to Foot Ulcerations

Different causes have been identified that serve as the fundamental pathways of foot ulcers. The first and the most significant cause include Diabetic Peripheral Neuropathy (DPN), which refers to different symptoms associated with the problems of the nervous system and diabetes mellitus. Boulton et al. [59] in their study provided the most common definition of diabetes mellitus, which states that "DPN refers to different symptoms that are caused due to the dysfunction of the peripheral nervous system among patients suffering from diabetes mellitus. These symptoms are studied by excluding other causes. In Western regions, peripheral neuropathy is further identified as the most commonly growing complication that are found among 50% patients with diabetic mellitus. The problem however is considered the most common type of peripheral neuropathy found in the given region. The most significant and commonly found diabetic neuropathies include symmetrical, distal, and sensorimotor neuropathy.

Diabetic neuropathy is further associated with the autonomic nervous system, while during the development of foot ulcers among diabetic patients' sympathetic peripheral autonomic neuropathy of lower limb is implied. DPN can be characterized through several symptoms depending upon the severity of the disease. The most extreme form of the disease involves symptoms where a high level of pain penetrates through the disease following various other problematic symptoms. These symptoms are in the form of different nociceptive that is usually in the form of pain held as a result of severe burning or fall from the height. The following symptoms have been presented by various diabetic patients who were attending clinical assistance as a result of severe inflammation, shooting pain, or even stabbing, freezing sensations along with minor but constant ache. Most of such patients experienced severe pain at night [60]. The symptoms however may vary from time to time and gradually take place. Shakiness or instability while standing is another important sign of DPN among patients with diabetes mellitus leading toward sensory dysfunction and subsequent variations taking place in motor response. Patient's unsteadiness in most of the severe cases leads toward trips and sudden falls, developing its association with severe depression [61].

Another cause of foot ulcer is the occurrence of several microvascular complications that are associated with patients' poor vision. The following symptoms take place as a consequence of diabetic retinopathy that is the most common predictor of developing foot ulcers among diabetic patient. In addition, patients who have undergone through dialysis treatment are more toward the development of foot ulcerations [62]. Furthermore, a direct association between dialysis and foot ulceration has been identified. The factor is crucial and serves as an independent risk factor for developing pathways for diabetic foot ulcerations [63].

Trauma serves as another major cause of developing foot ulcerations among patients. In various patients' trauma may occur as a consequence of the high pressure exerted on the affected foot, the presence of any foreign body inside the shoe, or due to an ill-fitting shoe. In most of the western regions, unfitting footwears serve as the most common cause of trauma leading toward the development of foot ulcers. A detailed analysis of pathways for foot ulceration is provided in Fig. 6.6.

6.7 Diagnosis of Foot Ulcerations

The detailed examination of the feet may help in the identification of the disease. Risks of foot ulcers are generally detected through the screening of the peripheral and neuropathy arterial diseases. Patients undergoing through the given disease are

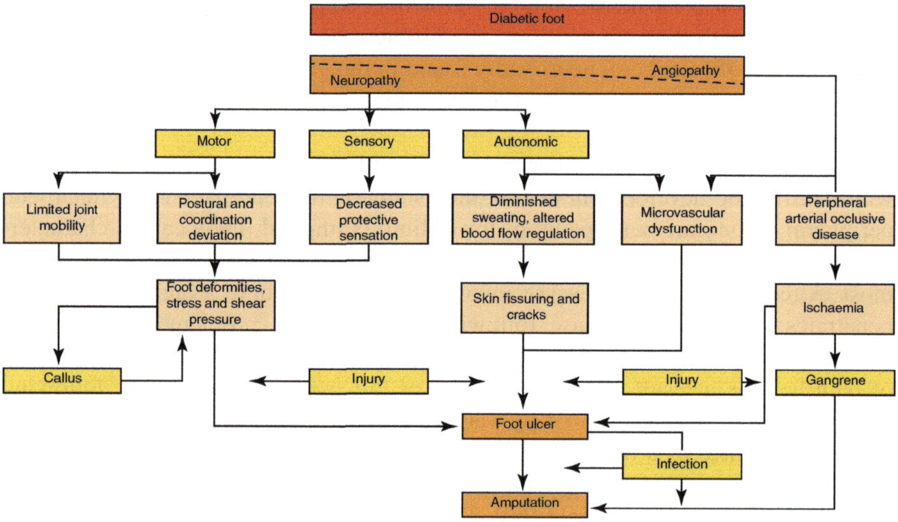

Fig. 6.6 Pathways for foot ulceration. (Adapted with license no. 4810921023311 from Ref. [91])

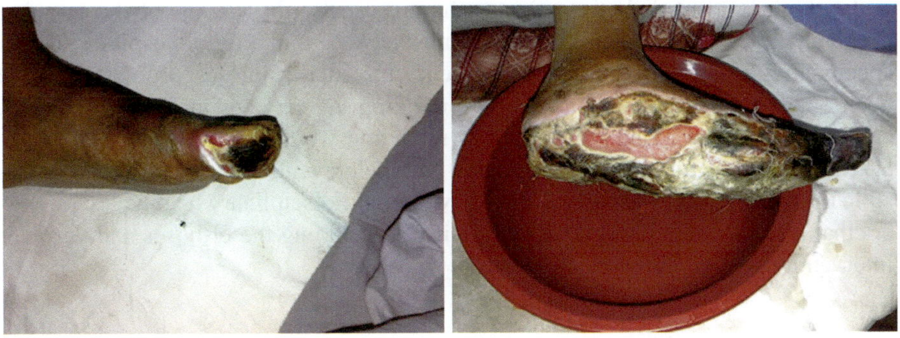

Fig. 6.7 Diabetic foot gangrene

initially assessed through the general symptoms of sepsis or toxicity of the disease, the conditions however include low responsiveness of patients, abnormal behavior of the body, patient looking severely sick, and reflecting abnormal behavior. Patients undergoing through foot ulcers tend to undergo through a strict examination of the disease along with the regular follow-ups for the diagnosis and the prevention of the disease including the gangrene and ulceration of foot (Fig. 6.7). Examination of the disease includes the detection of lesions including the fungal infections, deformation of nails, skin, and cracks fissures, calluses, macerated web spaces, and other types of deformities including the pes cavus, hammer, and claw toes that ultimately increase the possibilities of ulceration among diabetic patients. The temperature of the foot can be felt through the dorsum of the individual hand, where an extremely cold foot suggests the presence of ischemia while a warm foot followed by the increased redness and swelling might contribute to inflammation including the cellulitis and the acute Charcot foot [64].

In most of the middle and low incoming countries, almost 75% of patients are exposed to diabetes. As for instance; in India the ration of the diabetic patients increased up to 70 million individuals, the ration is further expected to rise up to 125 million in the proceeding years of 2040 [65]. According to the guideline provided by the National Institute for Foot Health and Care, the diabetic patients follow a system based on three different rankings, the first includes the preventive measures related to the diabetic foot, the next include the protection of foot from any such disease ranging from the community level for management and care of the simple foot-related problems followed by the tertiary care provided by the multidisciplinary health care providers that can appropriately handle the growing problems of the foot [64]. The cases are however different in most of the low and middle incoming countries, where primary care is often provided through the untrained doctors. In such areas, treatment measures are not undertaken by the multidisciplinary doctors and are available at minimal ratio in such tertiary care centers.

Therefore, in areas with a low level of preventive measures, it is highly recommended to have quality doctors that may provide quality care services related to the foot ulcerations. The following measures are particularly essential for countries with a high level of diabetic patients who are usually the victims of the growing problem. Other than this, such countries must have certain referral hospitals that are specifically designed to provide treatments for such injurious problems. These health care centers are responsible for providing the services including nail care, callus debridement along nail surgeries including wound debridement and major and minor amputations. The examination and the prevention of the disease are possible through the definite care provided by the multidisciplinary health care providers that are provided through various facilities including the orthoses and vascular intervention.

6.7.1 Common Diagnostic Techniques of Foot Ulcerations

6.7.1.1 Diagnosis Through Tests

Often, a common method that helps in the diagnosis of foot ulcerations includes the bedside tests that is the measurement of the pressure exerted on the ankle. The method is useful in estimating the ratio of the required pressure to obstruct the blood flow in the ankle in comparison to the brachial artery. These measurements are regarded as the ankle-brachial pressure index (ABPI) ratios. Clinical experts however suggested that the accuracy regarded the exerted pressure is found by the measurement of the toe pressure along with the toe brachial pressure index (TBPI). The following method is mainly used in cases with calcified crural vessels, which are mainly found among diabetic patients. The method is performed by the use of cuff that is tied around the toe to restrict the flow of blood in the given area. TBPI measurements that are attained <0.7 represents the normal conditions of the body. In addition, the degree of ischemia is measured through the microvascular transcutaneous oxygen pressure ($tcPO^2$) that provides major information regarding the microcirculation of blood in the affected area [66].

6.7.2 Radiological Tests

Another common source of collecting information about the given problem is the use of radiological tests. The use of radiological methods such as duplex ultrasonography is important in the identification of arterial lesions. The following examination is provided based on the hemodynamic values and anatomical evaluation to determine the level of stenosis. Collins et al. [67] provided important information in their study, according to which duplex ultrasonography occupies 88% sensitivity and 94% specificity levels. The levels increase when measuring lesions that are located above the knee. Similarly, CT angiography is another important method that is used for the imaging of the arterial tree measuring from heart to toe. Studies suggested the high accuracy levels of the given technique with sensitivity and specificity levels of 95% and 96% respectively. The specificity levels are expected to drop up to 91% when examining the imaging of tibial vessels [65, 68]. Certain adverse effects of the given techniques have been detected, including the impact of radiation and nephrotoxicity levels in the contrast dye. High levels of creatinine serum such as 44.20 μmol/l are commonly associated with the risk factors of nephropathy. However, in some rare cases, patients require the examination through renal replacement therapy during CT angiographies.

Another common radiological method includes the examination through magnetic resonance angiography (MRA) that provides imaging of the arterial system with a sensitivity and specificity ratio of 95% and 97% respectively [66]. Magnetic resonance angiography (MRA) in this regard is characterized in providing than worse imaging of tibial vessels in contrast to CT angiography. However, for certain researchers, MRA technique is still much better in the identification of the pedal vessels. This type of examination is mainly held among patients with diabetes mellitus who are undergoing through the critical limb ischemia. It was further suggested that the technique is safe, since it avoids the use of radiation. Another important method used in the identification of arterial lesion includes digital subtraction angiography (DSA), which is recognized as the top most preferred method for examination. The technique is comparatively much better than all other methods, due to its efficiency in providing the overall mapping of the arterial tree which can be easily analyzed by clinical experts. Since DSA serves as a 2D technique, therefore it lacks the ability to provide 3D imaging. Other drawbacks of DSA include the low accuracy levels in determining the eccentric lesions, pedal vessels, and patent distal crural.

Other complexities are in the form of inducing the ionizing radiations that result in renal failure and further require the use of costly tools that can be operated through highly experienced and skilled medical professionals. Norgren et al. [69] mentioned that DSA techniques involves minor probabilities of severe risks in the form of adverse reactions, and includes minimal chances of mortality. Treatment guidelines provided by the UK National Institute for Health and Care Excellence preferred the use of duplex ultrasonography in imaging the arterial tree among patients with diabetes mellitus. Similarly, MRI technique must be preferred when additional imaging is required for the examination. The process however must be integrated before revascularization. Lastly, CT angiography must be provided to individuals with weak metabolism and are unable to bear MRI.

6.7.3 Revascularization

Revascularization refers to the treatment that includes the preservation of cell tissues during severe ischemia conditions, since the excessive loss of tissue results in the form of amputation or even death. The important goal of the given treatment is to restore skin perfusion [69, 70]. The process is integrated through endovascular sources that include the stenting and balloon angioplasty through surgical measures. In most cases, bypass techniques are involved to create a segment around the disease. Studies suggested that most patients are not treated through revascularization treatments due to the presence of ischemic limb ulcers among diabetic patients. Such patients possess 53% chances of survival, i.e., wound healing. Others suggested that patients with diabetic mellitus and CLI are refrained from any such treatment, since the rate of amputation among such patients is 46% [71].

In contrast to this, patients suffering from the ischemic legs with normal glycemic levels when examined through revascularization resulted in reduced amputation rates [72]. The failure of bypass technique is associated with the excessive loss of tissue and high amputation rates. Another risk factor connected to the issue is the time duration involved between bypass and blood occlusions. The rate of amputation is said to be low among patients who have maximum time involved in the functionality of bypass. The most probable explanation, in this case, includes the loss of tissue, and the recovery of ulcer which contributes in posing minimum risks toward the consequences of bypass failure. In contrast to this, patients undergone through a first-line surgery supported by drug therapy usually results in providing improvised clinical outcomes by the involvement of revisualization. It is of greater significance that patients with diabetes mellitus need more critical care than those with normal glycemia levels.

6.7.4 Surgery

In most adverse conditions of foot ulcerations, surgical techniques are involved to cater to the disease. The first technique includes endarterectomy that is provided to patients undergoing through CLI. Another important technique includes the bypass surgery that is based on the use of prosthetic material or veins to recover from lesions. The techniques are of greater significance when performed under the controlled examination of anesthetics, since the disease takes a longer duration for recovery. Similarly, distal anastomosis that is usually much longer requires long duration in attaining the prevention from any further infections. Surgeries involving the prosthetic bypass below the knee involves greater patency levels than that provided in vein bypass. Patients suffering from diabetes usually involve distal bypasses covering the popliteal arteries that are reachable to the ankle.

6.8 Wound Healing Process

In most of the normal conditions, the wound healing process is mainly associated with the interplay among several types of cells that are often contacted through different hormonal and soluble chemical activities in the human body. In most of the infected areas, platelets are often gathered and combined leading toward different factors that are often responsible for the formation of clot and matrix within the human body. The fibrinogen found in the human body are often transformed into fibrins, this is due to the development of the thrombin that results in the formation of a network of various platelets that are often developed at the site of the injury.

Moreover, the growth factors and the cytokines make the blood vessels as permeable that in results allow that transfer or the movement of leukocytes that are attracted to the affected area in the human body. Furthermore, the formation of various products takes place here that are formed due to the decomposition of the elastin and collagens such as; cytokines interleukin-1 (IL-1), TGF-β, platelet factor IV along with TNF- α. Therefore, the accumulation of the macrophages and the neutrophils helps in the removal of contaminating bacteria along with other factors that are generally found at the affected part of the body. A significant role is played by the given factors that are responsible for the emancipation of several growth factors that are highly useful in the formation of tissue structures. The factors are often regarded as VEGF (vascular endothelial growth factors) and PDGF platelet-derived growth factors.

In addition, several factors are responsible for the proliferation and the migration of cells. These factors include keratinocytes and the epidermal growth factors. Cell migration is further developed through the secretion of the matrix metalloproteinases (MMP) that is essential for the degeneration of clot and extracellular matrix (ECM) that are generally found at the wound site. The incomplete digestion of the extracellular matrix generates long spaces in the migrating cells. The process is mainly regulated through the creation of a uniform balance between the development and the degradation of new tissues. Similarly, collagen synthesis is helpful in the formation of the tissue for the second time and is majorly stimulated through different growth factors including; platelet-derived growth factor (PGF), Transformation growth factor (TGF), and epidermal growth factor (EGF). The final stage of the wound healing process includes the contraction of wounds, that takes place through the activity of mesenchymal cells.

6.8.1 Process of Wound Healing Among Diabetic Patients

In diabetes, it has been noticed that all the stages of wound healing are often affected by the adverse effects of the diabetic foot syndrome. This leads toward the development of the final picture including the formation of a diabetic wound that serves as the fundamental mark of diabetic foot syndrome. Among diabetic patients, several growth factors including the chemokines and cytokines have different serum levels of macrophages, fibroblasts, keratinocytes, platelets, and endothelial cells. The following factors are mainly responsible for initiating the wound repair process along with its preservation leading toward the significant decrease in the inflammatory responses. In various diabetic patients most of the wounds are characterized through the decreased level of various growth and receptors including; nerve growth factors (NGF), transformation growth factor β (TGF- β1), keratinocyte growth factor (KGF), substance P, along with CGRP. Therefore, the minimal levels in the following growth factors contributes to the poor regeneration of tissue followed by the impaired recovery of wound (Fig. 6.8).

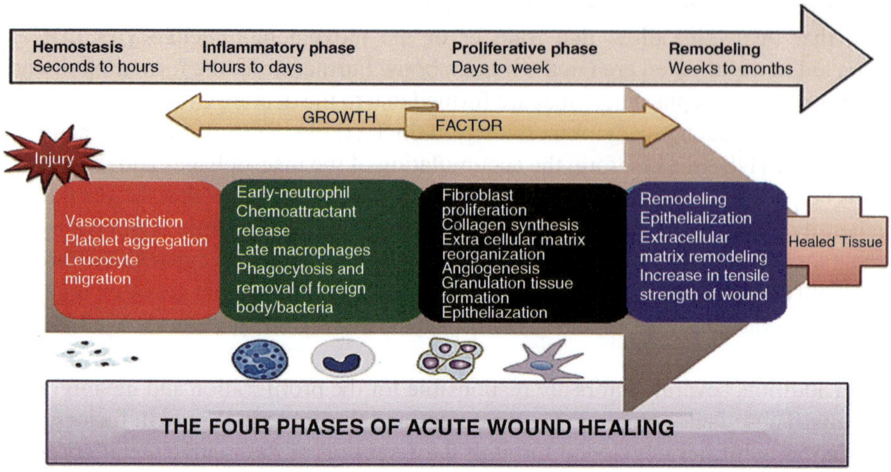

Fig. 6.8 Distinct and overlapping phases of wound healing (Adapted from Ref. [87])

6.8.2 Phases of Wound Healing

One of the most common reasons found among the diabetic patients is sepsis, leading toward the development of various infections including ulcers, chronic nonhealing wounds [73]. The general development in treatment measures is often associated with controlling diabetes, whereas among patients with foot ulcerations these treatments are associated with the general foot or wound care to refrain it from the development of any further disease in the human body. A significant focus is provided to the regeneration of different infections along with providing immunity in minimizing the growth of these infections [74]. In the treatment care of the diabetic foot, the wound healing processes are often followed by the impairment resulting in the development of different diseases including the anatomical changes. Whereas, in severe foot ulcerations among diabetic patients, most of the nonhealing wounds results in death. The wound healing processes are often dependent upon patient's health, the position or the location of wound, age, and other factors that are considerable in providing health-related treatments. For treating a wound, several processes are being presented to evolve the repair of wound in the human body. The healing process is initiated through various events; the first includes the hemostasis restorations, leading toward the formation of different clots in the affected area. It further includes the inflammation and proliferation of wounds, formation of tissues, epithelization, and the contraction of wounds. The final phase of the recovery includes the remodeling of the cutaneous tissues [75] (Fig. 6.8).

6.9 Management of Diabetic Foot Ulcers

6.9.1 Debridement

Management of the diabetic foot ulcerations requires maximum efforts. Debridement is one of such techniques that is used in conditions that involve the formation of the hyperkeratotic tissues over the plantar region of the foot. The problem is mainly caused due to the exertion of severe pressure. Regular debridement helps in reducing the exerted pressure which is due to the formation of excessive hyperkeratotic tissue, which creates a direct impact in the form of increased stress. The treatment methods are initial measures that are effectively reducing the probabilities of ulceration among diabetic patients. The process includes the removal of the layer that releases the gathered fluid in the affected area, while opening the ways for foot recovery. Wounds that are deep and are connected to both bones and the tissues require in depth debridement to remove the overall probabilities of the occurrence of non-viable tissue and toxic fluid. The effective and careful debridement is useful in decreasing the time duration required from the recovery.

6.9.2 Offloading

This is the most recommended method and often serve as the first choice of providing treatment for patients with foot ulcerations. The main goal of the method is to reduce the over loading of weight found in the affected area. The method is essential in redistribution of the weight in the overall affected area. Removable and unremovable casts are used to promote offloading through different orthotic devices including custom footwear and other fabricated shoes. The total contact cast is categorized as the most effective type of offloading and is determined as the gold standards in the clinical treatments. The main advantage of the process includes the short-term healing time of the given disease. Since the contact cast is non-removable, therefore patients might undergo through a rapid recovery due to continuous treatment.

6.9.3 Wound Dressings

The extremity of the disease is controlled through the regular wound dressing that helps in protecting the wounds from the external environment that carries poisonous or even the most harmful substances. The development of contact between such environmental elements with the wounded area promotes the extension of the problem resulting in the increased deformity of foot. Moist dressings are provided to such areas through the continuous maintenance of wound healing that promotes the migration of cells. Clinical experts regarded this method as one of the basic actions conducted at the time of identification of any such disease, which is not possible in dry dressings. Wound dressings that are provided by the incorporation of silver resulted in ineffective efforts in treating diabetic foot ulcers.

6.9.4 Negative Pressure Wound Therapy

In most of the clinical settings, negative wound therapy is the mostly used and recognized treatment method, that helps in the exemption of the wound fluid present in the sealed wound. The therapy is widely associated with the conditions that involve increased wound healing and have closure contact of wound. Besides, improvised perfusion and the development of new granulated tissues are the major benefits associated with the application of negative pressure at the central location of the disease [76].

6.10 Clinical Guidelines to Treatment

The current approaches to the treatment of the foot ulcerations among diabetic patients generally involve the combined efforts of physician, nurses, physio therapists, orthotist along with other care givers. The present practices in the treatment measures suggest that patients' education regarding the given problem is significant in this regard. Other important measures include patient's diet monitorization, foot inspection, maintenance of glucose levels up to normal, foot screening along with the modification of footwear is of greater significance [77]. Various researchers suggested that the interprofessional approach helps in the provision of significant improvements in the rate of amputation and foot ulcerations among diabetic patients [78]. The prevention of ulcer is still majorly dependent upon the interventions of footwear. Most of the care providers still follow the contemporary theory of ulcerations and is regarded as an important aspect of ulcer prevention. Furthermore, the intervention of footwear is commonly concerned with minimizing the exertion of increased weight over the affected area. It also contributes to minimizing the repetition of loadings.

Most of the researchers provided valuable suggestions in this regard. According to which, the goal of the footwear intervention must be to minimize the exerted pressure up to 30%. This is due to the fact that redistribution of the plantar pressure helps in breaking tissue [77]. Areas that are at greater risks of deformity and callusing foot can be easily addressed and recovered through the intervention of footwear People undergoing through diabetes mellitus and peripheral neuropathy (DMPN) accounts for majorly 53% variance in the plantar pressure of fore foot [79]. Other best practices include the provision of the improvised practices including the structural changes and centers of the elevated pressure that are specific to patients, followed by the examining of the impact created through the footwear. Researchers suggested that the intervention of footwear among diabetic patients is mainly dependent upon patient's adherence to the given treatment, as patients with the adherence level of below 80% usually create a negative impact over the efficacy of footwear among the target individuals [78, 80]. Moreover, the intervention of the footwear technique helps in providing a visible improvement in the rates of re-ulcerations. Therefore, the intervention of footwear must be in accordance with patients' physiological needs to observe definite results. Studies conducted through the randomized controlled trials suggested that in major cases people with DMPN provided minimal cases of foot re-ulcerations [77]. The results were common among patients who were suggested to wear the custom footwear with careful monitorization of the pressure relief. Findings indicated that the majority of the re-ulcerations were detected among patients who were recorded with a maximum adherence level. The idea is crucial as it demonstrates the value of both patient's adherence level and relief evaluation.

Recommendations regarding the prevention of ulceration majorly rely upon overloading factors. The development in the scientific interventions further suggested that diabetic patients must be liable to wear custom footwear to prevent the future developments of the disease. An RCT investigation conducted by Rizzo et al. [81] suggested that the ulceration incidence was least common among individuals that have undergone through the primary care in the form of custom footwear for 5 years. Therefore, it is considered that custom footwear serves as one of the most common treatment measures among patients either with or without history of ulcerations and diabetes. Despite the development of the risk factors, the need regarding the development of useful biomarkers is found to predict the future tissue damage. In addition, the development of more explicit screening practices is of greater need, as it may assist physicians and health care experts in the identification of the crucial time point for offloading the footwear interventions. Other important considerations include the interventions of footwear and screening processes that help in the prevention of deformity of tissues are important. The factors include the rate of foot bearing activity and the extent to which the affected foot efficiently functions.

A significant consideration is provided to the weight-bearing activities, since they are responsible for increasing the stress tolerance level of plantar tissues. Therefore, clinicians must incorporate such activities among the affected patients to refrain from various long-term damage in the tissues of the affected area. This helps in the prevention of the greater risks associated with different activities that are progressed through weight-bearing activities. Walking programs or weight controlling exercises are of critical value here as they might contribute to increasing the life expectancy of the affected area of diabetic patients [82]. Other important measures of the basic treatment include patient's knowledge regarding the stressed posed on the affected foot during everyday activities of patients. However, the abnormal stress that is provided to another foot may result in damaging the soft tissues. The basic guidelines are important and serve as an essential part of human knowledge, specifically for those suffering from major foot ulcerations. Patients following the given guidelines may prevent further damage to the affected foot area.

6.10.1 Advancing Clinical Methods

6.10.1.1 Weight-Bearing Activity

The primary focus in improving glycemic controls is significantly provided to glycemic control. For advanced clinical measures, the following guidelines seemed to be vague in the clinician's perspective of promoting the exercise among diabetic patients who are at greater risks of foot ulcerations. The functionality of the above-related activities includes maximum complications when applied to practical measures, due to the differences in the physical conditions of comorbidity among diabetic patients. This might be due to the fact that in most cases the plantar tissues lose the level of required fitness even before the occurrence of foot ulceration. In such cases, it has been suggested that extensive offloading in the prevention phase may result in the occurrence of foot ulcerations in the future. Individual and clinical efforts regarding the high weight-bearing activities and glycemic controls are effective techniques to develop resilience for the breakdown of soft tissues. The idea regarding the increased probability of ulcerations because of the increase in weight-bearing activities is still not clear and varies from cases to cases. Studies conducted in the given framework indicated that weight-bearing activities serve as a useful tool in developing maximum prevention against the occurrence of ulcerations [83]. It was further developed that DMPN patients provided positive results regarding the weight-bearing activities and thus indicated that the method is sufficiently effective in reducing the level of ulceration among such patients.

Researchers further examined the effect of weight-bearing and non-weight-bearing exercises and their effects on everyday activities along with the levels of HbA1C among people with DMPN. Visible improvements were detected in the weight-bearing individuals, which were related to the performance of everyday activities. However, no visible difference was observed in the rate of ulceration among both the groups. The results are specific to the type of activities performed including the walking, balancing, and length strengthening exercises. Therefore, it is suggested that weight-bearing activities may be considered as the mediating source of involving greater changes in the form of prevention of foot ulceration and thus can be viewed as an important guideline for patients with DMPN.

Clinical studies conducted in the given idea suggested the need for providing regular instructions to patients regarding the value of weight-bearing activities in controlling the glycemic levels and managing the integrity of plantar tissue. Notably, for some researchers, the development of the protocols related to the weight-bearing activity along with the practical implication of the exercises that help in promoting the management of patal tissues and ulceration are still questionable. This is due to the lack of effective biomarkers that help in providing extended knowledge in managing the integrity of plant tissue. Current treatment guidelines further include the adjustment of the treatment dosage that is provided with respect to patient's need. The inclusion of the weight-bearing activity serves as an additional factor here, that is related to the extent of providing stress over the affected area during the weight-bearing activities. Considering this, it is important to understand how often weight is being provided along with the way of creating stress among the given individuals.

Another important consideration includes the dynamic foot functions that specifically focus on the behavior of foot during a crucial period of foot ulceration. Dynamic foot functions are further assessed through different approaches. The first includes the single segment approach that focuses on modeling the complete foot while considering it a rigid body that moves with the ankle joint on the tibia. Though the approach is useful, it may cover the regional pathological characteristics of foot functions. Single segment modeling of foot among people with DMPN resulted in the development of mixed findings related to different factors that are potentially responsible for tissue breakdown. Different findings have been developed regarding the forefoot plantar pressure, joint mobility, and the motion of ankle during physical activity such as; walking. Researchers suggested no definite linkage between both dynamic and passive ankle motion. Similarly, no significant distinction was observed among individuals with or without DMPN [84]. Another study conducted by Sacco et al. [85] detected a significant decrease in the pressures exerted on the plantar tissue. The results were common among DMPN patients than in healthy patients. One probability for such types of different results may be due to the embedded motion of the mid foot and forefoot presented through the single segment model.

Another common approach is termed as the multi-segment approach that typically allows the evaluation of foot functions providing the explicit reality of the anatomical foot functions. The technique is useful in providing increased knowledge about the pathological and normal foot functions. Researchers identified significant alterations in the kinematics of people with the history of DM and ulcerations, by employing the multi-segment foot modeling approach. Comparative analysis of the given results concludes that the level of motion, when studied through multiple foot segments, is comparatively different among patients with DMPN than those with healthy foot. Other than this, the unlikeliness found in the metatarsal motion of individuals specifically in forefoot regions, provide greater contributions in increasing the pressure on plantar tissues toward certain locations.

6.11 Conclusion

Foot complications among diabetic individuals are developed through the complex interactions between macrovascular and microvascular irregularities. The development of diabetic foot ulcerations serves as the major contributor in promoting diseases including; peripheral neuropathy, ischemia, and foot lesions. The disease is highly risky as it reduces the individual ability to feel or respond to hurt or pain in the affected foot. External factors such as the inappropriate footwear, thermal injury along with the development of environmental contact with the disease lead toward the formation of complex conditions in diabetic foot ulcerations.

The preservation of the planter tissues among patients with diabetic foot ulcerations is indeed a challenging process for people that are exposed to high levels of diabetes. Similarly, the prevention of the neuropathic foot ulcerations serves as a greater challenge for care providers. The effectiveness of the preventive measures regarding the increase in foot ulcerations mostly depends on the glycemic controls, the management of the integrity of plantar tissues, as well as the intervention of the advance neuropathic process. It is highly critical for clinicians to provide developmental information regarding the interplay between different factors including the frequency of weight-bearing activity, the pressure exerted on the plantar tissues, and the quality of foot functions during the imposition of stress. Another important task includes the regulation of the effective balance between the required stress to overcome the consequences of ulcerations. Similarly, the effectiveness in loading parameters must be integrated through the evolved damage in the contingent tissues during and after the process of stressing.

Knowledge and the level of education of patients are equally important in controlling and preventing the foot from severe damages. Also, weight-bearing activities such as; balancing, walking, exercises related to the leg straightening are of greater importance in creating an influence over the health and functions of the affected person. A proper scheduling of such activities is important to minimize the effects of neuropathy along with the management of stress over the plantar tissue uploading. The dynamic foot function when integrated through the multi-segment modeling is important for the prevention of first-time ulcerations. Treatment-related to the foot ulceration requires regular screening to examine the strength of foot muscles. The overall information suggests that preventive measures can only be implemented by the development of the exercise programs that are functionally effective in improving the overall ulceration conditions of foot among diabetic patients.

References

1. Syafril S (2018) Pathophysiology diabetic foot ulcer. In: InIOP conference series: earth and environmental science, vol 125, no. 1. IOP Publishing, Philadelphia, PA, p 012161
2. Alexiadou K, Doupis J (2012) Management of diabetic foot ulcers. Diabetes Ther 3(1):4
3. Singh S, Pai DR, Yuhhui C (2013) Diabetic foot ulcer–diagnosis and management. Clin Res Foot Ankle 1(3):120
4. Armstrong DG, Boulton AJ, Bus SA (2017) Diabetic foot ulcers and their recurrence. N Engl J Med 376(24):2367–2375
5. Soewondo P, Suyono S, Sastrosuwignyo MK, Harahap AR, Sutrisna B, Makmun LH (2017) Prediction of wound healing in diabetic foot ulcers: an observational study in Tertiary Hospital in Indonesia. Acta Med Indones 49(1):41–51
6. Hoke GD, Ramos C, Hoke NN, Crossland MC, Shawler LG, Boykin JV (2016) Atypical diabetic foot ulcer keratinocyte protein signaling correlates with impaired wound healing. J Diabetes Res 2016:1. https://doi.org/10.1155/2016/1586927
7. Boulton AJ, Armstrong DG, Kirsner RS, Attinger CE, Lavery LA, Lipsky BA, Mills JL Sr, Steinberg JS (2018) Diagnosis and management of diabetic foot complications. American Diabetes Association, Arlington, VA
8. Gary Sibbald R, Woo KY (2008) The biology of chronic foot ulcers in persons with diabetes. Diabetes Metab Res Rev 24(S1):S25–S30. https://doi.org/10.1155/2016/1586927
9. Rafehi H, El-Osta A, Karagiannis TC (2011) Genetic and epigenetic events in diabetic wound healing. Int Wound J 8(1):12–21
10. Guyton GP, Saltzman CL (2001) The diabetic foot: basic mechanisms of disease. JBJS 83(7):1083–1096

11. Falanga V (2005) Wound healing and its impairment in the diabetic foot. Lancet 366(9498):1736–1743
12. Correa-Giannella ML, Vieira SM (2008) Genetic susceptibility to microangiopathy development in Type 1 diabetes mellitus. Arq Bras Endocrinol Metabol 52(2):375–386
13. Bassi R, Trevisani A, Tezza S, Ben Nasr M, Gatti F, Vergani A, Farina A, Fiorina P (2012) Regenerative therapies for diabetic microangiopathy. Exp Diabetes Res 2012:1. https://doi.org/10.1155/2012/916560
14. Frykberg RG, Zgonis T, Armstrong DG, Driver VR, Giurini JM, Kravitz SR, Landsman AS, Lavery LA, Moore JC, Schuberth JM, Wukich DK (2006) Diabetic foot disorders: a clinical practice guideline (2006 revision). J Foot Ankle Surg 45(5):S1–S66
15. Boulton AJ, Vileikyte L, Ragnarson-Tennvall G, Apelqvist J (2005) The global burden of diabetic foot disease. Lancet 366(9498):1719–1724
16. Nabuurs-Franssen MH, Huijberts MS, Kruseman AN, Willems J, Schaper NC (2005) Health-related quality of life of diabetic foot ulcer patients and their caregivers. Diabetologia 48(9):1906–1910
17. Martins-Mendes D, Monteiro-Soares M, Boyko EJ, Ribeiro M, Barata P, Lima J, Soares R (2014) The independent contribution of diabetic foot ulcer on lower extremity amputation and mortality risk. J Diabetes Complicat 28(5):632–638
18. Costa RH, Cardoso NA, Procópio RJ, Navarro TP, Dardik A, de Loiola Cisneros L (2017) Diabetic foot ulcer carries high amputation and mortality rates, particularly in the presence of advanced age, peripheral artery disease and anemia. Diabetes Metab Syndr Clin Res Rev 11:S583–S587
19. Sereday M, Damiano M, Lapertosa S, Cagide A, Bragagnolo JC (2009) Amputaciones de Miembros Inferiores en diabéticos y no diabéticos en el ámbito hospitalario. Asociacion latinoamericana de diabetes 17(1):9–15
20. Rezende KF, Nunes MA, Melo NH, Malerbi D, Chacra AR, Ferraz MB (2008) In hospital care for diabetic foot: a comparison between the estimated cost and the SUS reimbursement. Arq Bras Endocrinol Metab 52(3):523–530
21. Desormais I, Aboyans V, Bura A, Constans J, Cambou JP, Messas E, Labrunie A, Lacroix P (2014) Anemia, an independent predictive factor for amputation and mortality in patients hospitalized for peripheral artery disease. Eur J Vasc Endovasc Surg 48(2):202–207
22. Khanbhai ML, Wright JA, Hurel S, Richards T (2012) Anaemia, inflammation, renal function, and the diabetic foot: what are the relationships. Diabet Foot J 15(4):150–158
23. Obaid H, Eljedi A (2015) Risk factors for the development of diabetic foot ulcers in Gaza Strip: a case-control study. Int J Diabetes Res 4(1):1–6
24. Tesfaye S, Chaturvedi N, Eaton SE, Ward JD, Manes C, Ionescu-Tirgoviste C, Witte DR, Fuller JH (2005) Vascular risk factors and diabetic neuropathy. N Engl J Med 352(4):341–350
25. Zhou JF, Yan XF, Guo FZ, Sun NY, Qian ZJ, Ding DY (2000) Effects of cigarette smoking and smoking cessation on plasma constituents and enzyme activities related to oxidative stress. Biomed Environ Sci 13(1):44–55
26. Prasad C, Imrhan V, Marotta F, Juma S, Vijayagopal P (2014) Lifestyle and advanced glycation end products (AGEs) burden: its relevance to healthy aging. Aging Dis 5(3):212. https://doi.org/10.14336/ad.2014.0500212
27. Ogawa K, Tanaka T, Nagoshi T, Sekiyama H, Arase S, Minai K, Ogawa T, Yoshimura M (2015) Increase in the oxidised low-density lipoprotein level by smoking and the possible inhibitory effect of statin therapy in patients with cardiovascular disease: a retrospective study. BMJ Open 5(1):e005455
28. Choi S, Krishnan J, Ruckmani K (2017) Cigarette smoke and related risk factors in neurological disorders: an update. Biomed Pharmacother 85:79–86
29. Masayesva BG, Mambo E, Taylor RJ, Goloubeva OG, Zhou S, Cohen Y, Minhas K, Koch W, Sciubba J, Alberg AJ, Sidransky D (2006) Mitochondrial DNA content increase in response to cigarette smoking. Cancer Epidemiol Biomarkers Prev 15(1):19–24

30. Lindström D, Azodi OS, Wladis A, Tønnesen H, Linder S, Nåsell H, Ponzer S, Adami J (2008) Effects of a perioperative smoking cessation intervention on postoperative complications: a randomized trial. Ann Surg 248(5):739–745. https://doi.org/10.1097/sla.0b013e3181889d0d
31. Xia N, Morteza A, Yang F, Cao H, Wang A (2019) Review of the role of cigarette smoking in diabetic foot. J Diabetes Investig 10(2):202–215. https://doi.org/10.1111/jdi.12952
32. Pham H, Armstrong DG, Harvey C, Harkless LB, Giurini JM, Veves A (2000) Screening techniques to identify people at high risk for diabetic foot ulceration: a prospective multicenter trial. Diabetes Care 23(5):606–611. https://doi.org/10.2337/diacare.23.5.606
33. Ibrahim A (2017) IDF Clinical Practice Recommendation on the diabetic foot: A guide for healthcare professionals. Diabetes Res Clin Pract 127:285–287
34. Smith AG, Singleton JR (2013) Obesity and hyperlipidemia are risk factors for early diabetic neuropathy. J Diabetes Complicat 27(5):436–442
35. Armstrong DG, Lavery LA, Holtz-Neiderer K, Mohler MJ, Wendel CS, Nixon BP, Boulton AJ (2004) Variability in activity may precede diabetic foot ulceration. Diabetes Care 27(8):1980–1984. https://doi.org/10.2337/diacare.27.8.1980
36. Ross AJ, Mendicino RW, Catanzariti AR (2013) Role of body mass index in acute Charcot neuroarthropathy. J Foot Ankle Surg 52(1):6–8. https://doi.org/10.1053/j.jfas.2012.10.003
37. Payne CB (1998) The past, present, and future of podiatric biomechanics. J Am Podiatr Med Assoc 88(2):53–63
38. Prior TD (2011) The practical application of biomechanical theory for patient assessment. J Foot Ankle Res 4(S1):I9
39. Dinh T (ed) (2011) Global perspective on diabetic foot ulcerations. IntechOpen, London
40. Halawa MR, Eid YM, El-Hilaly RA, Abdelsalam MM, Amer AH (2018) Relationship of planter pressure and glycemic control in type 2 diabetic patients with and without neuropathy. Diabetes Metab Syndr Clin Res Rev 12(2):99–104
41. Nascimento OJ, Pupe CC, Cavalcanti EB (2016) Diabetic neuropathy. Rev Dor 17:46–51
42. Kim PJ (2013) Biomechanics of the diabetic foot: consideration in limb salvage. Adv Wound Care 2(3):107–111
43. Grant WP, Sullivan R, Sonenshine DE, Adam M, Slusser JH, Carson KA, Vinik AI (1997) Electron microscopic investigation of the effects of diabetes mellitus on the Achilles tendon. J Foot Ankle Surg 36(4):272–278
44. Birke JA, Cornwall MW, Jackson M (1988) Relationship between hallux limitus and ulceration of the great toe. J Orthop Sports Phys Ther 10(5):172–176
45. Wu S, Armstrong DG, Lavery LA, Harkless LB (2006) Clinical examination of the diabetic foot and the identification of the at-risk patient. In: The diabetic foot. Humana Press, Totowa, NJ, pp 201–226
46. Nonnekes J, Goselink RJ, Růžička E, Fasano A, Nutt JG, Bloem BR (2018) Neurological disorders of gait, balance and posture: a sign-based approach. Nat Rev Neurol 14(3):183
47. Nonnekes J, Snijders AH, Nutt JG, Deuschl G, Giladi N, Bloem BR (2015) Freezing of gait: a practical approach to management. Lancet Neurol 14(7):768–778
48. Nürnberger L, Klein C, Baudrexel S, Roggendorf J, Hildner M, Chen S, Kang JS, Hilker R, Hagenah J (2015) Ultrasound-based motion analysis demonstrates bilateral arm hypokinesia during gait in heterozygous PINK1 mutation carriers. Mov Disord 30(3):386–392
49. Araújo R, Ferreira JJ, Antonini A, Bloem BR (2015) "Gunslinger's gait": a new cause of unilaterally reduced arm swing. BMJ 351:h6141
50. Aminian K, Najafi B, Büla C, Leyvraz PF, Robert P (2002) Spatio-temporal parameters of gait measured by an ambulatory system using miniature gyroscopes. J Biomech 35(5):689–699
51. Mueller MJ, Minor SD, Sahrmann SA, Schaaf JA, Strube MJ (1994) Differences in the gait characteristics of patients with diabetes and peripheral neuropathy compared with age-matched controls. Phys Ther 74(4):299–308
52. Wrobel JS, Najafi B (2010) Diabetic foot biomechanics and gait dysfunction. J Diabetes Sci Technol 4:833
53. Duquette JJ, Grigg P, Hoffman AH (1996) The effect of diabetes on the viscoelastic properties of rat knee ligaments. J Biomech Eng 118:557

54. Armstrong DG, Lavery LA (1998) Elevated peak plantar pressures in patients who have Charcot arthropathy. JBJS 80(3):365–369
55. Hordon LD, Axford JS (2012) Limited joint mobility in diabetes mellitus. UpToDate, Inc., Seattle, WA
56. Fernando DJ, Masson EA, Veves A, Boulton AJ (1991) Relationship of limited joint mobility to abnormal foot pressures and diabetic foot ulceration. Diabetes Care 14(1):8–11
57. Doupis J, Veves A (2008) Classification, diagnosis, and treatment of diabetic foot ulcers. Wounds 20(5):117–126
58. Jain AK (2012) A new classification of diabetic foot complications: a simple and effective teaching tool. J Diab Foot Comp 4(1):1–5
59. Boulton AJ, Gries FA, Jervell JA (1998) Guidelines for the diagnosis and outpatient management of diabetic peripheral neuropathy. Diabet Med 15(6):508–514
60. Tesfaye S, Boulton AJ, Dickenson AH (2013) Mechanisms and management of diabetic painful distal symmetrical polyneuropathy. Diabetes Care 36(9):2456–2465
61. Abbott CA, Garrow AP, Carrington AL, Morris J, Van Ross ER, Boulton AJ (2005) Foot ulcer risk is lower in South-Asian and African-Caribbean compared with European diabetic patients in the UK: the north-west diabetes foot care study. Diabetes Care 28(8):1869–1875
62. Ndip A, Rutter MK, Vileikyte L, Vardhan A, Asari A, Jameel M, Tahir HA, Lavery LA, Boulton AJ (2010) Dialysis treatment is an independent risk factor for foot ulceration in patients with diabetes and stage 4 or 5 chronic kidney disease. Diabetes Care 33(8):1811–1816
63. Bowling FL, Rashid ST, Boulton AJ (2015) Preventing and treating foot complications associated with diabetes mellitus. Nat Rev Endocrinol 11(10):606
64. Mishra SC, Chhatbar KC, Kashikar A, Mehndiratta A (2017) Diabetic foot. BMJ 359:j5064
65. Atlas D (2015) International Diabetes Federation. IDF diabetes atlas, 7th edn. Brussels, Belgium, International Diabetes Federation
66. Cao P, Eckstein HH, De Rango P, Setacci C, Ricco JB, De Donato G, Becker F, Robert-Ebadi H, Diehm N, Schmidli J, Teraa M (2011) Chapter II: Diagnostic methods. Eur J Vasc Endovasc Surg 42:S13–S32
67. Collins R, Burch J, Cranny G, Aguiar-Ibáñez R, Craig D, Wright K, Berry E, Gough M, Kleijnen J, Westwood M (2007) Duplex ultrasonography, magnetic resonance angiography, and computed tomography angiography for diagnosis and assessment of symptomatic, lower limb peripheral arterial disease: systematic review. BMJ 334(7606):1257
68. Met R, Bipat S, Legemate DA, Reekers JA, Koelemay MJ (2009) Diagnostic performance of computed tomography angiography in peripheral arterial disease: a systematic review and meta-analysis. JAMA 301(4):415–424. https://doi.org/10.1001/jama.301.4.415
69. Norgren L, Hiatt WR, Dormandy JA, Nehler MR, Harris KA, Fowkes FG (2007) Inter-society consensus for the management of peripheral arterial disease (TASC II). J Vasc Surg 45(1):S5–S67
70. Bakker K, Apelqvist J, Schaper NC, International Working Group on the Diabetic Foot Editorial Board (2012) Practical guidelines on the management and prevention of the diabetic foot 2011. Diabetes Metab Res Rev 28:225–231
71. Benoit E, O'Donnell TF Jr, Kitsios GD, Iafrati MD (2012) Improved amputation-free survival in unreconstructable critical limb ischemia and its implications for clinical trial design and quality measurement. J Vasc Surg 55(3):781–789
72. Faglia E, Clerici G, Clerissi J, Gabrielli L, Losa S, Mantero M, Caminiti M, Curci V, Lupattelli T, Morabito A (2006) Early and five-year amputation and survival rate of diabetic patients with critical limb ischemia: data of a cohort study of 564 patients. Eur J Vasc Endovasc Surg 32(5):484–490. https://doi.org/10.1016/j.ejvs.2006.03.006
73. Bartus CL, Margolis DJ (2004) Reducing the incidence of foot ulceration and amputation in diabetes. Curr Diab Rep 4(6):413–418
74. Apelqvist J (2012) Diagnostics and treatment of the diabetic foot. Endocrine 41(3):384–397
75. Guo SA, DiPietro LA (2010) Factors affecting wound healing. J Dent Res 89(3):219–229
76. Krug E, Berg L, Lee C, Hudson D, Birke-Sorensen H, Depoorter M, Dunn R, Jeffery S, Duteille F, Bruhin A, Caravaggi C (2011) Evidence-based recommendations for the use of neg-

ative pressure wound therapy in traumatic wounds and reconstructive surgery: steps towards an international consensus. Injury 42:S1–S2
77. Bus SA, Van Netten JJ, Lavery LA, Monteiro-Soares M, Rasmussen A, Jubiz Y, Price PE, International Working Group on the Diabetic Foot (IWGDF) (2016) IWGDF guidance on the prevention of foot ulcers in at-risk patients with diabetes. Diabetes Metab Res Rev 32:16–24. https://doi.org/10.1002/dmrr.2696
78. Kennon B, Leese GP, Cochrane L, Colhoun H, Wild S, Stang D, Sattar N, Pearson D, Lindsay RS, Morris AD, Livingstone S (2012) Reduced incidence of lower-extremity amputations in people with diabetes in Scotland: a nationwide study. Diabetes Care 35(12):2588–2590. https://doi.org/10.2337/dc12-0511
79. Mueller MJ, Hastings M, Commean PK, Smith KE, Pilgram TK, Robertson D, Johnson J (2003) Forefoot structural predictors of plantar pressures during walking in people with diabetes and peripheral neuropathy. J Biomech 36(7):1009–1017. https://doi.org/10.1016/s0021-9290(03)00078-2
80. DiLiberto FE, Tome J, Baumhauer JF, Quinn JR, Houck J, Nawoczenski DA (2015) Multi-joint foot kinetics during walking in people with Diabetes Mellitus and peripheral neuropathy. J Biomech 48(13):3679–3684. https://doi.org/10.1016/j.jbiomech.2015.08.020
81. Rizzo L, Tedeschi A, Fallani E, Coppelli A, Vallini V, Iacopi E, Piaggesi A (2012) Custom-made orthesis and shoes in a structured follow-up program reduces the incidence of neuro-pathic ulcers in high-risk diabetic foot patients. Int J Low Extrem Wounds 11(1):59–64
82. DiLiberto FE, Baumhauer JF, Nawoczenski DA (2016) The prevention of diabetic foot ulceration: how biomechanical research informs clinical practice. Braz J Phys Ther 20(5):375–338
83. LeMaster JW, Mueller MJ, Reiber GE, Mehr DR, Madsen RW, Conn VS (2008) Effect of weight-bearing activity on foot ulcer incidence in people with diabetic peripheral neuropathy: feet first randomized controlled trial. Phys Ther 88(11):1385–1398. https://doi.org/10.2522/ptj.20080019
84. Rao S, Saltzman C, Yack HJ (2006) Ankle ROM and stiffness measured at rest and during gait in individuals with and without diabetic sensory neuropathy. Gait Posture 24(3):295–301
85. Sacco IC, Hamamoto AN, Gomes AA, Onodera AN, Hirata RP, Hennig EM (2009) Role of ankle mobility in foot rollover during gait in individuals with diabetic neuropathy. Clin Biomech 24(8):687–692. https://doi.org/10.1016/j.clinbiomech.2009.05.003
86. Shapiro J, Koshimune D, Moellmer R (2013) In: Masuo K (ed) Diabetic foot ulcers—treatment and prevention, in type 2 diabetes. IntechOpen, London. https://doi.org/10.5772/56400
87. Thiruvoth FM, Mohapatra DP, Sivakumar DK, Chittoria RK, Nandhagopal V (2015) Current concepts in the physiology of adult wound healing. Plast Aesthet Res 2:250–256. https://doi.org/10.4103/2347-9264.158851
88. Zubair M, Ahmad J (2019) Role of growth factors and cytokines in diabetic foot ulcer healing: a detailed review. Rev Endocr Metab Disord 20:207–217. https://doi.org/10.1007/s11154-019-09492-1
89. Bermudez DM, Herdrich BJ, Xu J, Lind R, Beason DP, Mitchell ME, Soslowsky LJ, Liechty KW (2011) Impaired biomechanical properties of diabetic skin: implications in pathogenesis of diabetic wound complications. Am J Pathol 178(5):2215–2223
90. Webster JB, Darter BJ (2019) 4—Principles of normal and pathologic gait. In: Atlas of orthoses and assistive devices, 5th edn. Elsevier, Amsterdam, pp 49–62.e1
91. Lepäntalo M, Apelqvist J, Setacci C, Ricco J-B, de Donato G, Becker F, Robert-Ebadi H, Cao P, Eckstein HH, De Rango P, Diehm N, Schmidli J, Teraa M, Moll FL, Dick F, Davies AH (2011) Chapter V: Diabetic foot. Eur J Vasc Endovasc Surg 42(Suppl 2):S60–S74

Foot Pressure Abnormalities, Radiographic, and Charcot Changes in the Diabetic Foot

7

Ahmad Faraz, Hamid Ashraf, Saifullah Khalid, and Razeen Fatima

7.1 Introduction

Diabetes Mellitus (DM) has become one of the biggest healthcare challenges of the twenty-first century and it has become one of the major causes of morbidity and mortality across the world. According to the International Diabetic Federation, 425 million had diabetes in the year 2016 and by the year 2045, the number will escalate to 629 million [1]. One of the most common complications of diabetes is Diabetic Neuropathy. According to the American Diabetic Association diabetic neuropathy is "the presence of symptoms and/or signs of peripheral nerve dysfunctions in people with diabetes after exclusion of other causes" '[2]. The prevalence of diabetic peripheral neuropathy can be as low as 16% to as high as 66% [3, 4]. While the incidence of amputation in diabetic patients is 10–20 times greater than in non-diabetic patients [5].

A. Faraz
Department of Physiology, Faculty of Medicine, J N Medical College & Hospital, Aligarh Muslim University, Aligarh, India

H. Ashraf (✉)
Rajiv Gandhi Center for Diabetes & Endocrinology, Faculty of Medicine, J N Medical College & Hospital, Aligarh Muslim University, Aligarh, India

S. Khalid
Department of Radio-diagnosis, Faculty of Medicine, J N Medical College & Hospital, Aligarh Muslim University, Aligarh, India

R. Fatima
Department of Medicine, Faculty of Medicine, J N Medical College & Hospital, Aligarh Muslim University, Aligarh, India

M. Zubair et al. (eds.), *Diabetic Foot Ulcer*,
https://doi.org/10.1007/978-981-15-7639-3_7

7.2 Forces on Foot During Weight-Bearing

During weight-bearing, foot is exposed to ground reaction forces (GRF), so while standing a person exerts a force equivalent to weight and an equal amount of force (GRF) is exerted by ground in opposite direction. GRF has a parallel component when a person is moving where a deformable force is present. Deformation forces can be categorized as Stress and Strain, stress is the force exerted on the body per unit area, and it is a measure of internal forces on surrounding particle. Stress perpendicular to the body is a compressive force, while stress parallel to the body is shear stress. A strain is the deformation of any material due to stress [6]. During standing stress is perpendicular to the body, so the pressure is greater at the heel than at the forefoot [7].

Weight is mainly distributed on three prominent points of the foot: 1. center of the heel, 2. the first and the 3. fourth–fifth metatarsal heads. Weight-bearing on foot while standing is evenly distributed on these three prominent points, thereby providing optimal stabilization. Distribution of pressure on the plantar surface depends mainly on body weight [8], age [9], and abnormalities of the foot secondary to any disease [10].

When a person is standing, weight is evenly distributed on both the feet but when a person is walking stress is much higher because of multiple reasons as follows: (1) During the gait cycle both the feet come in contact with the ground for only 22% of the cycle, hence one foot is exposed to force of weight for a longer period. (2) During walking GRF moves anteriorly from heel to forefoot and portions of the foot makes contact with the ground during different stages of gait cycle. The heel comes in contact with the ground during ~64% of the stance phase while the forefoot is in contact during the last 59% of the stance phase [11]. (3) GRF vary with the phases of gait, the peak pressure is exerted during the initial contact and loading and the push off phase of the terminal stance, so the heel and forefoot experience higher pressure [6].

7.3 Forces on Diabetic Foot

7.3.1 Disorder of Mobility

Decreased movement of ankle joint impedes the normal rollover of the sole throughout the stance phase of the gait cycle, it may be a result of early heel rise and early loading of the forefoot. During the push off phase, the altered mobility of the great toe can cause early landing of the great toe [12]. Altered movement of these joints can lead to increased plantar pressures and it further increases the risk of ulceration.

7.3.2 Structural Foot Changes

Neuropathy secondary to prolonged hyperglycemia leads to several structural changes in the foot of these patients. These include intrinsic muscle wasting, hammertoes, claw toes, hallux valgus, dislocation of a smaller toe, and changes in height of arches. The structural deformity may lead to increased plantar pressure by diminishing the support surface or by raising the prominence of bony points (metatarsal heads and bunions). Amputations of partial foot and Charcot fractures also decrease the support surface and may cause high plantar pressure [13]. Diabetic foot ulcer occurs most commonly on the site of maximal load, there was a lateral shift of pressure on the forefoot [14]. DPN patients often present with hammertoe deformity which may lead to increased plantar pressure at the lesser toe [15, 16]. In patients of diabetes with neuropathy, there is a regional difference in plantar shear values, therefore shear-forces can help in predicting the site of ulcer formation and in designing footwear [17]. Patients with multiple deformities are more prone to higher plantar pressure and ulceration. However, the repetition of stress on a particular site is a more important factor, than the magnitude of pressure or shear stress [18].

The lifetime risk of foot ulcer in patients with diabetes is 10–15% Barrett et al. [19] and Stokes et al. [14] found out that foot ulceration is common in areas of high foot pressure in patients of peripheral neuropathy. Due to peripheral motor neuropathy in diabetes, muscles of the foot like long and short flexors and intrinsic muscles become weak, which then causes decreased loading of toes. This leads to increased pressure on metatarsal heads. Seventy percent of normal toe loading is transmitted through the hallux, so when toe loading is decreased all the pressure is then transmitted by metatarsal instead of the hallux. This is why the first metatarsal is the most common site of neuropathic ulcers [20]. The mobility of subtalar joints is significantly reduced in patients of diabetic neuropathy with ulceration. The axis of the subtalar joint is oblique to all three body planes [21, 22]. When the heel strikes the ground, there is loading of the forefoot, with pronation of subtalar joint which allows molding of soft tissue to surface and absorption of shock. It is then followed by the supination of a subtalar joint which makes the foot rigid to enable leverage for stride. The reduced subtalar joint movement in the foot with ulceration will probably lead to uneven distribution of forces [23]. The presence of abnormal forces (both vertical weight-bearing and horizontal shearing) at the ulceration site is the key factor in the development of ulceration in the insensitive neuropathic foot [24]. Decreased joint mobility in association with neuropathy is the main etiological factor for high foot pressure that is often found in diabetes patients and is associated with foot ulceration.

7.3.3 Soft Tissue Abnormality

The diabetic patient often has stiffer and thinner plantar soft tissue especially in an elderly subject [25]. The soft tissue under the first metatarsal head most commonly has increased stiffness, which may lead to decreased shock absorption and increased peak pressures under dynamic conditions. Reduced thickness of plantar tissue is associated with an increase in peak plantar pressure [26]. The formation of calluses under the forefoot was also associated with an increase in plantar pressure and also increases the risk of ulceration [27].

7.4 Association of Neuropathy with Ulceration

Sensory neuropathy in diabetes lead to decreased sensation and loss of protective sensation, a patient may not be able to localize pain or discomfort due to overloading of plantar surface [28]. Ulcers and lesions remain undetected and may cause deterioration of trivial injury.

7.4.1 Altered Gait Pattern

There is a decrease in plantar pressure due to short steps with a shuffling gait, it would increase the duration of the foot flat and the area of weight-bearing [29]. Shuffling gait results in an increase in the foot to floor contact area and time. However, shuffling gait is an inefficient gait since patients get fatigued easily [30].

7.4.2 Pressure Changes with Ulceration

High plantar pressure in patients of diabetic peripheral neuropathy (DPN) cause diabetic foot ulcer (DFU). But plantar pressure during ulceration is not raised [31]. Forefoot plantar pressure is raised in patients of active ulceration despite the increased stance phase owing to slow walking speed. However, faster speed lead to increased pressure at the heel, medial, and forefoot while decreased pressure in the midfoot and lateral forefoot [32]. The extended stance phase is insufficient to decrease plantar pressure in an ulcerated foot [33]. In patients of diabetes with neuropathy previous history of ulceration demonstrates increased plantar pressure, but patients with active ulceration do not show higher plantar pressure which may be because these patients protect the part with ulceration [34]. Also, poor glycemic control in patients of diabetes may lead to abnormal plantar pressure [35]. Other factors like excess weight gain also play an important role in elevated plantar pressure [36].

7.5 Clinical Findings Predicting High Plantar Pressure [37]

- *History*
  - Prior ulceration
  - Prior surgery involving the metatarsal bones
- *Physical finding*
  - Callus*
  - Hemorrhagic callus*
  - Blister or macerated skin*
  - Limited hallux dorsiflexion (less than 30°)
  - Prominent metatarsal heads inadequately covered with soft tissue**
  - Other plantar bony prominences

- *Radiograph finding*: Charcot fracture
  - *High pressure or shear capable of injuring soft tissue is being generated.
  - **Detected by gently stroking a finger across the plantar surface of the forefoot.

7.6 Charcot Foot

One of the overwhelming complications of DPN is the development of Charcot foot (CF) or Charcot neuropathic osteoarthropathy (CN). CF is named after the famous French neurologist Jean-Martin Charcot, who first identified the neuroarthropathic changes in patients of tertiary syphilis [38]. William Riley Jordan in 1936, first depicted the connection between Diabetes Mellitus and painless neuropathic arthropathy of the ankle [39]. It is an uncommon issue that is characterized by the destruction of bones and joints prompting fractures, dislocation, deformity, and amputation. CF is frequently associated with DM, alcoholic peripheral neuropathy, tertiary syphilis, leprosy, spinal cord injury, Charcot-Marie-Tooth disease, and idiopathic neuropathy. Currently, the number of patients of diabetes is increasing worldwide, and these patients are living longer because of better diabetes care. This has prompted a circumstance where DM is the most common reason for CN and the number of patients with CN is expected to rise. The reported incidence of CF varies widely in the literature from 0.1–7.5%, because of different diagnostic criteria used, different inclusion criteria, and different duration of diabetes [40]. Recently, a study from India revealed a high prevalence of CN (9.8%) in patients of type 2 DM with DPN [41].

7.7 Pathogenesis of Charcot Foot

The exact pathogenesis of CF is not yet clear, and there is no single factor for CF development, some neuropathic DM patients develop CF while others do not. Several factors predispose an individual to the development of Charcot Foot. The popular explanations for the production of CF include the "neurovascular" hypothesis suggested by Charcot himself, which indicates that there is a lack of vasoregulation resulting in high flow state and opening of arteriovenous shunting due to underlying autonomic neuropathy [38]. Such increased blood flow contributes to increased flux of monocytes and osteoclast, resulting in the bone washout of structural calcium. The net result is localized osteopenia and continuous weight-bearing resulting in deformation. The hypothesis of "neurotraumatic" proposed by Volkmann and Virchow indicated that repetitive microtrauma to the foot induces an uncontrolled inflammatory cascade in the absence of protective sensation, resulting in collapse and joint destruction in CN [42]. Most likely CF occurs because of combination of these factors. The discomfort is not experienced by patients in the presence of sensory neuropathy and chronic microtrauma continues unabated. Motor neuropathy affects the foot stress mechanisms resulting in irregular plantar tension and deformation. Autonomic neuropathy contributes to local osteopenia by increasing the local blood flow. If fracturing occurs in healthy people, it results in the release of pro-inflammatory cytokines like tumor necrosis factor α (TNF α) Interleukin 1β (IL-1β) and Interleukin 6 (IL-6). This, in turn, leads to enhanced expression of receptor activator the nuclear factor kβ ligand (RANKL) [43]. This pro-inflammatory cytokine state promotes osteoclast formation from the precursor cells to mature and activate. NF kB also stimulates osteoprotegerin synthesis from osteoblast that antagonizes RANKL [44]. In normal individual fracturing is compounded with pain, it contributes to bone splinting, and with time the pro-inflammatory condition may relieve. Unlike a normal person, when an individual with severe DPN experiences an acute Charcot foot impairment of pain sensation allows for sustained ambulation with repeated injury, resulting in persistent pro-inflammatory condition, contributing to chronic local osteolysis [45]. All these factors lead to bone destruction, fracture, dislocation at the foot, and ankle joint.

Hyperglycemia results in excessive nonenzymatic collagen glycation and binds to other protein molecules with the amino groups, contributing to the development of advanced glycation end products (AGEs). Binding of AGEs to their receptor (RAGE) prevents the differentiation of human mesenchymal stem cells [46]. They induce apoptosis of osteoblast and results in increased osteoclastogenesis through the RANKL/NF-kβ pathway. All these factors together with neuropathy lead to the continuance of inflammation and death. Calcitonin gene-related peptide (CGRP) normally secreted from the nerve terminals, has been documented to be critical in maintaining the integrity of joint capsules, as well as inhibiting RANKL synthesis. Any reduction of CGRP from the nerve terminals would affect the health of the bone and the strength of the joint. Both peripheral and autonomic neuropathy was shown to be linked with decreased release of CGRP, resulting in persistent RANKL action [47].

7.8 Clinical Presentation

The diagnosis of CF in acute stages requires a high index of suspicion. Patients are ordinarily present in the sixth or seventh decade. CF can have both acute and chronic presentations. The early symptoms of acute CF include mild to moderate discomfort, swelling of the affected limb, increased local temperature, and erythema [48]. The difference in temperature between the two limbs is ≥ 2 °C, which can be determined by an infrared thermometer. Pain is less when compared to cellulitis. At this stage, it can mimic cellulitis, deep vein thrombosis, or acute gout (Table 7.1). Clinical features such as raised temperature and increased heart rate are absent, peripheral pulses are well maintained in the diseased limb or it can be bounding also [49]. Elevation of the affected leg leads to a substantial reduction in the edema and erythema. Imaging studies like X-ray is not useful at this juncture as they may not reveal any changes (Fig. 7.1). Nevertheless, magnetic resonance imaging can provide some evidence for early diagnosis [50]. If proper diagnosis and treatment are not made at this stage, it may lead to additional destruction of bone and subsequent permanent damage.

Table 7.1 Difference between cellulitis and acute stage of Charcot foot

Features	Cellulitis	Acute Charcot foot
Age	Any	5–7 decade
History of diabetes	+/–	+
Neuropathy	+/–	+
Deformity	–	+/–
Pedal pulses	Normal/reduced	Bounding
Pain	+++	+/–
Fever/tachycardia	+	–
Pus discharge	+/–	–
WBC count	↑	Normal
MRI (low intensity on T1 and T2 hyperintensity)	Absent	Present
Calcaneal BMD	Normal	Reduced

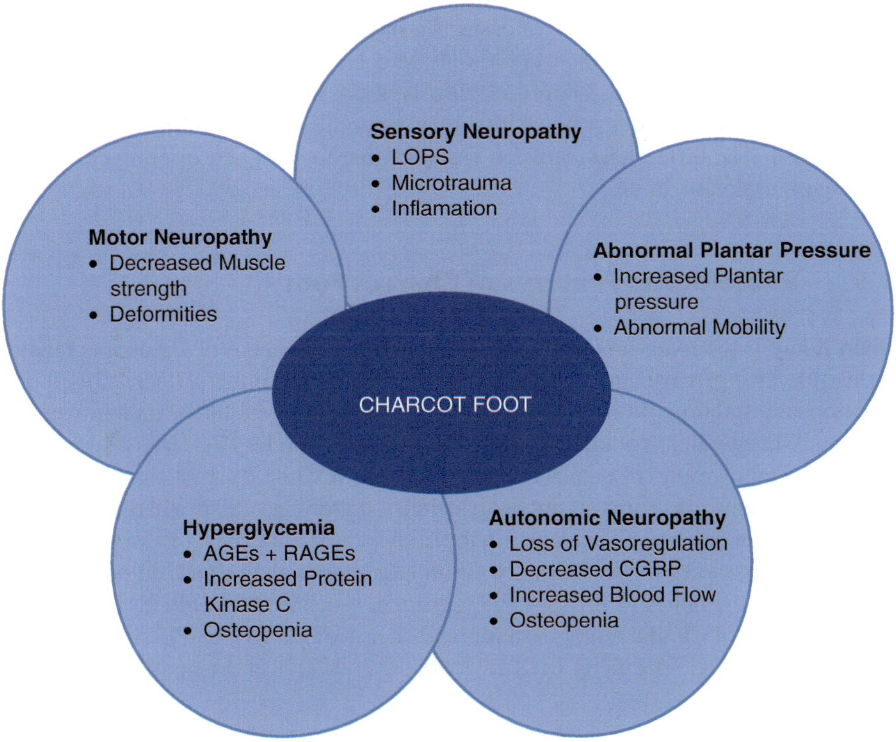

Fig. 7.1 Pathogenesis of Charcot foot. (*AGEs* advanced glycation end products, *CGRP* calcitonin gene-related peptide, *LOPS* loss of protective sensation, *RAGEs* receptor of advanced glycation end products)

Following the resolution of acute stage patients often land in chronic CF in which residual deformity has developed. Breakdown of the midfoot arch leads to the development of Rocker bottom foot which is the characteristic of chronic CF. Patients present clinically with features suggestive of neurological, vascular, musculoskeletal, and radiographic abnormalities [51].

Neuropathy is present in all patients with CF, and this can be detected by five simple clinical tests. During the screening exam, two of these should be used regularly, typically the 10 g monofilament and one other test. Four remaining tests comprise, vibration test using 128 Hz tuning fork, ankle reflex, pinprick sensation, and biothesiometry. Though patients have insensate foot, up to 50% of them give a history of preceding trauma, which is often trivial [50]. Deformities in CF can be varying from trivial to grossly evident deformity (Fig. 7.1). Feet deformities result in irregular high-pressure on the plantar surface weight-bearing area, rendering it vulnerable to ulceration.

Involvement in CF is unilateral in most of the cases, but the bilateral presentation has also been reported in 9–75% of cases. An Indian study revealed bilateral presentation in 16% of cases. The most commonly affected site is midfoot in the literature, while an Indian study revealed midfoot involvement in 43% of patients. If the sinus tract is present or probe test is positive than osteomyelitis should be strongly suspected [49]. The differences between chronic Charcot foot and osteomyelitis have been enumerated in Table 7.2.

7.9 Radiological Features of Charcot Foot

Plain X-ray is the main imaging tool for the initial assessment of CF as it is readily accessible, inexpensive, and provides information on bone mineral density, joint orientation, and stability. While taking a radiograph, emphasis should be on non-weight-bearing A-P, lateral and oblique X-rays of the foot and ankle. The earliest sign of CF on a plain radiograph is Localized demineralization, while the first sign of diabetic neuroarthropathy on X-ray is metatarsal head flattening. CF is characterized by Subchondral or periarticular changes in the midfoot and multiple joints were involved without soft tissue changes. X-Ray of CF in later stages shows marked periarticular osteopenia in the bones of the foot and periosteal reaction. It is difficult to visualize trivial changes of CF like minor fractures and edema of marrow on Plain Radiograph. The sensitivity and specificity of X-rays are around 50% in the acute phase of CF

Table 7.2 Difference between osteomyelitis and chronic Charcot foot

Features	Osteomyelitis	Chronic Charcot foot
Location	Toes and metatarsal heads	Commonly midfoot
Distribution	Multiple bones/joints	Focal
Deformity	Absent	Present
Soft tissue changes	Inflamed, sinus tracts, abscess formation	Subcutaneous tissue edema
Bone marrow edema	Periarticular	Around ulcers, fistula tracts

Table 7.3 Classification of Charcot foot

Eichenholtz classification	Sanders and Frykberg
Natural history and radiological	Anatomical
Stage I: Developmental; redness, swelling, and raised temperature	Pattern 1: Forefoot involvement; phalanges, interphalangeal, and the metatarsophalangeal joints
Stage II: Coalescence; active period of the disease process when bony destruction and deformity occur	Pattern 2: Tarsometatarsal
Stage III: Stage of reconstruction; commencing when the destructive process "burns out" and the bone consolidates with the resulting deformity	Pattern 3: Cuneonavicular, talonavicular, and calcaneocuboid articulations
	Pattern 4: Talocrural joint
	Pattern 5: Involves the posterior calcaneus

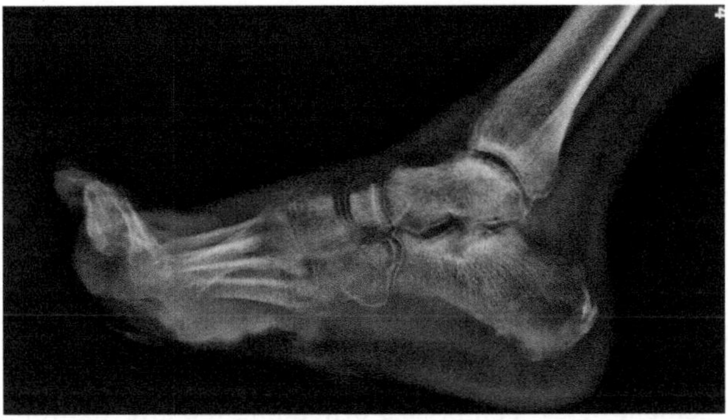

Fig. 7.2 X-ray foot lateral view: shows diffuse osteopenia and marked periarticular osteopenia in the bones of the foot, and subtle periosteal reaction with cortical irregularity in the lateral aspect of first metatarsal with extension to all metatarsophalangeal joints. Deformed contours at the distal end of the proximal phalanx with medial flexion deformity at the interphalangeal joint. Skin and subcutaneous tissue edema are also present

[50]. Eichenholtz classifies CF based on X-Ray. He divides CF into three stages: bone dissolution (stage I), bone coalescence (stage II), and bone remodeling (stage III) (Table 7.3). X-Ray in chronic stages of CF, shows decreased inclination angle of calcaneum, obliteration of the first talo-metatarsal angle (Fig. 7.2) [48]. Since the sensitivity and specificity of X-Ray are low in acute CF, magnetic resonance imaging (MRI) is an investigation of choice in the initial stage of CF. MRI offers exceptional details about the anatomy and pathological changes in both soft tissue and bone. MRI has high sensitivity and specificity for diagnosing osteomyelitis, it can also help in distinguishing between osteomyelitis and diabetic foot. Further, it is the first-line investigation for the assessment of diabetic patients with a complicated foot [52]. MRI shows soft tissue edema, joint effusion, interruption of Lisfranc ligament, and subchondral bone marrow edema in the acute phase of CF. MRI shows low signal intensity on T1W and high signal intensity on T2W images of bone marrow edema. The subchondral region shows characteristic differential signal enhancement of bone

marrow [52]. Radionuclide study can be used in CF. The sensitivity of Triple phase technetium-99m methylene diphosphonate (Tc-99m MDP) is high but specificity is low for the diagnosis of osteomyelitis (95–100% and 25–38%, respectively). Since the site of infection involves the recruitment of white blood cells (WBC), labeled white cell scans (In-WBC) provide a very precise diagnosis of osteomyelitis with an accuracy level of 80–90%. Both In-WBC scans and three phases of Tc-99m MDP can be used to diagnose patients with high suspicion of osteomyelitis. Nowadays positron emission tomography (PET) scanning has been used to differentiate between osteomyelitis and Charcot foot. According to a few studies PET scan has better sensitivity and specificity than MRI [53].

7.10 Management of Charcot Foot

CF care aims to provide a healthy, plantigrade foot that works in a shoe and also to avoid persistent ulceration. Factors affecting CF treatment include the disease phase, the presence or absence of deformity, infection, and comorbidity. Depending on the severity of the disease, the goals of the treatment should be personalized and realistic. CF treatment may vary from modified footwear to limb amputation [52].

7.10.1 Medical Management

Medical management of CF comprises, offloading the affected foot, correction of bony abnormalities, and reducing additional foot fractures. Acute phases of CF typically need medical management. Such management protocols are generally based on expert opinions since the evidence from randomized control trials are lacking.

7.10.2 Offloading

Offloading is the most important component of management in acute CF. Offloading could slow the progression to deformity. The gold standard for offloading of affected foot is the total contact cast (TCC). Application of TCC decrease the physical stress, it further reduces the inflammation and edema, thereby decreasing the bone and joint destruction. TCC providing cover to the entire foot, including the ankle joint, also providing an adequate cushion with cotton-based bandages over a bony prominence to avoid ulceration, should be used. The patients should be kept under close monitoring, and a new cast should be applied, at a regular interval of 3–7 days [54]. The application of TCC leads to perseveration of the plantigrade foot, which enables it for weight-bearing in a shoe or brace. Usually, in the first few weeks, there is a significant decline in the edema. Repeated cast change is necessary, to avoid "pistoning" with declining edema. The use of crutches or wheelchair should be encouraged, thereby preventing weight-bearing on the affected limb. The cast needs to apply until the edema has subsided and the temperature variance among the two limbs is less than 2 °C. The average time of cast application in chronic CF with ulceration is 5 weeks, with progression to therapeutic footwear at 3 months. An alternative device for offloading the active stage of CF is a prefabricated removable walker brace. The advantage is the low cost in comparison to TCC, but it has a problem of inability to fit severe deformities and possibly incomplete compliance [52].

7.10.3 Antiresorptive Therapy

Bisphosphonate, due to its anticlastic activity is an appealing treatment method for acute CF. Among the bisphosphonate, Pamidronate has been the most commonly used agent. Bisphosphonate decreases the Charcot foot activity, which is evident by a decrease in skin temperature, pain, and edema. They can be used besides immobilization and offloading. The adverse effects of bisphosphonates and their contraindications for use should be kept in mind before prescribing them [55].

7.10.4 Bone Growth Stimulation

Ultrasonic bone stimulation is a newer technique, which has been used for the healing of new fractures in acute CF. In patients of CF with arthrodesis, direct current electrical bone growth stimulators were used. Findings were encouraging, but more evidence is required before its routine use. At this point, it is at best an adjuvant to the established treatment [52].

7.11 Surgical Treatment

Surgical treatment of CF is primarily dependent on the expert opinion of treating surgeons. Surgery has been utilized for removal of infected bone in osteomyelitis, correction of prominent bony points to accommodate the foot in the therapeutic footwear. This decision is primarily based on expert opinion and small, uncontrolled retrospective case series. Before surgical treatment patient's other comorbidities, compliance, site, and severity of deformity, infection, or joint instability should be considered. The surgical procedure includes release and augmentation of Achilles tendon, plantar osteotomy, debridement of the osseous points, arthrodesis, and open reduction with several methods of internal fixation with or without external fixation. Currently, we do not have enough evidence for the superiority of any procedure. Now there is a group that has suggested earlier surgical repair of deformity and arthrodesis, based on the idea that it will contribute to an improved patient-perceived quality of life [56].

References

1. IDF atlas (2017). Available from: http://www.idf.org/e-library/epidemiology-research/diabetes-atlas.html
2. American Diabetes Association (2007) Standards of medical care in diabetes—2007 [Position statement]. Diabetes Care 30:S4–S41
3. Boulton AJ, Vileikyte L, RagnarsonTennvall G et al (2005) The global burden of diabetic foot disease. Lancet 366:1719–1724. https://doi.org/10.1016/S0140-6736(05)67698-2
4. Boulton AJM, Armstrong DG, Albert SF et al (2008) Comprehensive foot examination and risk assessment. Diabetes Care 31:1679–1685. https://doi.org/10.2337/dc08-9021
5. Moxey PW, Gogalniceanu P, Hinchliffe RJ et al (2011) Lower extremity amputations – a review of global variability in incidence. Diabet Med 28(10):1144–1153. https://doi.org/10.1111/j.1464-5491.2011.03279.x
6. van Deursen R (2004) Mechanical loading and off-loading of the plantar surface of the diabetic foot. Clin Infect Dis 39:S87–S91
7. Cavanagh PR, Rodgers MM, Iiboshi A (1987) Pressure distribution under symptom-free feet during barefoot standing. Foot Ankle 5:262–276
8. Hotfiel T, Carl HD, Wendler F, Jendrissek A, Heiß R, Swoboda B (2017) Plantar pressures increase with raising body weight: a standardised approach with paired sample using neutral shoes. J Back Musculoskelet Rehabil 30(3):583–589
9. Martinez-Nova A, Huerta JP, Sánchez-Rodriguez R (2008) Cadence, age, and weight as determinants of forefoot plantar pressures using the biofoot in-shoe system. J Am Podiatr Med Assoc 98(4):302–310
10. Rao S, Saltzman C, Yack HJ (2006) Ankle ROM and stiffness measured at rest and during gait in individuals with and without diabetic sensory neuropathy. Gait Posture 24(3):295–301
11. Blanc Y, Balmer C, Landis T, Vingerhoets F (1999) Temporal parameters and patterns of the foot roll over during walking: normative data for healthy adults. Gait Posture 10:97–108
12. Mueller MJ, Diamond JE, Delitto A, Sinacore DR (1989) Insensitivity, limited joint mobility, and plantar ulcers in patients with diabetes mellitus. Phys Ther 69:453–459
13. Armstrong DG, Lavery LA (1998) Plantar pressures are higher in diabetic patients following partial foot amputation. Ostomy Wound Manage 44:30–32. 34, 36
14. Stokes IA, Faris IB, Hutton WC (1975) The neuropathic ulcer and loads on the foot in diabetic patients. Acta Orthop Scand 46:839–847
15. Barn R, Waaijman R, Nollet F, Woodburn J, Bus SA (2015) Predictors of barefoot plantar pressure during walking in patients with diabetes, peripheral neuropathy and a history of ulceration. PLoS One 10:e0117443
16. Ledoux WR, Shofer JB, Smith DG, Sullivan K, Hayes SG, Assal M, Reiber GE (2005) Relationship between foot type, foot deformity, and ulcer occurrence in the high-risk diabetic foot. J Rehabil Res Dev 42:665–672
17. Yavuz M (2014) Plantar shear stress distributions in diabetic patients with and without neuropathy. Clin Biomech (Bristol, Avon) 29:223–229
18. Lavery LA, Armstrong DG, Wunderlich RP, Tredwell J, Boulton AJM (2003) Predictive value of foot pressure assessment as part of a population-based diabetes disease management program. Diabetes Care 26:1069–1073
19. Barrett JP, Mooney V (1973) Neuropathy and diabetic pressure lesions. Orthop Clin North Am 4:43–47
20. Ctercteko GC, Dhanendran M, Hutton WC, Le Quesne LP (1981) Vertical forces acting on the feet of diabetic patients with neuropathic ulceration. Br J Surg 68:608–614
21. Root ML, Weed JH, Sgarlato TE, Bluth DR (1966) Axis of motion of the sub-talar joint. Am Pod Ass 56:149–155
22. Lnman VT (1976) The sub-talar joint. In: Lnman VT (ed) The joints of the ankle. Williams and Wilkins, Baltimore, pp 35–43

23. Delbridge L, Perry P, Marr S, Arnold N, Yue DK, Turtle JR, Reeve TS (1988) Limited joint mobility in the diabetic foot: relationship to neuropathic ulceration. Diabet Med 5:333–337
24. Delbridge L, Ctercteko G, Fowler C, Reeve TS, LeQuesne LP (1985) The aetiology of neuropathic ulceration in the diabetic foot. Brit Surg 75:1–6
25. Gefen A, Megido-Ravid M, Azariah M, Itzchak Y, Arcan M (2001) Integration of plantar soft tissue stiffness measurements in routine MRI of the diabetic foot. Clin Biomech (Bristol, Avon) 16:921–925
26. Abouaesha F, van Schie CH, Griffths GD, Young RJ, Boulton AJ (2001) Plantar tissue thickness is related to peak plantar pressure in the high-risk diabetic foot. Diabetes Care 24:1270–1274
27. Murray HJ, Young MJ, Hollis S, Boulton AJ (1996) The association between callus formation, high pressures, and neuropathy in diabetic foot ulceration. Diabet Med 13:979–982
28. van Deursen RW, Sanchez MM, Derr JA, Becker MB, Ulbrecht JS, Cavanagh PR (2001) Vibration perception threshold testing in patients with diabetic neuropathy: ceiling effects and reliability. Diabet Med 18:469–475
29. Brand PW (1983) The diabetic foot. In: Ellenberg M, Rifkin H (eds) Diabetes mellitus: theory and practice, 3rd edn. Medical Examination Publishing, New York, pp 829–849
30. Zhu H, Wertsch JJ, Harris GF, Lofisgaarden JD, Price MB (1991) Foot pressure distribution during walking and shuffling. Arch Phys Med Rehabll 72:390–397
31. Fernando ME, Crowther RG, Pappas E, Lazzarini PA, Cunningham M, Sangla KS, Buttner P, Golledge J (2014) Plantar pressure in diabetic peripheral neuropathy patients with active foot ulceration, previous ulceration and no history of ulceration: a meta-analysis of observational studies. PLoS One 9:e99050
32. Rosenbaum D, Hautmann S, Gold M, Claes L (1994) Effects of walking speed on plantar pressure patterns and hindfoot angular motion. Gait Posture 2:191–197
33. Fernando M, Crowther R, Lazzarini P, Sangla K, Cunningham M, Buttner P, Golledge J (2013) Biomechanical characteristics of peripheral diabetic neuropathy: a systematic review and meta-analysis of findings from the gait cycle, muscle activity and dynamic barefoot plantar pressure. Clin Biomech (Bristol, Avon) 28(8):831–845
34. Fernando ME, Crowther RG, Pappas E et al (2014) Plantar pressure in diabetic peripheral neuropathy patients with active foot ulceration, previous ulceration and no history of ulceration: a meta-analysis of observational studies. PLoS One 9(6):e99050
35. Couppé C, Svensson RB, Kongsgaard M et al (2016) Human Achilles tendon glycation and function in diabetes. J Appl Physiol 120(2):130–137
36. Cavanagh PR, Sims DS Jr, Sanders LJ (1991) Body mass is a poor predictor of peak plantar pressure in diabetic men. Diabetes Care 14:750–755
37. Caputo GM, Cavanagh PR, Ulbrecht JS et al (1994) Assessment and management of foot disease in patients with diabetes. N Engl J Med 331:854–860
38. Charcot JM (1868) Sur quelques arthropathies qui paraiise d'ependre d' une l'esion du cerveau ou de la mouelle épini'ere. Arch Physiol Norm Pathol 1:161–178
39. Jordan WR (1936) Neuritic manifestations in diabetes mellitus. Arch Intern Med 57:307–366
40. Rajbhandari SM, Jenkins RC, Davies C, Tesfaye S (2002) Charcot neuroarthropathy in diabetes mellitus. Diabetologia 45:1085–1096
41. Salini D, Harish K, Minnie P et al (2018) Prevalence of Charcot arthropathy in type 2 diabetes patients aged over 50 years with severe peripheral neuropathy: a retrospective study in a tertiary care South Indian Hospital. Indian J Endocrinol Metab 22:107–111
42. Ramanujam CL, Zgonis T (2017) The diabetic Charcot foot from 1936 to 2016: eighty years later and still growing. Clin Podiatr Med Surg 34:1–8
43. Jeffcoate WJ, Game F, Cavanagh PR (2005) The role of proinflammatory cytokines in the cause of neuropathic osteoarthropathy (acute Charcot foot) in diabetes. Lancet 366:2058–2061
44. Boyce BF, Xing L (2008) Functions of RANKL/RANK/OPG in bone modeling and remodeling. Arch Biochem Biophys 473:139–146
45. Larson SA, Burns PR (2012) The pathogenesis of Charcot neuroarthropathy: current concepts. Diabet Foot Ankle 3

46. Katayama Y, Akatsu T, Yamamoto M et al (1996) Role of nonenzymatic glycosylation of type I collagen in diabetic osteopenia. J Bone Miner Res 11:931–937
47. Jeffcoate WJ, Game FL (2010) New theories on the causes of the Charcot foot in diabetes. In: Frykberg RG (ed) The diabetic Charcot foot: principles and management. Data Trace Publishing Company, Brooklandville, MD, pp 29–44
48. Eichenholtz SN (1966) Charcot joints. Charles C. Thomas, Springfield, IL
49. Cofield RH, Morrison MJ, Beabout JW (1983) Diabetic neuroarthropathy in the foot: patient characteristics and patterns of radiographic change. Foot Ankle 4:15–22
50. Morrison WB, Ledermann HP (2002) Work-up of the diabetic foot. Radiol Clin North Am 40:1171–1192
51. Caputo GM, Ulbrecht J, Cavanagh PR et al (1998) The Charcot foot in diabetes: six key points. Am Fam Physician 57:2705–2710
52. Rogers LC, Frykberg RG, Armstrong G, Boulton AJM, Edmonds M, Ha Van G et al (2011) The Charcot foot in diabetes. Diabetes Care 34(9):2123–2129
53. Keidar Z, Militianu D, Melamed E et al (2005) The diabetic foot: initial experience with 18F-FDG PET/CT. J Nucl Med 46:444–449
54. Armstrong DG, Lavery LA (1997) Monitoring healing of acute Charcot's arthropathy with infrared dermal thermometry. J Rehabil Res Dev 34:317–321
55. Durgia H, Sahoo J, Kamlanathan S et al (2018) Role of bisphosphonates in the management of acute Charcot foot. World J Diabetes 9(7):115–126
56. Dhawan V, Spratt KF, Pinzur MS et al (2005) Reliability of AOFAS diabetic foot questionnaire in Charcot arthropathy: stability, internal consistency, and measurable difference. Foot Ankle Int 26:717–731

Aerobic and Anaerobic Bacterial Infections and Treatment Strategies

8

Tarek Hassan M. Kabil

8.1 Introduction

The wound infections are defined by the classical findings of inflammation or the presence of purulence. The wounds Infections are classified into mild (superficial and limited in size and depth), moderate (deeper or more extensive), or severe (accompanied by systemic signs or metabolic disturbances) [1].

Diabetic foot ulcers (DFU) and its infections are usually inadequately managed due to poor knowledge of the microbial agents associated with the ulcers [2]. Therefore, diabetic foot ulcers should be evaluated for microbial agents before treatment is instituted. The study of microbial infection and investigating the pathogens infecting diabetic foot ulcers and their susceptibility pattern in uncontrolled diabetes mellitus can help in the improvement of the patient's management and reduce the frequency of amputation [3].

8.2 The Microbiology and Rate of Infection in DFU

Wounds and other soft tissues can be infected by a variety of aerobic and anaerobic species of bacteria, either singly or in combination. The diabetic foot infection is mostly mixed infection, and polymicrobial involving both aerobic and anaerobic bacteria but mono-microbial infection can occur. A study recorded 100% infection rate with mono-microbial infection occurred among 28.0% of the subjects while polymicrobial infection affected 72.0% of the subjects [3–7]. On the other hand, Pal and Gupta reported that patients with very long hospital stay had negative culture reports [8]. The knowledge of the contribution of the entire microbiome to clinical outcomes is limited. However, the development of complex microbial communities,

T. H. M. Kabil (✉)
Department of Medical Microbiology & Immunology, Faculty of Medicine, University of Tabuk, Tabuk, Kingdom of Saudi Arabia

M. Zubair et al. (eds.), *Diabetic Foot Ulcer*,
https://doi.org/10.1007/978-981-15-7639-3_8

that involve strict anaerobes and Enterobacteriaceae, may contribute to poor clinical outcomes in DFUs. DFUs which fail to heal are likely to be persistently colonized with heterogeneous microorganisms including anaerobes and Enterobacteriaceae [9]. The aerobic bacteria associated with diabetic foot infection include Gram-positive cocci such as *Staphylococcus aureus*, *Staphylococcus saprophyticus*, *Staphylococcus epidermidis*, *Streptococcus pyogenes*, pneumococci, *Streptococcus mutans*, Gram-positive rods as *Bacillus subtilis*, and Gram-negative rods as *Pseudomonas aeruginosa*, Proteus *species*, *Escherichia coli* and *Klebsiella pneumoniae* [10]. Ramakant et al., reported *P. aeruginosa* as the most common gram-negative isolate in diabetic foot ulcer patients in their study [11].

Anaerobic organisms, such as *Clostridium* species, *Bacteroides* species as *Bacteroides fragilis*, and anaerobic *Streptococci* such as *Peptostreptococcus*, may be present in infections of wounds, such as lacerated wounds and soiled deep wounds [1, 10, 12]. Mixed infections, in DFU, with Gram-positive cocci and coliform bacilli, are frequent. Polymicrobial infections with anaerobes include fusiforms or fusospirochete associations [5]. This was confirmed by other studies that showed that the diabetic foot ulcer severity of grade 4 is commonly infected with mixed bacteria including Methicillin-resistant *Staphylococcus aureus* (MRSA), and ESBL *Klebsiella* species [8, 13]. The polymicrobial nature of the infection was demonstrated, in a study, with 84% aerobic and 16% anaerobic species of bacteria were isolated. *Pseudomonas aeruginosa* (26.98%) followed by *Staphylococcus aureus* and *Klebsiella* sp. (16.66%) were the more frequently isolated aerobic bacteria. The anaerobic isolates were *Bacteroides* species (62.5%). *Peptostreptococcus* sp. (29.16%) and *Clostridium* sp. (8.3%) [6]. Another study was carried out to isolate and identify the microorganisms infecting DFUs. Seventy percent of these infections were polymicrobial. *Staphylococcus aureus* was the only Gram-positive bacterial isolate, 31.9%, and the most prevalent isolate. Regarding Gram-negative isolates, the study showed a dominance of Gram-negative bacteria among the isolates with *Pseudomonas aeruginosa,* 24.7%, the most common Gram-negative isolate, and *Klebsiella pneumoniae* the least isolated pathogen [3].

The patients who have chronic diabetic foot wounds or who have recently received antibiotic therapy may be infected with Gram-negative rods. Patients with diabetic foot accompanied by foot ischemia or gangrene may be colonized with obligate anaerobic pathogens [14]. There is no significant relationship between the duration of diabetic foot ulcers and infection rates. Also, infection rates are not significantly associated with gender [3, 14].

8.3 Pathogenesis of Infection

Peripheral vascular disease in the form of macro and microangiopathy of DM will lead to the decreased blood supply of foot tissues and when a wound occurs, it will become more susceptible to infection than nondiabetic wound where the infection rate coincides with blood sugar levels. Also, various immunological disturbances play a secondary role in DM foot infections [6, 14–16]. Foot infections in diabetic persons are common and form a serious problem. Typically, diabetic foot infections begin in a neuropathic ulceration wound [1]. The major predisposing factor to mixed infections of diabetic foot with more than one bacterial species is foot ulceration, which is usually related to peripheral neuropathy. In some of these mixed infections, a pathogenic synergy may be evident with two or more species acting in concert to cause more damage to the tissues than would be caused by either alone. The presence of devitalized tissues provides suitable conditions for the growth of anaerobic organisms. In addition, the preliminary infection with aerobic bacteria leads to the consumption of the available oxygen, which may encourage the growth of clostridia and other anaerobic bacteria [6]. Cellulitis, necrotizing cellulitis, and wet gangrene are deep diabetic foot infections that drag the patient to the option of amputation [3]. Besides, osteomyelitis can occur in many diabetic foot wound patients [1].

8.4 Laboratory Examination

The sending of specimens for culture may not be required in patients with mild or previously untreated DFUs. Generally, for the examination of wound swabs, specimens of pus, exudate, or tissue for detection of the common pathogens, a panel of basic procedures are to be applied. The obtained specimens are to be sent for culture before starting empirical antibiotic therapy in all cases of infection [14]. The basic procedures include a naked-eye examination of the specimen, the microscopical examination of a Gram-stained film, and culture on aerobic and anaerobic blood agar plates, on MacConkey agar and in Robertson cooked-meat broth. The growth seen on the plates is to be identified and, if significant, it should be tested for antibiotic susceptibility.

8.4.1 Sample Collection and Processing of the Sample

The debrided tissue sample from deep sites of DFU is used for smear preparation. The tissue samples, whatever obtained by biopsy or ulcer curettage identify pathogens more frequently, and non-pathogens less frequently when compared with wound swab samples [14, 17, 18]. A sterile container without fixative reagent is to be used for the sample curetted from infected tissue and for fragments of an excised tissue. Pus or exudate should be submitted in a small screw-capped bottle, a firmly stoppered tube or syringe, or a sealed capillary tube [19]. If there is a suspected delay in the transit of specimens to the laboratory, the samples should be placed in the appropriate transport media. Brain heart infusion broth is used as transport media for aerobic culture to be incubated overnight at 37 °C. For anaerobic culture, the sending of pus in oxygen-free gassed-out vials or special transport media as Robertson cooked-meat media is recommended. In the case of sample by swabbing, the swab is to be dropped into a cooked-meat broth. The pathogens may grow in the directly seeded broth and in its subcultures when they cannot be recovered in culture from the conventional swabs. Therefore, the arrangement of an immediate extra swab taken from the lesion in the clinical setting dropped into a cooked-meat broth, and send to the laboratory with the collected packaged swabs is recommended [6, 19, 20].

Gram-stained film of the sample is to be examined for the presence of pus cells, bacteria, and morphology, arrangement, and spore formation [6]. The samples should be homogenized in a tissue grinder with a little sterile broth, then cultured [19]. The culture plates have to be overnight incubated at 37 °C for 18—24 h, then examined for the relative numbers and types of the colonies. In addition, the performance of the tests for the identification and the determination of the antibiotic sensitivities is required. In case of absence of growth on the plates, or no growth of an organism seen in the Gram-stained film, the blood agars should be reincubated both aerobically and anaerobically for another 24 h. If the plates still showed no growth, they can be discarded. However, if there is a suspicion of the presence of a slow-growing pathogen such as some species of Bacteroides, a longer incubation up to 7 days is recommended. The growth in the cooked-meat broth after 24–48 h is indicated by turbidity in its appearance [21].

The preliminary performance of antibiotic sensitivity tests to give an early indication of an aspect of antibiotic sensitivity will assist in the identification of colonies of species with constant sensitivities. Also, it can help in the isolation of resistant strains from mixed cultures by selecting the colonies from the inhibition zones. Therefore, it is a good practice to apply one or two antibiotic discs on the inoculum areas of the aerobic blood agar plates before incubation as 1-unit benzylpenicillin disc and a 10 mg gentamicin disc. Also, it is wise to place a 5-pg. metronidazole disc and a 50-pg. neomycin disc on the anaerobic blood agar plates. The use of the metronidazole discs, differentiate strict anaerobes to be inhibited rather than aerobes or facultative bacteria. In addition, the inhibition of most aerobes caused by neomycin discs can help the identification of many anaerobes that are resistant to it [19].

8.4.2 For Aerobic Culture

For aerobic culture, the broth showing growth has to be subcultured on Blood agar, Chocolate agar (both incubated in presence of 5–10% CO_2), and MacConkey agar. The identification of the growth of organisms is to be made by Gram staining, colonial morphology, and biochemical tests [19, 22].

8.4.2.1 For Cultivation of Anaerobic Bacteria

The specimens for culture of anaerobes require complete absence of oxygen from the atmosphere and using media that allow the growth of anaerobes in these strict anaerobic conditions.

8.4.2.2 Anaerobic Incubation

For cultures of anaerobes, oxygen must be removed from the atmosphere, either by using it for combustion or by replacing it with an inert gas. It is recommended that all media for the growth of anaerobes should be incubated under strictly anaerobic conditions. The technique of repeated evacuation of jars and filling with nitrogen tends to dehydrate cultures and unsuitable for very strict anaerobes. The hydrogen and carbon dioxide, single or a mixture is commercially available, where, cylinders of the compressed gases are fitted with valves to deliver the gases at low pressure. Commercially available Hydrogen generators are a safer technique than holding hydrogen-containing gas cylinders in the laboratory. After putting the plates into the jar, the lid is clamped on. Approximately 6/7 of the air is evacuated (pressure is monitored on a vacuum gage). The pump is disconnected and the pressure is increased to 160 mmHg with $C0_2$ and then to 760 mmHg with hydrogen. The oxygen-adsorbing envelope (AnaeroGen) removes oxygen from the atmosphere in anaerobic jars. The process does not produce hydrogen and does not require catalysts. It produces 10% CO_2 in the anaerobic atmosphere [19]. Petri dishes with the medium uppermost and lid downwards has to be placed inside the jar. Vented Petri dishes should be used, like sealing of the lid to the bottom of the unvented Petri dish interferes with the removal of oxygen inside the Petri dish.

A smear from the inoculated Robertson cooked-meat broth showing turbidity, is to be subcultured on Neomycin Blood agar plate with the addition of metronidazole disc to identify anaerobic bacteria. Neomycin Blood agar plate is incubated for 2–3 days at 37 °C in an anaerobic jar with Gaspaks. The organisms are to be identified using Gram staining and colony morphology [6].

8.5 Antibiotic Sensitivity Testing and the Susceptibility Pattern of the Bacterial Isolates in DFU

Applying Clinical Laboratory Standards Institute (CLSI) guidelines is recommended during performing the antibiotic susceptibility testing by Kirby Bauer method of disk diffusion, following the culture of a smear prepared from 24 h cultured broth [23]. Many studies reported that *Staphylococcus aureus* and *Pseudomonas aeruginosa* exhibit a low susceptibility and a high resistance to ampicillin, cotrimoxazole, and gentamycin [24, 25]. The antibiotic susceptibility profile of the Gram-positive and Gram-negative bacteria isolated from D.M. patients with foot ulcers was investigated. Gram-positive bacteria were sensitive to Vancomycin (100%) and Gram-negative bacteria were sensitive to Imipenem, Meropenem, and Levofloxacin. Aerobic bacteria showed resistance to the cephalosporin group of antibiotics. *Pseudomonas* aeruginosa was found sensitive to Levofloxacin, less sensitive to Meropenem and Imipenem, but displayed resistance to cephalosporins [6]. A study showed that the susceptibility of the isolates to the used antibiotics in DFU, was low and none of the isolates showed 100% susceptibility to any of the tested antibiotics. A low level of antibiotic susceptibility of the isolates tested was observed with ampicillin and cotrimoxazole. The Gram-positive isolate, *Staphylococcus aureus*, was more susceptible to erythromycin (67.7%), followed by amoxicillin (61.2%). The Gram-negative isolate, *Pseudomonas aeruginosa*, was more susceptible to ciprofloxacin (80.4–100%), followed by zinacef (25.0–66.7%), and amoxicillin (50.0–64.7%). Erythromycin was the most effective antibiotic against *Staphylococcus aureus*. Augmentin and ciprofloxacin were effective against Gram-negative rods [3].

8.6 The Treatment Strategies of Diabetic Foot Ulcer

The infection of diabetic foot ulcers can be prevented by practicing good hygiene measures in and around the foot ulcer [2]. The early observation and careful follow-up of diabetic patients with infected wounds are required to ensure the appropriateness and effectiveness of the applied medical and surgical treatment regimens [14]. In addition, the clinicians and healthcare organizations are required to monitor the outcomes of management to improve the processes carried out during care for diabetic foot infections [1]. Diabetic foot infections require coordinated management with a multidisciplinary foot-care team that should include a medical microbiologist or an infectious disease specialist. The foot-care team should, also, recruit surgeons with experience and interest. This team takes attention of both local (foot) and systemic (metabolic) issues of the DFU [26–31]. The improvement of the patient's management and reduction of the frequency of amputation can be achieved through the clear knowledge of the microbial agents associated with the diabetic foot ulcers. This can be done by investigating the pathogens infecting the ulcers and testing their antimicrobial susceptibility pattern [32–34].

Chronic wounds in D.M. patients are associated with high morbidity and healthcare expenditures. A study of neuropathic diabetic foot ulcer (DFU) patients explored the role of colonizing microbiota in wound healing, clinical outcomes, and response to interventions. The strain-level variation of *Staphylococcus aureus* and genetic signatures of biofilm formation was found to be associated with poor clinical outcomes. Therefore, the DFU microbiota may be used as a marker for clinical outcomes and response to therapeutic interventions. *Corynebacterium striatum* and *Alcaligenes faecalis* isolated from the chronic wounds in D.M. patients were previously considered commensals or contaminants, but surprisingly they are found to significantly impact wound severity and healing [35].

Regarding treatment, no available evidence to support antibiotic use in treating clinically uninfected ulcers. It is not known whether systemic or local antibiotic treatment can lead to better outcomes or if a particular agent can be more effective in this regard. Also, there is no particular antimicrobial agent to be recommended for resolution of diabetic foot infection, ulcer healing, or the prevention of amputation [36–39]. However, antibiotic therapy is necessary for all infected wounds, not alone, but in combination with appropriate wound care. The strategy is to select an empirical antibiotic based on the suspected microorganisms and the grade of severity of the infection. The definitive use of chemotherapy should be based on the clinical response to the empirical antibiotic used and on both the culture results and susceptibility testing profile. The local antibiotic susceptibility testing data, as the occurrence of prevalent methicillin-resistant *S. aureus* (MRSA) or any other resistant bacteria and the recent use of antibiotics, must be considered [40–42]. Regarding to the treatment of most of the mild diabetic foot infections, oral antibiotics of appropriate bioavailability can be used, usually, for a period of 12 weeks but some may require treatment extension to another 12 weeks. On the other hand, the treatment of some of the mild superficial infections is just, topical chemotherapy [43, 44].

In DFU patients who have mild-to-moderate infections and do not receive antibiotic therapy, chemotherapy can be sufficient for aerobic Gram-positive cocci [36].

In many of the moderate infections, and some cases of osteomyelitis, appropriate oral antibiotics with adequate bioavailability can be used. A period of 24 weeks is usually enough for treating moderate and severe infections. This period depends on the structures involved in DFU infection, wound vascularity, the adequacy of debridement, and the type of soft-tissue wound cover [45]. Usually, broad-spectrum antibiotic regimens are required for diabetic patients at risk for infection with antibiotic-resistant organisms or with chronic infections, previously treated, or severe infections. In case of severe infections with pending culture results and antibiotic susceptibility, the empirical treatment with broad-spectrum antibiotic is indicated [1]. The failure of response of DFU infection to the prescribed antibiotic courses in a clinically stable patient drags the attention to the need of discontinuing all antimicrobials and after a few days, new specimens are to be collected for another optimal culture [14].

Treatment of diabetic patients with osteomyelitis requires a duration of treatment for at least 46 weeks that probably becomes longer with the presence of the infected bone, but shorter on entire infected bone removal. The antibiotic therapy should be continued until there is an evidence of resolution of the infection but not until a wound healing occur [43, 44, 46, 47].

Surgical consultation and intervention ranging from debridement to resection or amputation may be needed in diabetic foot infections [45, 48–52]. These diabetic foot infections are specially accompanied by a deep abscess, extensive bone, joint involvement, crepitus, substantial necrosis, gangrene, or necrotizing fasciitis. Evaluation of the limb's arterial supply and revascularizing is indicated in cases with ischemic foot in these infections [15, 16]. The debridement, rather than antibiotic treatment, significantly shifts the microbiota in DFU patients to favorable outcomes [35, 53–57]. The healing of DFU infection requires the provision of optimal wound care in the form of proper wound cleansing, debridement of any callus and necrotic tissue, and off-loading of pressure, together with the appropriate antibiotic treatment [45, 48, 50–52]. The regular follow-up of the patients is needed with proper dressing of the wounds and off-loaded of pressure. There is no evidence for recommending the use of wound healing agents or products for infected foot wounds or a specific wound dressing [58–60].

8.7 The Role of Adjunctive Therapies for Diabetic Foot Infections

Selected adjunctive measures may be useful for some nonresponding DFU patients [1]. Trials were carried out by systematic reviews to define the role of adjunctive therapies for diabetic foot infections. They suggested that applying systemic hyperbaric oxygen therapy and granulocyte colony-stimulating factors may help in preventing amputations in patients with severe infections or in patients with inadequate response to chemotherapy, despite the correction of their local and systemic adverse factors [61–64].

Interestingly, the development of diabetic foot ulceration can result from the increased magnitude of the local mechanical repetitive stresses on the foot by the use of inappropriate footwear or walking barefoot [65–68]. DFUs are one of the leading causes of lower extremity amputations, therefore, it is of paramount importance to prevent DFUs [69–73]. To help prevent diabetic foot ulceration, it is recommended that diabetic patients wear appropriate footwear designed to reduce repetitive stresses at all times. The adherence and prescription of wearing footwear has been studied, and evidenced effective and important maneuvers for ulcer prevention in diabetic people [67, 68, 74–83]. In this regard, ten key recommendations were published in Australia guidelines to guide the health professionals to select the most appropriate footwear for an individual with D.M. to meet the specific foot risk needs.

Updated Australia recommendations for selection of the footwear for diabetic patients are:

1. Wearing footwears that fit, protect, and accommodate the feet shape.
2. Always wear socks within footwear to reduce friction and shear.
3. Education to diabetics, their relatives, and caregivers about the importance of foot ulcer prevention by wearing the appropriate footwear.
4. In intermediate- or high-risk diabetic foot ulceration, the diabetic is instructed to obtain the footwear that fits, protects, and accommodates the shape of feet from a trained professional.
5. Diabetics with intermediate- or high-risk of foot ulceration are motivated to wear their footwear both indoors and outdoors.
6. In intermediate- or high-risk of foot ulceration, diabetic patients, or their relatives and caregivers are motivated to check the feet after footwear removal to ensure there are no trauma, ulceration or signs of abnormal pressure, and check their footwear before wearing, to ensure that there are no foreign objects in, or penetrating the footwear.
7. Prescription of medical grade footwear with custom-made in-shoe orthoses or insoles should be considered for people with a pre-ulcerative lesion or a foot deformity.
8. Prescription of medical grade footwear with custom-made in-shoe orthoses or insoles with a demonstrated plantar pressure-relieving effect at high-risk areas for healed plantar diabetic foot ulcer patients.
9. The prescribed footwear should be reviewed every 3 months to guarantee it still fits adequately, protects, and supports the foot.
10. Prescription of appropriate off-loading devices to heal plantar diabetic foot ulcers [84].

8.8 Summary

This chapter:

- Emphasizes the importance of the knowledge of microorganisms associated with diabetic foot ulcer (DFU) infections in the management of these infections and the prevention of their suspected complications.

- Discuss the microbiology and rate of infection in DFU, the various pathogens and colonizers associated with DFU infection.
- Outlines the pathogenesis process in infections of DFU.
- Demonstrates the laboratory examination procedures, starting from sample collection and processing, passing through the methods of cultivation aerobically and anaerobically, and finally testing the susceptibility pattern of significant isolates from DFU.
- Maps the treatment strategies of DFU, and drawing the attention to the coordinated management of DFU with a foot-care team.

References

1. Lipsky BA, Berendt AR, Cornia PB, Pile JC, Peters EJ, Armstrong DG, Deery HG, Embil JM, Joseph WS, Karchmer AW, Pinzur MS, Senneville E (2013) 2012 Infectious Diseases Society of America clinical practice guideline for the diagnosis and treatment of diabetic foot infections. J Am Podiatr Med Assoc 103(1):2–7
2. Singh N, Armstrong DG, Lipsky BA (2015) Preventing foot ulcers in patients with diabetes. JAMA 293:217–228
3. Ogba OM, Nsan E, Eyam ES (2019) Aerobic bacteria associated with diabetic foot ulcers and their susceptibility pattern. Biomed Dermatol 3:1
4. Altrichter LC, Legout L, Assal M, Rohner P, Hoffmeyer P, Bernard L (2015) Severe *Streptoccocus agalactiae* infection of the diabetic foot. Presse Med 34:491–494
5. Chin J (2013) The bacteriology of diabetic foot ulcers with a special reference to multidrug resistant strains. J Clin Diagn Res 7(3):441–445
6. Halpati A, Desai KJ, Ravindra J, Mayur P (2014) A study of aerobic and anaerobic bacteria in diabetic foot ulcer and in vitro sensitivity of antimicrobial agent. Int J Med Sci Public Health 3:818. https://doi.org/10.5455/ijmsph.2014.220420145
7. Wheat J, Allen SD, Henry M, Kernek CB (1986) Diabetic foot infections—bacteriological analysis. Arch Intern Med 146:1935–1940
8. Pal B, Gupta SK (2016) A study on the relation of the severity of diabetic foot ulcers with the type of bacterial flora isolated from the wounds. Int Surg J 3(1):189–194. https://doi.org/10.18203/2349-2902.isj20160224
9. Sloan TJ, Turton JC, Tyson J, Musgrove A, Fleming VM, Lister MM, Loose MW, Sockett RE, Diggle M, Game FL, Jeffcoate W (2019) Examining diabetic heel ulcers through an ecological lens: microbial community dynamics associated with healing and infection. J Med Microbiol 68(2):230–240. https://doi.org/10.1099/jmm.0.000907
10. Richard JL, Lavigne JP, Sotto A (2012) Diabetes and foot infection: more than double trouble. Diabetes Metab Res Rev 28:46–53
11. Ramakant P, Verma A, Misra R, Prasad K (2011) Changing microbiological profile of pathogenic bacteria in diabetic foot ulcer. Diabetologia 54(1):58–64
12. Lipsky BA, Berewdt AR, Cornia PB, Pile JC, Peters EY, Armstrong DG, Deery HG, Embil JM, Joseph WS, Karchmer HW, Pinzur MS, Sennevilk E (2012) 2012 Infectious Diseases Society of America clinical practices guideline for the diagnosis and treatment of diabetic foot infections. Clin Infect Dis 54:e132–e173
13. Raja NS (2007) Microbiology of diabetic foot infections in a teaching hospital in Malaysia: a retrospective study of 194 cases. J Microbiol Immunol Infect 40(1):39–44
14. Lipsky BA, Berendt AR, Deery HG, Embil JM, Joseph WS, Karchmer AW, LeFrock JL, Lew DP, Mader JT, Norden C, Tan JS, Infectious Diseases Society of America (2006) Diagnosis and treatment of diabetic foot infections. Plast Reconstr Surg 117(7 Suppl):212S–238S

15. American Diabetes Association (2003) Peripheral arterial disease in people with diabetes. Diabetes Care 26:3333–3341
16. Bridges RM Jr, Deitch EA (1994) Diabetic foot infections: pathophysiology and treatment. Surg Clin North Am 74:537–555
17. Nelson A, Wright-Hughes A, Backhouse MR, Lipsky BA, Nixon J, Bhogal MS, Reynolds C, Brown S, CODIFI Collaborators (2018) CODIFI (Concordance in Diabetic Foot Ulcer Infection): a cross-sectional study of wound swab versus tissue sampling in infected diabetic foot ulcers in England. BMJ Open 8(1):e019437. https://doi.org/10.1136/bmjopen-2017-019437
18. Pellizzer G, Strazzabosco M, Presi S et al (2001) Deep tissue biopsy vs. superficial swab culture monitoring in the microbiological assessment of limb-threatening diabetic foot infection. Diabet Med 18:822–827
19. Collee JG, Duguid JP, Fraser AG, Marmion BP, Simmons A (1989) Mackie and Mccarteny practical medical microbiology, 14th edn. Churchill Livingstone, Singapore
20. Sapico FL, Witte JL, Canawati HN, Montgomerie JZ, Bessman AN (1984) The infected foot of the diabetic patient: quantitative microbiology Guidelines for Diabetic Foot Infections • CID 2004:39 (1 October) • 905 and analysis of clinical features. Rev Infect Dis 6(Suppl 1):S171–S176
21. Ogba OM, Olorode OA, Adie GA (2014) Bacterial pathogens associated with wound infections in Calabar, Nigeria. J Med 13(1):26–33
22. Carvalho CB, Neto RM, Aragoa LP, Oliveira MM, Nogueira MB, Forti AC (2014) Diabetic foot ulcer infection, bacteriological analysis of 141 patients. Arq Bras Endocrinol Metabol 48:398–405
23. CLSI (2011) Performance standards for antimicrobial susceptibility testing; 21st informational supplement. CLSI document M100–S21. Wayne, Clinical and Laboratory Standards Institute
24. Anguzu JR, Olila D (2007) Drug sensitivity patterns of bacterial isolates from septic post-operative wounds in a regional referral hospital in Uganda. Afr J Health Sci 7(3):148–154
25. Ogba OM, Udo NI, Inyang-Etoh PC, Olorode OA (2017) Evaluation of the potency of commercial and locally prepared antibiotic discs on clinical bacterial isolates in Calabar, Nigeria. Int J Biomed Life Sci 2(1):1–7
26. Armstrong DG, Harkless LB (1998) Outcomes of preventative care in a diabetic foot specialty clinic. J Foot Ankle Surg 37:460–466
27. Crane M, Werber B (1999) Critical pathway approach to diabetic pedal infections in a multidisciplinary setting. J Foot Ankle Surg 38:30–33. discussion 82–83
28. Dargis V, Pantelejeva O, Jonushaite A, Vileikyte L, Boulton AJ (1999) Benefits of a multidisciplinary approach in the management of recurrent diabetic foot ulceration in Lithuania: a prospective study. Diabetes Care 22:1428–1431
29. Ragnarson Tennvall G, Apelqvist J (2001) Prevention of diabetes-related foot ulcers and amputations: a cost-utility analysis based on Markov model simulations. Diabetologia 44:2077–2087
30. Schaper NC, Apelqvist J, Bakker K (2003) The international consensus and practical guidelines on the management and prevention of the diabetic foot. Curr Diab Rep 3:475–479
31. Todd WF, Armstrong DG, Liswood PJ (1996) Evaluation and treatment of the infected foot in a community teaching hospital. J Am Podiatr Med Assoc 86:421–426
32. Armstrong DG, Liswood PJ, Todd WF (1995) Prevalence of mixed infections in the diabetic pedal wound: a retrospective review of 112 infections. 1995 William J. Stickel bronze award. J Am Podiatr Med Assoc 85:533–537
33. Calhoun JH, Cantrell J, Cobos J et al (1988) Treatment of diabetic foot infections: Wagner classification, therapy, and outcome. Foot Ankle 9:101–106
34. Edelson GW, Armstrong DG, Lavery LA, Caicco G (1996) The acutely infected diabetic foot is not adequately evaluated in an inpatient setting. Arch Intern Med 156:2373–2378
35. Kalan LR, Meisel JS, Loesche MA, Horwinski J, Soaita I, Chen X, Uberoi A, Gardner SE, Grice EA (2019) Strain- and species-level variation in the microbiome of diabetic wounds is associated with clinical outcomes and therapeutic efficacy. Cell Host Microbe 25(5):641–655.e5. https://doi.org/10.1016/j.chom.2019.03.006

36. Lipsky BA, Pecoraro RE, Larson SA, Hanley ME, Ahroni JH (1990) Outpatient management of uncomplicated lower-extremity infections in diabetic patients. Arch Intern Med 150:790–797
37. Nelson EA, O'Meara S, Craig D, Iglesias C, Golder S, Dalton J, Claxton K, Bell-Syer SE, Jude E, Dowson C, Gadsby R, O'Hare P, Powell J (2006) A series of systematic reviews to inform a decision analysis for sampling and treating infected diabetic foot ulcers. Health Technol Assess 10(12):iii–iv. ix–x, 1–221
38. Piwernetz K, Home PD, Snorgaard O, Antsiferov M, Staehr-Johansen K, Krans M (1993) Monitoring the targets of the St. Vincent Declaration and the implementation of quality management in diabetes care: the DIABCARE initiative. The DIABCARE Monitoring Group of the St. Vincent Declaration Steering Committee. Diabet Med 10:371–377
39. Wright PR, Roye GK, Bodonaik N (2011) The medical management of diabetes mellitus with particular reference to lower extremity: the Jamaican experience. West Indian Med J 50(1):46–49
40. Asfar SK, al-Arouj M, al-Nakhi A, Baraka A, Juma T, Johny M (1993) Foot infections in diabetics: the antibiotic choice. Can J Surg 36:170–172
41. Cunha BA (2000) Antibiotic selection for diabetic foot infections: a review. J Foot Ankle Surg 39:253–257
42. West NJ (1995) Systemic antimicrobial treatment of foot infections in diabetic patients. Am J Health Syst Pharm 52:1199–1207. quiz, 1239–1240
43. Lipsky BA, McDonald D, Litka P (1997) Treatment of infected diabetic foot ulcers: topical MSI-78 vs. oral ofloxacin. Diabetologia 40:482
44. Lipsky BA (1999) Evidence-based antibiotic therapy of diabetic foot infections. FEMS Immunol Med Microbiol 26:267–276
45. American Diabetes Association (1999) Consensus development conference on diabetic foot wound care: 7–8 April 1999, Boston, Massachusetts. Diabetes Care 22:1354–1360
46. Grayson ML, Gibbons GW, Habershaw GM et al (1994) Use of ampicillin/sulbactam versus imipenem/cilastatin in the treatment of limb-threatening foot infections in diabetic patients. Clin Infect Dis 18:683–693
47. Lobmann R, Ambrosch A, Seewald M et al (2004) Antibiotic therapy for diabetic foot infections: comparison of cephalosporins with quinolones. Diabetes Nutr Metab 17:156–162
48. Armstrong DG, Nguyen HC (2000) Improvement in healing with aggressive edema reduction after debridement of foot infection in persons with diabetes. Arch Surg 135:1405–1409
49. Chaytor ER (2000) Surgical treatment of the diabetic foot. Diabetes Metab Res Rev 16(Suppl 1):S66–S69
50. Jones V (1998) Debridement of diabetic foot lesions. Diabet Foot 1:88–94
51. Rauwerda JA (2000) Foot debridement: anatomic knowledge is mandatory. Diabetes Metab Res Rev 16(Suppl 1):S23–S26
52. Smith J, Thow J (2001) Is debridement effective for diabetic foot ulcers? A systematic review: 1. Diabet Foot 1:10–14
53. Gill LH (1994) Foot surgery in the patient with diabetes. J South Orthop Assoc 3:261–267
54. Giurini JM, Rosenblum BI (1995) The role of foot surgery in patients with diabetes. Clin Podiatr Med Surg 12:119–127
55. Pinzur MS, Sage R, Abraham M, Osterman H (1988) Limb salvage in infected lower extremity gangrene. Foot Ankle 8:212–215
56. Steffen C, O'Rourke S (1998) Surgical management of diabetic foot complications: the Far North Queensland profile. Aust N Z J Surg 68:258–260
57. Tan JS, Friedman NM, Hazelton-Miller C, Flanagan JP, File TM Jr (1996) Can aggressive treatment of diabetic foot infections reduce the need for above-ankle amputation? Clin Infect Dis 23:286–291
58. Embil JM, Papp K, Sibbald G et al (2000) Recombinant human platelet-derived growth factor-BB (becaplermin) for healing chronic lower extremity diabetic ulcers: an open-label clinical evaluation of efficacy. Wound Repair Regen 8:162–168

59. Nagai MK, Embil JM (2002) Becaplermin: recombinant platelet derived growth factor, a new treatment for healing diabetic foot ulcers. Expert Opin Biol Ther 2:211–218
60. Robson MC, Mustoe TA, Hunt TK (1998) The future of recombinant growth factors in wound healing. Am J Surg 176:80S–82S
61. Bakker DJ (2000) Hyperbaric oxygen therapy and the diabetic foot. Diabetes Metab Res Rev 16(Suppl 1):S55–S58
62. Kalani M, Jorneskog G, Naderi N, Lind F, Brismar K (2002) Hyperbaric oxygen (HBO) therapy in treatment of diabetic foot ulcers: long-term follow-up. J Diabetes Complicat 16:153–158
63. Wang C, Schwaitzberg S, Berliner E, Zarin DA, Lau J (2003) Hyperbaric oxygen for treating wounds: a systematic review of the literature. Arch Surg 138:272–279
64. Wunderlich RP, Peters EJ, Lavery LA (2000) Systemic hyperbaric oxygen therapy: lower-extremity wound healing and the diabetic foot. Diabetes Care 23:15515
65. Crawford F, Cezard G, Chappell FM, Murray GD, Price JF, Sheikh A, Simpson CR, Stansby GP, Young MJA (2015) Systematic review and individual patient data meta-analysis of prognostic factors for foot ulceration in people with diabetes: the international research collaboration for the prediction of diabetic foot ulcerations (PODUS). Health Technol Assess 19(57):1–210
66. Monteiro-Soares M, Boyko EJ, Ribeiro J, Ribeiro I, Dinis-Ribeiro M (2012) Predictive factors for diabetic foot ulceration: a systematic review. Diabetes Metab Res Rev 28(7):574–600
67. Schaper NC, Van Netten JJ, Apelqvist J, Lipsky BA, Bakker K, International Working Group on the Diabetic Foot (2016) Prevention and management of foot problems in diabetes: a Summary Guidance for Daily Practice 2015, based on the IWGDF Guidance Documents. Diabetes Metab Res Rev 32(Suppl 1):7–15
68. Waaijman R, de Haart M, Arts ML, Wever D, Verlouw AJ, Nollet F, Bus SA (2014) Risk factors for plantar foot ulcer recurrence in neuropathic diabetic patients. Diabetes Care 37(6):1697–1705
69. Boulton AJ, Vileikyte L, Ragnarson-Tennvall G, Apelqvist J (2005) The global burden of diabetic foot disease. Lancet 366(9498):1719–1724
70. Jupiter DC, Thorud JC, Buckley CJ, Shibuya N (2016) The impact of foot ulceration and amputation on mortality in diabetic patients. I: From ulceration to death, a systematic review. Int Wound J 13(5):892–903
71. Lazzarini PA, Hurn SE, Fernando ME, Jen SD, Kuys SS, Kamp MC, Reed LF (2015) Prevalence of foot disease and risk factors in general inpatient populations: a systematic review and meta-analysis. BMJ Open 5(11):e008544
72. Lazzarini PA, Hurn SE, Kuys SS, Kamp MC, Ng V, Thomas C, Jen S, Wills J, Kinnear EM, d'Emden MC, Reed LF (2017) The silent overall burden of foot disease in a representative hospitalized population. Int Wound J 14(4):716–728
73. Tapp RJ, Shaw JE, De Courten MP, Dunstan DW, Welborn TA, Zimmet PZ (2003) Foot complications in type 2 diabetes: an Australian population-based study. Diabet Med 20(2):105–113
74. Arts ML, de Haart M, Waaijman R, Dahmen R, Berendsen H, Nollet F, Bus SA (2015) Data-driven directions for effective footwear provision for the high-risk diabetic foot. Diabet Med 32(6):790–797
75. Bus SA, van Deursen RW, Armstrong DG, Lewis JE, Caravaggi CF, Cavanagh PR (2016) International working group on the diabetic foot. Footwear and offloading interventions to prevent and heal foot ulcers and reduce plantar pressure in patients with diabetes: a systematic review. Diabetes Metab Res Rev 32(Suppl 1):99–118
76. Bus SA, van Netten JJ, Lavery LA, Monteiro-Soares M, Rasmussen A, Jubiz Y, Price PE (2016) International working group on the diabetic foot. IWGDF guidance on the prevention of foot ulcers in at-risk patients with diabetes. Diabetes Metab Res Rev 32(Suppl 1):16–24
77. Bus SA, Waaijman R, Arts M, de Haart M, Busch-Westbroek T, van Baal J, Nollet F (2013) Effect of custom-made footwear on foot ulcer recurrence in diabetes: a multicenter randomized controlled trial. Diabetes Care 36(12):4109–4116

78. Healy A, Naemi R, Chockalingam N (2013) The effectiveness of footwear as an intervention to prevent or to reduce biomechanical risk factors associated with diabetic foot ulceration: a systematic review. J Diabetes Complicat 27:391–400
79. Lewis J, Lipp A (2013) Pressure-relieving interventions for treating diabetic foot ulcers. Cochrane Database Syst Rev 1:CD002302
80. Morona JK, Buckley ES, Jones S, Reddin EA, Merlin TL (2013) Comparison of the clinical effectiveness of different off-loading devices for the treatment of neuropathic foot ulcers in patients with diabetes: a systematic review and meta-analysis. Diabetes Metab Res Rev 29(3):183–193
81. Paton J, Bruce G, Jones R, Stenhouse E (2011) Effectiveness of insoles used for the prevention of ulceration in the neuropathic diabetic foot: a systematic review. J Diabetes Complicat 25(1):52–62
82. Ulbrecht JS, Hurley T, Mauger DT, Cavanagh PR (2014) Prevention of recurrent foot ulcers with plantar pressure-based in-shoe orthoses: the careful prevention multicenter randomized controlled trial. Diabetes Care 37(7):1982–1989
83. van Netten JJ, Price PE, Lavery LA, Monteiro-Soares M, Rasmussen A, Jubiz Y, Bus SA (2016) International working group on the diabetic foot. Prevention of foot ulcers in the at-risk patient with diabetes: a systematic review. Diabetes Metab Res Rev 32(Suppl 1):84–98
84. van Netten JJ, Lazzarini PA, Armstrong DG, Bus SA, Fitridge R, Harding K, Kinnear E, Malone M, Menz HB, Perrin BM, Postema K, Prentice J, Schott K-H, Wright PR (2018) Diabetic Foot Australia guideline on footwear for people with diabetes. J Foot Ankle Res 11(2). https://doi.org/10.1186/s13047-017-0244-z

MRSA, EBSL, and Biofilm Formation in Diabetic Foot Ulcer Infections

9

Fohad Mabood Husain, Mohammad Shavez Khan, Mohammad Zubair, Altaf Khan, Saba Noor, Iftekhar Hassan, Mohammed Arshad, Mohd Shahnawaz Khan, Faizan Abul Qais, and Salman Al-Amery

9.1 Introduction

Diabetes and its related complications are considered as one of the major causes of morbidity and mortality round the globe [1]. Diabetes is a noncommunicable metabolic syndrome may either characterized by defective or decreased level of insulin secretion [2]. The current estimate on global diabetes epidemiology reveals that

F. M. Husain (✉)
Department of Food Science and Nutrition, College of Food and Agriculture Sciences, King Saud University, Riyadh, Kingdom of Saudi Arabia
e-mail: fhusain@ksu.edu.sa

M. S. Khan · F. A. Qais
Department of Agricultural Microbiology, Aligarh Muslim University, Aligarh, India

M. Zubair
Department of Medical Microbiology, Faculty of Medicine, University of Tabuk, Tabuk, Kingdom of Saudi Arabia

A. Khan
Department of Pharmacology and Toxicology, Central Laboratory, College of Pharmacy, King Saud University, Riyadh, Kingdom of Saudi Arabia

S. Noor
National Institute of Cancer Prevention and Research, Noida, Uttar Pradesh, India

I. Hassan
Department of Zoology, College of Science, King Saud University, Riyadh, Kingdom of Saudi Arabia

M. Arshad
Department of Clinical Laboratory Sciences, College of Applied Medical Sciences, King Saud University, Riyadh, Kingdom of Saudi Arabia

M. S. Khan · S. Al-Amery
Department of Biochemistry, College of Science, King Saud University, Riyadh, Kingdom of Saudi Arabia

M. Zubair et al. (eds.), *Diabetic Foot Ulcer*,
https://doi.org/10.1007/978-981-15-7639-3_9

roughly under half of billion population is affected by diabetes and associated pathologies and is projected to increase by around 50% by 2045 [3].

One of the most severe and dreadful complications of diabetes mellitus is diabetic foot infections (DFIs). These infections are consequent to skin ulceration characterizes with loss of peripheral neuropathy (protective sensation) and also with some forms of trauma. The developed wounds serve as ideal spot for the colonization and multiplication of a wide range of pathogenic microorganisms and facilitate their entry into tissues leading to the inflammatory response [4]. Infectious disease society of America classified diabetic foot infections as mild, moderate, and severe subject to extent of damage been done to infected foot [5]. However, the majority of infections are superficial while about quarter of total infection is deep enough which spread from epidermal layer to inner regions including subcutaneous tissues and bones leading to necrotic fasciitis, osteomyelitis, and septic arthritis [6]. Patients with DFIs are also shown to develop some level of peripheral arterial disease as describe with restriction in blood supply to tissues and causing oxygen deficit needed for cellular metabolism (Ischemia) which results into peripheral tissue dysfunction [7]. These types of invasive infections are the most frequent and severe in patients with diabetes mellitus [8]. It has been estimated that nearly one-third of patients with diabetes develop a diabetic foot ulcer at one or other stage of disease progression [9]. Furthermore, diabetic foot infection/diabetic foot ulceration exponentially increases the probability of amputations, with a factor of 155 times higher than those patients having no diabetes [10]. Recent study also has shown that patient anxiety related to amputation is extremely high, a person with diabetes and associated foot infection feared amputation more than death, as compared to diabetic patients without foot infection/foot ulceration pathologies [11]. Death risk associated with diabetic foot infection is also significant when infection runs deep into the internal tissues [12]. It has been estimated that 5 year mortality rate of patients with diabetic foot infection/ulceration is about 50% that is higher than those of different types of cancer including prostate cancer, breast cancer, and Hodgkin lymphoma [13, 14].

Since DFI/DFU are colonized with numerous pathogenic microorganism, the problem is further compounded with increasing incidence of antimicrobial resistance among them [10]. Progression in colonization of these microorganism leads to the development of biofilm, a self-embedded bacterial community with altered metabolic and physical parameters [15]. These microbial biofilms when formed and specially reached to internal tissues possess great difficulty in the removal and subsequent getting rid of infections [16]. Antimicrobial therapy constitute a major component of DFIs management practices, however injudicious and inappropriate use of antibiotics make it difficult to eliminate multidrug-resistance bacteria. Thus it is indispensable to have a broader and subjective understanding of drug resistance among the microbial community with special focus drug resistant biofilm formation in infected feet for successful treatment regimen. In this chapter, an attempt has been made to present a brief review of different type multidrug-resistance bacteria (MRSA and ESβL) associated with diabetic foot infections with special focus on biofilms formation.

9.2 Microbiology of DFIs/DFUs

The microbiological profile of DFIs/DFUs is varied and depend upon specific geographical/environmental setting, duration, and stage of progression of the disease, antibiotic use history, and significance of infections [17]. Further, the development of infection varied with aspects such as microbial load at specific time, diversity among the colonized microbial population, presence of pathogenic/invasive microorganism, and synergistic association between the populations [18]. Once the microbial load reaches greater value than 105 organisms per gram of tissue, the infection is considered to be initiated [2]. As evident from a different culture and non-culture based techniques, different aerobic and non-aerobic bacterial communities have been identified. At initial stage of simple epidermal infection, Gram-positive cocci (*Staphylococcus* and *Streptococcus* spp.) were mainly found to colonize. While, in case of chronic infections/ulcerations may be characterized with predominantly polymicrobial communities of different type of aerobic pathogens such as *Staphylococcus*, *Streptococcus*, *Enterococcus*, *Pseudomonas* spp. along with pathogenic anaerobes [19, 20]. *Pseudomonas aeruginosa* and *S. aureus* are predominant Gram-negative and Gram-positive bacterial species present in feet infections/ulcers [21, 22]. Studies carried out at tertiary care center in developing countries revealed that infections caused multidrug-resistant aerobic microbes, as mention above, are predominant [23, 24]. Moreover, in these geographical regions with warm climates, *P. aeruginosa* is more prevalent while *S. aureus* is less prevalent [25, 26], which may be attributed to environmental factors, footwear, personal hygiene, antibiotic treatment history, etc. [19]. Whereas, in colder regions, Gram-positive aerobes predominantly *S. aureus* is more common than members of Enterobacteriaceae and *Pseudomonas* [4]. Deeper chronic DFIs associated with ischemia, necrosis, foul odor, or gangrene are predominantly occupied with anaerobes [27]. The most abundant anaerobic bacterial pathogens found in infected feet is *Bacteroides fragilis,* which has been reported in various studies [28, 29]. Although it was also evident from these studies that the abundance of anaerobic microflora is low and also have a lesser impact on the progression of infection or their significance in the infection is not clearly understood [29].

Recent studies highlighted the increasing incidence of multidrug-resistance pathogens in DFIs and resultant grave outcomes [30]. *Staphylococcus aureus* is one of the major causative organisms in the majority of all clinical DFIs associated with clinical phenotypes ranging from acute paronychia to deeper chronic osteomyelitis and severe soft tissue necrosis [30, 31]. Methicillin-resistant *Staphylococcus aureus* (MRSA) is now considered as a chief infectious agent in the feet infections of diabetic persons specifically for skin and soft tissues. These MRSA associated skin and soft tissue infections are more difficult to eradicate in diabetic patients when compare to those having no diabetes at all [32]. However, there is still a need for objective research to attribute the consequences that MRSA has on other clinical outcomes in patients with diabetes-associated foot infection [33]. Continues progression of antimicrobial resistance (AMR) in Gram-negative bacteria have now encompassed nearly all the available representative of present antibiotic arsenal. Resistants have been emerged against advanced generation cephalosporins which are attributed to the emergence of extended-spectrum beta-lactamases (ESβL) and AmpC-β-lactamases [34]. "Pan resistant" isolates of Gram-negative bacterial species of Pseudomonas and Acinetobacter are of severe life-threatening nature which is being reported in DFIs [35]. Among other factors responsible for the development of AMR in microbial communities residing in diabetic foot settings, biofilm formation is considered as a major driving force. Biofilms provide protective barriers against antibiotics treatment, moreover, the altered metabolic rate of bacteria enclosed in bacteria also supplement their resistance potential [10, 15, 36]. Biofilms formation is multistage process and well-known virulence factors enabling the bacterial community to cope with challenging environmental stresses such as the presence of antimicrobial in the settings. As mention above, it is well known that microbial cells in surface-attached biofilms are physiologically distinct from their planktonic counterparts residing in the liquid medium [37]. The overall resistance observed in biofilms is different from than those of planktonic cells, sometimes 1000 times higher [38]. Since DFIs are associated with polymicrobial drug resistance microbial communities, polymicrobial biofilms further complicate the problem of drug resistance and possess an even greater challenge for effective antibiotic therapy [15, 36].

9.3 Methicillin-Resistant *Staphylococcus aureus* (MRSA) and Diabetic Foot Ulcers

Methicillin was the first synthetic penicillin introduced in 1960 to treat the infection caused by *S. aureus*. However, the joy was short-lived as methicillin-resistant strains of *S. aureus* (MRSA) surfaced in hospitals [39]. This was followed by several outbreaks of MRSA leading to severe morbidity as well as high mortality [40].

There are kinds of MRSA, one is hospital-acquired (HA-MRSA) and the second one is community-acquired (CA-MRSA). HA-MRSA is also known as nosocomial infection as it acquired from hospital and other medical settings while CA-MRSA as the name suggests is acquired from the community. Diabetic people are prone to both HA and CA-MRSA due to the presence of pores and ulcerations [41].

MRSA produces a penicillin-binding protein PBP2a having low binding affinities for most of the penicillin as well as cephalosporins/cephamycins. Methicillin resistance in *S. aureus* is attributed to the presence of Staphylococcal cassette chromosome mec (SCCmec) element, that carries methicillin-resistance determinant mecA. CA-MRSA carries *SCCmecA type IV* or *V* elements while HA-MRSA carries larger *SCCmecA type I, II, III* elements along with multidrug resistance (MDR) genes [41].

In the current review, we discuss the reports on MRSA infection in diabetic foot infection published in the last 10 years. Centre for Disease Control (CDC) recognizes MRSA as microorganisms having a serious threat level. Incidence and prevalence of MRSA differ in different geographical zones. According to a report published by US military Health system for a period of 5 years (2005–2010), HA-MRSA bacteremia decreased from 0.7 to 0.4 cases per 100,000 patients per year while CA-MRSA bacteremia came down from 1.7 cases per 100,000 patients per year to 1.4 cases per year [42]. In a retrospective case-control study conducted in China on 118 type 2 diabetes patients with DFI, *S. aureus* was found to be the most common pathogen (25.6%). High percentage of *S. aureus* was found to be MRSA (63.4%) and a high proportion of these MRSA satisfied the criteria for hospital-acquired MRSA (HA-MRSA) infection [43]. Lavery et al. [44] did a cohort study to evaluate the risk factors for MRSA in patients admitted with DFIs. They reported the presence of MRSA in 29.8% infections and risk factors for MRSA diabetic foot infections were history of MRSA foot infection, MRSA nasal colonization, and multidrug-resistant organisms ($p < 0.05$). Positive predictive value (PPV) and negative predictive value (NPV) of nasal colonization with MRSA to identify MRSA diabetic foot infections were 66.7% and 80.0% (sensitivity 41%, specificity 90%). In another study conducted on 318 patients in a USA hospital, around 46% patients with diabetic foot infection (DFI) had *S. aureus* infection of which 15% had MRSA infection [45]. In a similar investigation, 80 DFI specimen were collected in a hospital in Iran over a period of 1 year. Phenotypic identification resulted in 35% MRSA and 32% *S. aureus* were found to be resistant to methicillin carrying *mecA* gene by PCR [46]. In Korea, a pilot study on 737 patients with DFUs admitted between January 2012–December 2016 was conducted. Among 832 microbial isolates, 13.7% (114) were identified as MRSA [47].

In a study in Southwest China, 428 patients were enrolled and 555 strains were cultivated. Among isolated bacteria, 85 were *S. aureus,* of which 17 were MRSA [48]. A prospective investigation of 261 with DFIs in intensive care unit of a tertiary care hospital was performed over a 2-year period. A total of 289 isolates were cultivated and the most abundant bacteria were found to be *S. aureus* (26.9%). Among *S. aureus*, 23.7% were resistant to methicillin [24]. Recently, in Kenya, a cross-sectional study was conducted to identify bacteria in DFUs and to compare conventional microbiological methods with RT-PCR for the detection of MRSA. RT-PCR based identification of MRSA was accomplished in isolated bacteria whereas, culture methods could not identify MRSA among isolated bacteria [49].

9.4 Extended Spectrum Beta-Lactamases and Diabetic Foot Infection

Extended-spectrum beta-lactamases (ESβL) are enzymes produce by certain bacteria that can hydrolyze cephalosporins like ceftazidime, ceftriaxone, cefotaxime, and oxyiminomonobactum [50]. Gram-negative bacteria, especially Enterobacteriaceae and *Pseudomonas aeruginosa* are known to produce ESβLs [50]. Most ESβLs are derivatives of TEM or SHV enzymes. There are now >90 TEM-type β-lactamases and >25 SHV-type enzymes. With both of these groups of enzymes, a few point mutations at selected loci within the gene give rise to the extended-spectrum phenotype. TEM- and SHV-type ESβLs are most often found in *E. coli* and *K. pneumoniae*; however, they have also been found in *Proteus* spp., *Providencia* spp., and other genera of Enterobacteriaceae. In recent years a new family of plasmid-mediated ESBLs, called CTX-M, that preferentially hydrolyze cefotaxime has arisen. They have mainly been found in strains of *Salmonella* enterica serovar Typhimurium and *E. coli*, but have also been described in other species of Enterobacteriaceae [51].

The emergence of ESβLs has rendered the current antimicrobial therapy ineffective as they make infection-causing bacteria resistant to cephalosporins, the "workhorse" antibiotics. ESβL producers often are associated with multidrug resistance, so any delay in the identification and failure to treat infections caused by ESβL producing pathogen can lead to severe morbidity as well as mortality [52]. It is therefore imperative to review the prevalence of ESβL producers in patients with DFUs in order to control the spread of infection. In India, over a period of 1 year 191 samples were collected from indoor patients with DFIs in a tertiary care hospital. ESβL production was observed in 46.51% of the 43 isolated *E. coli* strains and 44.44% of the 27 *K. pneumoniae* isolated [53]. Zubair et al. [54] studied 60 patients with DFI. They found that 23.3% patients were infected by multidrug-resistant (MDR) strains and 45% of the isolated Gram-negative bacteria were ESβL producers. The prevalence of $bla_{CTX\text{-}M}$ (33%) gene was highest followed by bla_{SHV} and least was bla_{TEM} gene. In another study conducted by the same group in a tertiary care hospital of North India over a period of 3 years, it was found that out of 127 isolates belonging to Enterobacteriaceae, 81.9% were found to be positive for the bla gene, of which $bla_{CTX\text{-}M}$ showed 81.8% positivity, followed by bla_{TEM} (50%) and bla_{SHV} (46.9%) [55]. Similarly, a retrospective study was carried out between June 2007 to July 2008 in Kuwait on the microbiological profile of DFIs and their drug susceptibility. ESβL producers were identified from the 777 pathogens isolated. Double disk synergy and ESβL test revealed 11% and 14% of the *E. coli* and *K. pneumoniae* were producing extended-spectrum beta-lactamases, respectively [56].

In Egypt, 91 patients with DFUs were examined and a total of 135 Gram-negative bacteria was recovered from ulcer specimens. Initial screening results demonstrated 114 bacteria as ESβL producers but confirmatory test revealed that 58 of these 114 bacteria produced ESβL and 8 of these were plasmid mediated. Majority of these 8 strains carried 2 or more ESβL genes on the same plasmid. The most common combination was $bla_{CTX\text{-}M}$ and bla_{TEM} (n = 3/8; 37.5%), followed by bla_{SHV} and $bla_{CTX\text{-}M}$ (n = 2/8; 25%) and $bla_{CTX\text{-}M}$ + bla_{TEM} + bla_{SHV} (n = 1/8;12.5%). One strain of harbored a plasmid (pECDF16) coding for the three ESβL genes [57].

Clinical samples from 150 patients were collected over a period of 1 year and examined for the incidence of ESβL, AmpC, and MBL producing *Pseudomonas* spp. Majority (80%) of the isolated *Pseudomonas* spp. were multidrug resistant and 22.9%, 42.8% and 14.4% of the Pseudomonads produced ESβL, AmpC, and MBL, respectively. Mortality was found to be 20% in these patients [58]. In a study conducted in Pakistan, among the isolated bacteria 66% of the *K. pneumoniae* were found to produce ESβL. Overall prevalence of β-lactamase (bla)-CTX-M, bla-CTX-M-15, bla-TEM, bla-OXA, and bla-SHV genes was found to be 76.9%, 76.9%, 75.0%, 57.7% and 84.6%, respectively, in Gram-negative DFI isolates. The prevalence of antibiotic resistance genes was considered alarmingly high in the studied DFIs [59]. In a recent report, a pilot study was conducted across 19 centers in

Turkey, between May 2011 and December 2015. In total, 791 patients with DFIs were included in the investigation and 536 microorganisms were isolated. Antibiotic resistance profiling revealed that 21% *Pseudomonas aeruginosa* were multidrug resistant and 38% *E. coli* and *K. pneumoniae* were found to be ESβL positive. Further, 3% [24] mortality was also reported [30].

9.5 Biofilm and Diabetic Foot Infections

Biofilms are a complex structure of microorganisms encapsulated in a matrix of exo-polysaccharides or exo-polymeric substances that attach to living or inert surface [60]. Most biofilms are polymicrobial and consist of bacteria, fungi, viruses, protein, extracellular DNA, and several biological factors. Biofilms not only confers resistance to the microbes residing in biofilm mode but protects the microbes and helps survive in hostile environmental conditions [61]. Several reports have emerged that studied the formation of biofilm and the presence of multidrug-resistant microorganisms in DFIs [62, 63].

9.5.1 Biofilm Formation

Biofilm formation takes place by the reversible attachment of the microbe as the first step. This attachment is facilitated by pili, flagella, surface appendages, or specific receptors. This is followed by EPS mediated irreversible attachment to the substratum. In the third stage, cells multiply and microcolony formation takes place. In the fourth step, biofilm matures by the growth and differentiation of the cells, and finally in the fifth stage biofilm cells disperse actively or by passive detachment [64]. EPS plays a key role in the formation and maintenance of biofilm. EPS protects the cells from the harsh environment, prevents the entry of antimicrobials, and protects from the action of the immune system. EPS also protects the biofilm cells from dessication, facilitates ion exchange, houses, and maintains degradation enzymes and carries nutrients [65].

9.5.2 Biofilm Virulence and Wound Care

Diabetic foot ulcers/infections are included in the class of chronic wounds. The annual incidence of foot ulcers in diabetic patients is 1–4% in the USA, with a lifetime risk of occurrence of between 15% and 25%. In 2006, the total cost of treatment, amputation, rehabilitation, and long-term care of diabetic foot ulcers in the USA totaled $10.9 billion [66]. Therefore, it is very important to study how biofilms are the cause of persistent infections and hamper effective wound care. Cells residing in the biofilm mode are sessile and in comparison to their free-living planktonic counterparts are metabolically less active. Reduced metabolic activity increases resistance to antimicrobials as most antibiotics are effective against actively dividing cells as, for example, beta-lactams target peptidoglycan, aminoglycosides disrupt the protein synthesis and quinolones interfere with DNA replication [67]. Further, EPS prevents the entry of antimicrobials and protects from the action of the immune system [65]. Stimulation of the immune system without effectively curing the infection causes collateral damage to the surrounding tissues and inflammation becomes chronic. This not only aggravates the wounds but impedes the healing action considerably [61].

Biofilm increases the probability for the transfer of drug resistance genes carried on mobile genetic elements like plasmids. This transfer of resistance genes can be intraspecies as well as interspecies, thus making the infections more virulent and persistent [68].

In addition to the drug resistance, tolerance to antibiotics is another property of the biofilm cells. Tolerance is not plasmid mediated but is believed to be a result of metabolically inactive biofilm cells [69]. Tolerance to drugs is a transient phenotype that allows the maintenance of a subpopulation of cells in the wounds, called *persister* cells. Upon suspension of the drug therapy, the persister cells regenerate to give rise to biofilm cells that retain the similar susceptibility profile of the original biofilm, so the persister cells are maintained. Drug therapy is rendered ineffective, treatment failure of the wound occurs and infections become persistent [70].

Removal of necrotic tissues and microbial load through debridement is an essential and important part of the wound care [71]. Since EPS facilitates irreversible attachment of the biofilm cells to the wound bed, it makes debridement rather difficult and incomplete as some cells remain attached to the wound bed and are not removed. These leftover cells regenerate and form biofilms again leading to recurrent infections [72].

Biofilm formation is a dangerous property of the microbiome that colonizes diabetic foot wounds. Consequently, the last few decades have seen a major problem in treating DFU infections due to the ever-increasing rate of colonization by drug-resistant pathogens. The presence of MRSA, ESβL, and MβL producing bacteria along with the formation of polymicrobial biofilms are some of the major causes of the DFI/Us healing impediment [15].

9.6 Conclusion

The severity of the diabetic foot infections and the huge amount of money that is involved in the prevention, treatment, and control have made researchers as well as medical practitioners to understand the mechanisms involved and device strategies to interfere with them. Diabetic foot infections caused by biofilm-forming bacteria that produce mecA and ESβL enzymes are on the upsurge and are very much responsible for the increasing amputations. The resistance of DFIs to antimicrobials has made treatment very challenging. Further, dissemination of the resistant strains coupled with the slow development of new antibiotics has made the task of treating DFIs herculean. Therefore, new alternative approaches are required to combat the problem of drug resistance.

Acknowledgments The authors extend their appreciation to Research Centre, College of Food and Agriculture Sciences, Deanship of Scientific Research at King Saud University for funding this work.

References

1. WHO (2018). Available from: https://www.who.int/news-room/fact-sheets/detail/diabetes
2. Noor S, Zubair M, Ahmad J (2015) Diabetic foot ulcer – a review on pathophysiology, classification and microbial etiology. Diabetes Metab Syndr Clin Res Rev 9(3):192–199. https://doi.org/10.1016/j.dsx.2015.04.007
3. Saeedi P, Petersohn I, Salpea P, Malanda B, Karuranga S, Unwin N et al (2019) Global and regional diabetes prevalence estimates for 2019 and projections for 2030 and 2045: results from the international diabetes federation diabetes atlas, 9th edition. Diabetes Res Clin Pract 157:107843. https://doi.org/10.1016/j.diabres.2019.107843
4. Kwon KT, Armstrong DG (2018) Microbiology and antimicrobial therapy for diabetic foot infections. Infect Chemother 50(1):11–20
5. Lipsky B (2001) Infectious problems of the foot in diabetic patients. In: Bowker J, Pfeifer M (eds) The diabetic foot. Mosby, St. Louis, pp 467–480
6. Lipsky BA, Berendt AR, Deery HG, Embil JM, Joseph WS, Karchmer AW et al (2004) IDSA guidelines: diagnosis and treatment of diabetic foot infections. Clin Infect Dis 39:885–910
7. Lipsky BA, Berendt AR, Cornia PB, Pile JC, Peters EJG, Armstrong DG et al (2012) 2012 infectious diseases society of America clinical practice guideline for the diagnosis and treatment of diabetic foot infections. Clin Infect Dis 54(12):132–173
8. Alves C, Casqueiro J, Casqueiro J (2012) Infections in patients with diabetes mellitus: a review of pathogenesis. Indian J Endocrinol Metab 16(7):27
9. Commons RJ, Raby E, Athan E, Bhally H, Chen S, Guy S et al (2018) Managing diabetic foot infections: a survey of Australasian infectious diseases clinicians. J Foot Ankle Res 11(1):1–8
10. Chastain CA, Klopfenstein N, Serezani CH, Aronoff DM (2019) A clinical review of diabetic foot infections. Clin Podiatr Med Surg 36(3):381–395. https://doi.org/10.1016/j.cpm.2019.02.004
11. Wukich DK, Raspovic KM, Suder NC (2018) Patients with diabetic foot disease fear major lower-extremity amputation more than death. Foot Ankle Spec 11(1):17–21
12. Fincke BG, Miller DR, Turpin R (2010) A classification of diabetic foot infections using ICD-9-CM codes: application to a large computerized medical database. BMC Health Serv Res 10:192
13. Armstrong DG, Wrobel J, Robbins JM (2007) Guest editorial: are diabetes-related wounds and amputations worse than cancer? Int Wound J 4(4):286–287
14. Robbins JM, Strauss G, Aron D, Long J, Kuba J, Kaplan Y (2008) Mortality rates and diabetic foot ulcers: is it time to communicate mortality risk to patients with diabetic foot ulceration? J Am Podiatr Med Assoc 98(6):489–493
15. Santos R, Veiga AS, Tavares L, Castanho M, Oliveira M (2016) Bacterial biofilms in diabetic foot ulcers: potential alternative therapeutics. In: Microbial Biofilms – Importance and Applications. IntechOpen, London
16. Kalan LR, Brennan MB (2019) The role of the microbiome in nonhealing diabetic wounds. Ann N Y Acad Sci 1435(1):79–92
17. Uçkay I, Gariani K, Pataky Z, Lipsky BA (2014) Diabetic foot infections: state-of-the-art. Diabetes Obes Metab 16(4):305–316. Available from: http://doi.wiley.com/10.1111/dom.12190
18. Rao N, Lipsky BA (2007) Optimising antimicrobial therapy in diabetic foot infections. Drugs 67(2):195–214

19. Lipsky BA, Aragón-Sánchez J, Diggle M, Embil J, Kono S, Lavery L et al (2016) IWGDF guidance on the diagnosis and management of foot infections in persons with diabetes. Diabetes Metab Res Rev 32:45–74. Available from: http://doi.wiley.com/10.1002/dmrr.2699
20. Jneid J, Lavigne JP, La Scola B, Cassir N (2017) The diabetic foot microbiota: a review. Hum Microbiome J 5–6:1–6. Available from: https://linkinghub.elsevier.com/retrieve/pii/S2452231717300076
21. Mendes JJ, Leandro C, Mottola C, Barbosa R, Silva FA, Oliveira M et al (2014) In vitro design of a novel lytic bacteriophage cocktail with therapeutic potential against organisms causing diabetic foot infections. J Med Microbiol 63(8):1055–1065. Available from: https://www.microbiologyresearch.org/content/journal/jmm/10.1099/jmm.0.071753-0
22. Spichler A, Hurwitz BL, Armstrong DG, Lipsky BA (2015) Microbiology of diabetic foot infections: from Louis Pasteur to 'crime scene investigation'. BMC Med 13(1):2. Available from: http://bmcmedicine.biomedcentral.com/articles/10.1186/s12916-014-0232-0
23. Miyan Z, Fawwad A, Sabir R, Basit A (2017) Microbiological pattern of diabetic foot infections at a tertiary care center in a developing country. J Pak Med Assoc 67(5):665–669
24. Saseedharan S, Sahu M, Chaddha R, Pathrose E, Bal A, Bhalekar P et al (2018) Epidemiology of diabetic foot infections in a reference tertiary hospital in India. Braz J Microbiol 49(2):401–406. https://doi.org/10.1016/j.bjm.2017.09.003
25. Ramakant P, Verma AK, Misra R, Prasad KN, Chand G, Mishra A et al (2011) Changing microbiological profile of pathogenic bacteria in diabetic foot infections: time for a rethink on which empirical therapy to choose? Diabetologia 54(1):58–64. Available from: http://link.springer.com/10.1007/s00125-010-1893-7
26. Hatipoglu M, Mutluoglu M, Uzun G, Karabacak E, Turhan V, Lipsky BA (2014) The microbiologic profile of diabetic foot infections in Turkey: a 20-year systematic review. Eur J Clin Microbiol Infect Dis 33(6):871–878. Available from: http://link.springer.com/10.1007/s10096-014-2047-5
27. Charles PGP, Uçkay I, Kressmann B, Emonet S, Lipsky BA (2015) The role of anaerobes in diabetic foot infections. Anaerobe 34:8–13. Available from: https://linkinghub.elsevier.com/retrieve/pii/S1075996415300019
28. Abdulrazak A, Ibrahim Bitar Z, Ayesh Al-Shamali A, Ahmed Mobasher L (2005) Bacteriological study of diabetic foot infections. J Diabetes Complications 19(3):138–141. Available from: https://linkinghub.elsevier.com/retrieve/pii/S105687270400073X
29. Sadeghpour Heravi F, Zakrzewski M, Vickery K, Armstrong DG, Hu H (2019) Bacterial diversity of diabetic foot ulcers: current status and future prospectives. J Clin Med 8(11):1935
30. Saltoglu N, Ergonul O, Tulek N, Yemisen M, Kadanali A, Karagoz G et al (2018) Influence of multidrug resistant organisms on the outcome of diabetic foot infection. Int J Infect Dis 70:10–14
31. Uçkay I, Gariani K, Dubois-Ferrière V, Suvà D, Lipsky BA (2016) Diabetic foot infections. Curr Opin Infect Dis 29(2):145–152. Available from: http://content.wkhealth.com/linkback/openurl?sid=WKPTLP:landingpage&an=00001432-201604000-00008
32. Lipsky BA, Itani KMF, Weigelt JA, Joseph W, Paap CM, Reisman A et al (2011) The role of diabetes mellitus in the treatment of skin and skin structure infections caused by methicillin-resistant Staphylococcus aureus: results from three randomized controlled trials. Int J Infect Dis 15(2):e140–e146. Available from: https://linkinghub.elsevier.com/retrieve/pii/S1201971210025269
33. Zenelaj B, Bouvet C, Lipsky BA, Uçkay I (2014) Do diabetic foot infections with methicillin-resistant *Staphylococcus aureus* differ from those with other pathogens? Int J Low Extrem Wounds 13(4):263–272. Available from: http://journals.sagepub.com/doi/10.1177/1534734614550311
34. Xie X, Bao Y, Ni L, Liu D, Niu S, Lin H et al (2017) Bacterial profile and antibiotic resistance in patients with diabetic foot ulcer in Guangzhou, Southern China: focus on the differences among different Wagner's grades, IDSA/IWGDF grades, and ulcer types. Int J Endocrinol 2017:1–12. Available from: https://www.hindawi.com/journals/ije/2017/8694903/

35. Sekhar S, Vyas N, Unnikrishnan M, Rodrigues G, Mukhopadhyay C (2014) Antimicrobial susceptibility pattern in diabetic foot ulcer: a pilot study. Ann Med Health Sci Res 4(5):742. Available from: http://www.amhsr.org/text.asp?2014/4/5/742/141541
36. Mottola C, Matias CS, Mendes JJ, Melo-Cristino J, Tavares L, Cavaco-Silva P et al (2016) Susceptibility patterns of Staphylococcus aureus biofilms in diabetic foot infections. BMC Microbiol 16(1):1000
37. Bridier A, Dubois-Brissonnet F, Greub G, Thomas V, Briandet R (2011) Dynamics of the action of biocides in *Pseudomonas aeruginosa* biofilms. Antimicrob Agents Chemother 55(6):2648–2654. Available from: http://aac.asm.org/lookup/doi/10.1128/AAC.01760-10
38. Ceri H, Olson ME, Stremick C, Read RR, Morck D, Buret A (1999) The Calgary Biofilm Device: new technology for rapid determination of antibiotic susceptibilities of bacterial biofilms. J Clin Microbiol 37(6):1771–1776. Available from: http://www.ncbi.nlm.nih.gov/pubmed/10325322
39. Eriksen KR, Erichsen I (1964) Resistance to methicillin, l soxazolyl penicillins, and cephalothin in staphylococcus aureus. Acta Pathol Microbiol Scand 62:255–275
40. O'Toole RD (1970) An outbreak of methicillin-resistant *Staphylococcus aureus* infection. JAMA 213(2):257
41. Viswanathan V, Pendsey S, Radhakrishnan C, Rege TD, Ahdal J, Jain R (2019) Methicillin-resistant *Staphylococcus aureus* in diabetic foot infection in India: a growing menace. Int J Low Extrem Wounds 18(3):236–246
42. Landrum ML, Neumann C, Cook C, Chukwuma U, Ellis MW, Hospenthal DR et al (2012) Epidemiology of *Staphylococcus aureus* blood and skin and soft tissue infections in the US Military Health System, 2005–2010. JAMA 308(1):50–59
43. Wang SH, Sun ZL, Guo YJ, Yang BQ, Yuan Y, Wei Q et al (2010) Meticillin-resistant *Staphylococcus aureus* isolated from foot ulcers in diabetic patients in a Chinese care hospital: risk factors for infection and prevalence. J Med Microbiol 59(10):1219–1224
44. Lavery LA, La Fontaine J, Bhavan K, Kim PJ, Williams JR, Hunt NA (2014) Risk factors for methicillin-resistant *Staphylococcus aureus* in diabetic foot infections. Diabet Foot Ankle 5. https://doi.org/10.3402/dfa.v5.23575
45. Reveles KR, Duhon BM, Moore RJ, Hand EO, Howell CK (2016) Epidemiology of methicillin-resistant *Staphylococcus aureus* diabetic foot infections in a large academic hospital: implications for antimicrobial stewardship. PLoS One 11(8):1–8
46. Akhi MT, Ghotaslou R, Memar MY, Asgharzadeh M, Varshochi M, Pirzadeh T et al (2017) Frequency of MRSA in diabetic foot infections. Int J Diabetes Dev Ctries 37(1):58–62. https://doi.org/10.1007/s13410-016-0492-7
47. Lee JS, Son ST, Han S-K (2017) Risk factors of methicillin-resistant *Staphylococcus aureus* and pseudomonas infection in diabetic foot ulcers in Korea. J Wound Manag Res 13(2):29–34
48. Wu M, Pan H, Leng W, Lei X, Chen L, Liang Z (2018) Distribution of microbes and drug susceptibility in patients with diabetic foot infections in Southwest China. J Diabetes Res 2018:1–9
49. Mutonga DM, Mureithi MW, Ngugi NN, Otieno FCF (2019) Bacterial isolation and antibiotic susceptibility from diabetic foot ulcers in Kenya using microbiological tests and comparison with RT-PCR in detection of S. aureus and MRSA. BMC Res Notes 12(1):1–6. https://doi.org/10.1186/s13104-019-4278-0
50. Bradford PA (2001) Extended-spectrum beta-lactamases in the 21st century: characterization, epidemiology, and detection of this important resistance threat. Clin Microbiol Rev 14(4):933–951
51. Shaikh S, Fatima J, Shakil S, Rizvi SMD, Kamal MA (2015) Antibiotic resistance and extended spectrum beta-lactamases: types, epidemiology and treatment. Saudi J Biol Sci 22(1):90–101. https://doi.org/10.1016/j.sjbs.2014.08.002
52. Ghafourian S, Sadeghifard N, Soheili S, Sekawi Z (2014) Extended spectrum beta-lactamases: definition, classification and epidemiology. Curr Issues Mol Biol 17(1):11–22

53. Varaiya A, Dogra J, Kulkarni M, Bhalekar P (2008) Extended spectrum beta lactamase (ESBL) producing *Escherichia coli* and *Klebsiella pneumoniae* in diabetic foot infection. Indian J Med Microbiol 26(3):281–282
54. Zubair M, Malik A, Ahmad J (2010) Clinico-bacteriology and risk factors for the diabetic foot infection with multidrug resistant microorganisms in North India. Biol Med 2(4):22–34
55. Zubair M, Malik A, Ahmad J (2012) Study of plasmid-mediated extended-spectrum β-lactamase-producing strains of enterobacteriaceae, isolated from diabetic foot infections in a north indian tertiary-care hospital. Diabetes Technol Ther 14(4):315–324
56. Benwan KA, Mulla AA, Rotimi VO (2012) A study of the microbiology of diabetic foot infections in a teaching hospital in Kuwait. J Infect Public Health 5(1):1–8. https://doi.org/10.1016/j.jiph.2011.07.004
57. Kamel NA, Aboshanab KM, Abouelwafa MM, El-tayeb WN (2013) Plasmid mediated extended spectrum beta-lactamase producing strains of enterobacteriaceae isolated from diabetic foot infections in Egypt. Arch Clin Microbiol 4(4):1–8
58. Gupta R, Malik A, Rizvi M, Ahmed SM (2016) Incidence of multidrug resistant *Pseudomonas* spp. in ICU patients with special reference to ESBL, AMPC, MBL and biofilm production. J Glob Infect Dis 8(1):25–31
59. Chaudhry WN, Badar R, Jamal M, Jeong J, Zafar J, Andleeb S (2016) Clinico-microbiological study and antibiotic resistance profile of meca and ESBL gene prevalence in patients with diabetic foot infections. Exp Ther Med 11(3):1031–1038
60. Costerton JW, Stewart PS, Greenberg EP (1999) Bacterial biofilms: a common cause of persistent infections. Science 284:1318
61. Clinton A, Carter T (2015) Chronic wound biofilms: pathogenesis and potential therapies. Lab Med 46(4):277–284
62. Malik A, Mohammad Z, Ahmad J (2013) The diabetic foot infections: biofilms and antimicrobial resistance. Diabetes Metab Syndr Clin Res Rev 7(2):101–107
63. Banu A, Noorul Hassan MM, Rajkumar J, Srinivasa S (2015) Spectrum of bacteria associated with diabetic foot ulcer and biofilm formation: a prospective study. Australas Med J 8(9):280–285
64. Purevdorj-Gage B, Costerton WJ, Stoodley P (2005) Phenotypic differentiation and seeding dispersal in non-mucoid and mucoid Pseudomonas aeruginosa biofilms. Microbiology 151(5):1569–1576
65. Flemming HC, Neu TR, Wozniak DJ (2007) The EPS matrix: the "House of Biofilm Cells". J Bacteriol 189(22):7945–7947
66. Driver VR, Blume PA (2014) Evaluation of wound care and health-care use costs in patients with diabetic foot ulcers treated with negative pressure wound therapy versus advanced moist wound therapy. J Am Podiatr Med Assoc 104(2):147–153
67. Peterson LR (2005) Squeezing the antibiotic balloon: the impact of antimicrobial classes on emerging resistance. Clin Microbiol Infect Suppl 11(5):4–16. https://doi.org/10.1111/j.1469-0691.2005.01238.x
68. James GA, Swogger E, Wolcott R, Pulcini ED, Secor P, Sestrich J et al (2008) Biofilms in chronic wounds. Wound Repair Regen 16(1):37–44
69. Keren I, Kaldalu N, Spoering A, Wang Y, Lewis K (2004) Persister cells and tolerance to antimicrobials. FEMS Microbiol Lett 230(1):13–18
70. Fauvart M, de Groote VN, Michiels J (2011) Role of persister cells in chronic infections: clinical relevance and perspectives on anti-persister therapies. J Med Microbiol 60(6):699–709
71. Wolcott RD, Cox SB, Dowd SE (2010) Healing and healing rates of chronic wounds in the age of molecular pathogen diagnostics. J Wound Care 19(7):272–281
72. Falanga V, Brem H, Ennis W, Wolcott R, Gould L, Ayello E (2008) Maintenance debridement in the treatment of difficult-to-heal chronic wounds. Recommendations of an expert panel. Ostomy Wound Manage 2:2–13

Fungal Infection: The Hidden Enemy? 10

Mohammad Oves, Mohd Ahmar Rauf,
Fohad Mabood Husain, Mohammad Zubair,
Iqbal M. I. Ismail, and Arun Iyer

10.1 Introduction

In the current years, reports on the fungal infections are increasing in the human population. The eradication of disease provides a challenging task to health care researches and doctors [1]. Fungal infection is occurring in humans and animals when and invasive fungal sp. attached to the body parts and controlled enough immune systems for its growth. The reports on fungal Infection is increasing due to the increasing the human population and lifestyle become modernize resulting in changing medical practice and require intensive care of emerging disease which mostly leads to the immunocompromised in the patient [2].

Fungi can make alive in the air, soil, water, plants, and animals and live naturally in the human body, and it exists in two forms fungi molds [3–5]. Mold colonies

M. Oves (✉)
Department of Biological Science, Faculty of Science, King Abdulaziz University, Jeddah, Kingdom of Saudi Arabia

Center of Excellence in Environmental Studies, King Abdul Aziz University, Jeddah, Kingdom of Saudi Arabia

M. A. Rauf · A. Iyer
Use-Inspired Biomaterials & Integrated Nano Delivery (U-BiND) Systems Laboratory, Department of Pharmaceutical Sciences, Eugene Applebaum College of Pharmacy and Health Sciences, Wayne State University, Detroit, MI, USA

F. M. Husain
Department of Food Science and Nutrition, College of Food and Agriculture Sciences, King Saud University, Riyadh, Kingdom of Saudi Arabia

M. Zubair
Department of Medical Microbiology, Faculty of Medicine, University of Tabuk, Tabuk, Kingdom of Saudi Arabia

I. M. I. Ismail
Department of Chemistry, King Abdulaziz University, Jeddah, Kingdom of Saudi Arabia

M. Zubair et al. (eds.), *Diabetic Foot Ulcer*,
https://doi.org/10.1007/978-981-15-7639-3_10

consist of filamentous strands called hyphae, whereas yeasts are typically single, small, oval cells. Some fungi are dimorphic, existing as either yeasts or molds depending on the external environment. Like other microbes, some fungi are helpful and some harmful. Whenever harmful fungi invade the body, they can be challenging to kill, as they can survive in the environment and reinfect the person trying to get better. Superficial and subcutaneous fungal infections can affect the surface skin, keratinous tissues, and mucous membranes and cause irritation and abruptness [6]. Worldwide, millions of people suffering from skin diseases caused by the fungal infection. However, superficial fungal infection is rarely life-threatening while debilitating effects on a person's quality of life. But sometimes it becomes highly contagious and spread to other individuals or become an invasive and systemic infection. Systemic fungal infections can be life-threatening and are associated with high morbidity and mortality [6, 7]. In a specific geographical location, some fungal infections may cause by either an opportunistic microorganism that infects an at-risk host or may be associated with a more invasive organism. The diagnosis of systemic Infection is difficult, and the exact incidence determination is difficult and the causative agent could be confirmed by autopsy. The count of fungal species in millions, but only a few of them can make people sick. Fungi can cause the number of different types of infection and disorders such as allergies or asthma, skin rushes, nails and lungs infection, meningitis sometimes bloodstream infections [8]. The most fungal infection recurrently comes across result from the inhalation of conidia, which can intensify allergic response atopic and nonatopic animals and humans [9, 10]. Sometimes the primary source of infection is inhalation by immunocompromised patients, which cause invasive pulmonary disease. Another primary source of infection is gastrointestinal routes due to eating of contamination foods [11, 12]. *Aspergillus fumigatus* and *Aspergillus flavus* cause the most significant fungal infection which leads to invasive aspergillosis [13, 14]. *A. niger*, *A. terreus*, and *A. nidulans* species of fungi also cause severe infection and lead to the mortality of immunocompromised patients [14–17]. The high number of fungal infections are not reportable and unrecorded due to lack of knowledge of fungal taxonomy. However, the researcher estimated appoximetly1.5 million species exist globally while only ~70,000 have described formally by the features [18]. Near about 300 fungal species have virulence factor may because disease and harmful to humans, only a few of them able to influence the central nervous system of human [19, 20].

In general, the filamentous fungi are characterized by branching hyphae, with septate hyphae containing species *Aspergillus* spp., *Fusarium* spp. and Mucoromycetes with non-septate hyphae containing species are *Rhizopus*, *Rhizomucor*, and *Mucor*, and additionally moniliaceous species with light-colored as molds. Dark pigmented molds are seen less common and include species which are considered as true neurotropic fungi [20, 21]. Dark pigmented fungi *Cladophialophora bantiana* are most commonly find in India, *Verruconis gallopava* was recovered worldwide while, *Exophiala dermatitidis* was also encountered worldwide but most common in East Asia, *Rhinocladiella mackenziei* is mainly recovered from the Middle East [21, 22]. The dimorphic fungi grow well in two morphological stages at lower temperature below 25 °C as a molds in environment and higher temperature up to 37 °C as a yeast-like *Blastomyces*, *Histoplasma*, *Coccidioides*, and *Paracoccidioides* are restricted to specific endemic areas [23–25]. This book chapter focuses on the unique hidden infections caused by fungus in humans. Number of localized opportunistic fungal infections that affect any human not only in older adults but in older people age-related physiological changes and some fungal infection becomes more serious. Here we discussed only hidden infection caused by fungus in neonatal to old age humans and required protection and treatment.

10.2 Mycobiont Reservoir in the Human Body

10.2.1 Fungal Infection in the Oral Cavity and Treatment

Fungal infection in the mouth to gastrointestinal (GI) tract may occur due to overgrowth of invasive mycobiota, sometimes high exposure to the contaminated consumable items and water [26, 27]. The degree of the disease be contingent on the primary risk factors of an individual body, such as immunosuppression by the different diseases like diabetes, and ranges from colonization, localized Infection, or fungemia, to aggressive life-threatening. The oral cavity is one of the primary mucosal locales where asymptomatic carriage of fungi was exposed [28]. The diversity in the oral mycobiota is low and controlled by the *Ascomycota phylum* species, such as *Candida* spp. [29]. While in culture-independent strategies have uncovered the nearness of a few individuals from the Saccharomycetaceae family (*Candida albicans*, *Candida dubliniensis*, *Candida rugosa Candida pararugosa*, *Saccharomyces cerevisiae*, *Hanseniaspora uvarum*, and *Pichia* spp.), and *Fusarium* species, that speaks to most of the parasitic species found in the oral cavity [29]. During the dysbiosis, the oral mucosa is less identified, and most of the studies focused on the overgrowth of *Candida albicans* upon immunosuppression and diabetes [30]. During the culture-independent investigation of the oral cavity sample of HIV-infected patients, mycobiota revealed the overgrowth of *C. albicans* while other species *Dothideomycetes* spp. and *Leotiomycetes* spp., related to the phylum Ascomycota, was also increased [29–32]. Although, oral mucosa is easily infected by the *Candida albicans* because of its adherence properties and high level of adherence properties and found 40–65% of healthy adult mouths as oral commensalism. In the mouth, papillated dorsal surface of the tongue and beneath a maxillary denture and palatal mucosa are preferred reservoir sites for Candida [33]. Such type of infection become pathogenic and increased due to compromised host interaction. These interactions between host and organism may be local or systemic. The salivation decreasing and weaning of dentures are considered local factors, while Infection during diabetes mellitus, pernicious anemia, and AIDS is known as systemic infection [34]. *C. albicans* infection can cause the weak immune system of its host and cause oral candidiasis, and it occurs in different form denture erythematous, pseudomembranous, erythematous, hyperplastic [35, 36]. Median rhomboid glossitis is a form of oral candidiasis was investigated by researchers. The number of drugs is available in the market for the treatment of oral candidiasis, such as nystatin, clotrimazole, ketoconazole, and fluconazole. Three times oral rinse with the Chlorhexidine as a disinfectant for dentures [37].

10.2.2 Gastrointestinal Tract Fungal Infection and Treatment

The lower gastrointestinal tract is containing more diverse fungal communities than the mouth or upper gastrointestinal tract. Here most of the species are belongs to the genera of *Candida*, *Saccharomyces*, *Aspergillus*, *Cryptococcus*, *Malassezia*, *Cladosporium*, *Galactomyces*, and *Trichosporon* [38]. However, some commensalism fungi able to influence host immunity, but it is not the only way of fungi infection. Some commensal fungi species are present in the food items, and air and the environmental source might activate the immune response in the gut—for example, *Histoplasma* spp., *Blastomyces* spp. and *Coccidioides* species cannot colonize the mucosal surfaces, but they can cause severe infections in the lung [39, 40]. In some studies observed temporal instability in fungal variability of the intestinal mycobiota, due to most of the infection based studies rely on the sampling of fecal and other materials. While in recent studies, from the mucosa-associated fungi suggest that a more stable community, the intestinal mycobiota [41, 42]. Sometimes this mycobiota perturbed by the intestinal disease [43]. These intestinal fungi are reservoirs in the proximity of the intestinal mucosa, and it might be interacting with the epithelium and the mucosal immune system. During bacterial dysbiosis, target lower gastrointestinal tract, and an inflammatory condition is known as inflammatory bowel disease (IBD) [44]. Recently, observed the fungal burden in the colonic mucosa become increased during the IBD, such as Crohn's disease and ulcerative colitis [45, 46] During the chronic intestinal inflammation, exits, the number of fungal species has reported in several studies [45–47]. It is confirmed and recovered a high number of cultivable *C. albicans* from the feces of IBD patients [48]. In Crohn's disease, the patient observed the inflamed mucosa of the intestine due to the high growth of *Candida albicans* and *Candida parapsilosis* [49]. The continuous increasing inflammation in the gut mucosa of mice due to the high rate of colonization of *Candida* sp. [50]. In a few investigations, find the Ascomycota phylum decrease and expansion of *Basidiomycota* spp. [51], while in another study, contradictory results observed in IBD patients. The development of clone libraries based on the 18S rDNA denaturing gradient gel electrophoresis (DGGE) from patients with Crohn's disease [52]. They have to find a high number of fungal diversity and richness in the feces and the mucosa when compared to the healthy individuals or colitis induced intestinal inflammation of individuals [53, 54]. In a study, immunocompromised patients have found 41% of individuals gastrointestinal infected while 22% affecting the lower part of the track and mostly infection caused by the *Aspergillus* or *Candida* sp. [55]. Candida infections in the mucosa/submucosa of the intestine where the organisms preferentially colonize the previously infarcted bowel [56]. In several studies, pathologists considered the sepsis caused a major role in mortality; sometimes, fungemia was paying a contributory role in many cases, and combined infection of Candida and Aspergillus in jejunal caused fatal gastrointestinal hemorrhage [57–59].

German Society for Hygiene and Microbiology (DGHM) has defined the intestinal fungal Infection based on symptoms and enumeration of yeast up to, or >1 × 10^5 cells/g of stool consider pathogenic colonization and causing diarrhea and require specific medical treatment [60].

Antifungal agents such as amphotericin B, ketoconazole, fluconazole, and the various formulations of itraconazole are effective in most cases [61]. During intestinal infection, dietary supplements and measures are essential to control the colonization of fungal pathogens. To control the intestinal yeast infection, the patient should avoid the consumption of refining sugar and carbohydrates because Yeast cells metabolize a high rate in the presence of low molecular weight carbohydrates. Recommended foods are fiber-containing vegetables and roughage, which provide little nutrients for yeasts cell development and promote gut motility and support the natural flora of the intestine, which have natural antagonistic activity toward yeasts [62]. As such, food rich in roughage contributes to fortifying the body's defense system and to healing mycoses of the gastrointestinal tract [60].

10.2.3 Lung Infection Caused by the Fungal Pathogen

Lung infection caused by fungal pathogen mainly by Aspergillus and Cryptococcus, both are widespread mold species which can appropriately sporulate and released conidia [9, 63]. These conidia are air born and dispersed in the air and arrive in the human airways and enter into the pulmonary alveoli [64]. In a healthy human, inhaled conidia are engulfed by alveolar macrophages and destroyed in the phagocyte oxidase-dependent pathways [14]. While in immunocompromised individuals, these conidia not able to destroy by phagocytosis, and here the attached to the mucous and spreading and tissue invasion by fungal hype, they caused several human diseases like asthma allergies and lethal infections [65, 66]. Sometimes, the fungal infection site makes granulomas that occur due to the integration of different immune cells later it degenerate to scars and calcified; it can be detected by the X-ray imaging analysis. Whenever the cellular immunity becomes impaired due to some immunosuppressive disease, then fungal infection control is too difficult. Airborne fungus and its spore are inhibiting in dust and avian, it inhalation causes *Cryptococcosis*. It mainly caused by *Cryptococcus neoformans* and *Cryptococcus gattii* [67]. Cryptococcal meningitis is the most severe outcome of the Cryptococcus infection because it invades the blood-brain barrier, and fungal cells directly penetrate the endothelial cells on the blood vessels of the brain [68]. In some reports, *C. neoformans* find in the brain cells and sometimes caused severe colonization [68]. *Pneumocystis jirovecii* causes lung infection and induced Pneumocystis pneumonia and Endemic mycosis, it is also found in non-HIV immunocompromised patients with a deficiency in adaptive immunity, or individuals taking prolonged high-dose systemic glucocorticoids [69, 70]. Worldwide most of the region's incidents of endemic mycoses are increasing due to rapidly growing the immunocompromised population. Exposure to the soil containing bat or bird droppings causes *Histoplasma capsulatum* infection with patients also present pneumonia symptoms described as acute/chronic pulmonary histoplasmosis, and severe cases may culminate in respiratory failure and death [9, 71].

10.2.4 Fungal Infection Stimulus of Age, Sex, Diet, and Environment

The number of studies reveals the high variability in the mycobiota between different individuals, and this distinction leads to the dysbiosis between healthy and infected ones [43]. In general, the mycobiota in a human body or animal significantly influenced by the environment, gender, age, diet, and geographical location [72, 73]. According to gender-wise male individual mycobiota contain a high number of *Aspergillus* spp. and *Tremellomycetes* spp. while a female has *Candida* spp. [74, 75]. In most cases, some mycobiota decease age-wise, and some increase, for example, during the infant stage, the genera such as *Aspergillus*, *Tremellomycetes*, and *Penicillium* are abundant and fungal diversity overall decreases with age [73–76]. Likewise, the mycobiota of the skin decreases with age, and it may happen due to the high rate of sebaceous gland secretion in the skin that favors the colonization by lipophilic fungi species *Malassezia* [75]. The fungal diversity exists among different ethnicities due to variables in consumer behavior and lifestyle. Diet also significantly influences the fungal and bacterial diversity in humans; it depends on specific vegetables, cereals, fruits, and dairy products consumption [77–79]. If any individual feed on the animal-derived diet or cheese, then fugal load increase in human faces [38]. The based on DNA sequencing human gut microbiome study reveals each person has a unique microbial gut profile that influenced by lifestyle and diet [80, 81]. If avoid a vegetarian diet and high consumption of sugar contains food, which leads to an increase in *Candida* sp. in the gut [80–82]. Based on the commensal relationship, individual human fungal diagnosis is too tricky and isolation of fungi from different body parts does not indicate pathogenicity [76].

10.2.5 Auditory Infections

In the mid ear, fungal infection occurrence is sporadic, but sometimes otitis media case serious problems [83]. In the immunocompetent children are facing ear problems by Infection of *Candida albicans* [83]. In the warm, humid climates, *Aspergillus* sp. is the most common pathogen and case otomycosis or external otitis sometimes [84, 85]. These symptoms resemble bacterial otitis and pruritis pain more prominent than pain.

10.2.6 Neuroinfections Caused by Fungi

The rate of fungal infections is expanding each year, with more noteworthy quantities of infections noted among patients having a place with high-chance gatherings, for example, HIV-infected people and AIDS patients, transplant beneficiaries, and immunosuppressed patients treated with chemotherapeutics or corticosteroids, just as those experiencing hematological sicknesses and incessantly sick patients [86] Certain conditions may incline the patient to the improvement of a particular etiological specialist: ailment/treatment-related and hereditary elements (delayed anti-infection treatment, neutropenia, steroid treatment, transplantation, ceaseless granulomatous sickness, CARD9 lack, neurosurgery, and rashness in babies—Candida; diabetic ketoacidosis, necrotic consumes, renal disappointment, and intravenous medication use—Mucoromycetes; birds contact—Cryptococcus and Histoplasma; deferoxamine treatment and iron over-burden—Mucoromycetes [87–90]. Some fungi's like Cryptococcus, Coccidioides, and Histoplasma, can likewise cause disease in immunocompetent patients. In USA, it was evaluated that intrusive mycoses brought about by *Candida* spp. are accountable for about 2–228 infections for each million populace every year, while *Cryptococcus neoformans* is liable for 30–66 infections and *Aspergillus* spp., 12–34 infections [91, 92]. The most well-known CNS fungal contamination overall is cryptococcal meningoencephalitis. Dispersed mycosis is frequently connected with CNS inclusion. It is evaluated that somewhere in the range of 67% and 84% of patients with intrusive cryptococcosis create CNS mycosis, 3–64% create obtrusive candidiasis, 40% blastomycosis, 25% dispersed coccidioidomycosis, and 5–20% scattered histoplasmosis, while 12% produce mucormycosis and 4–6% obtrusive aspergillosis [93–95]. Remember that in clinical presentation, cases of FIsCNS differ depending on the form of etiological factors. Diverse methods of CNS sore that occur, depending on the size of the fungal structures that build in the human body, for example, blastospores or hyphae. Blastomyces, Histoplasma, Coccidioides, Paracoccidioides, Cryptococcus, and Candida enters the blood vessels and causes local necrotic lesions, with meningitis and subpial ischemic lesions, while Aspergillus, Cladosporium, and Mucoromycetes infiltrate large blood vessels and can cause strokes [96–98].

10.2.7 Fungal Cooperation with the BBB and CNS Attack

The pathogenesis of FIs-CNS is not yet completely comprehended. Infiltration of the pathogen over the blood-brain barrier (BBB) is a fundamental advance for CNS attack. The coursing pathogens in the blood should initially be captured in the brain microvasculature and afterward transmigrate into the brain parenchyma over the blood-brain barrier BBB. Three components have been depicted for pathogens to cross the BBB. transcellular movement, paracellular relocation, and the Trojan Horse Mechanism [99–101]. Those instruments are best comprehended for Cryptococcus and Candida. *C. neoformans* precisely captured in the brain vasculature can cross the BBB by both immediate and circuitous components. Direct mode of incorporating BBB section through transcytosis of endothelial cells, while indirect mode incorporates movement within phagocytes as Trojan Horse Mechanism. Likewise, the paracellular section of the *C. neoformans* between endothelial cells has been additionally recommended. To trigger the translocation forms, chiefly through paracellular and transcellular systems, connections between pathogen protein atoms and BBB are essential. Ongoing examinations show that utilizing the transcellular component by *C. neoformans* in brain microvascular endothelial cells (BMECs) requires protein kinase C-alpha actuation. The CPS1 quality is required for *C. neoformans* adherence to the surface protein CD44 of human BMECs. The dispersal of the pathogen into the brain is constrained by Isc1 quality encoding a chemical that hydrolyzes inositol [102, 103].

As of late, Huang et al. demonstrated that the attack of *Cryptococcus neoformans* into human BMECs is interceded through the lipid raft endocytic pathway by means of the intracellular kinase-DYRK3 [104, 105]. Adherence of *C. albicans* to the extracellular lattice is encouraged by fibronectin, laminin, and vitronectin. It was shown that *C. albicans* intrusion of brain endothelial cells is intervened by the fungal attacks Als3 and Ssa1 [106, 107]. Als3 ties to the gp96 heat shock protein that is communicated explicitly on brain endothelium, advancing endothelial transcytosis by the growth [108–110].

Trojan horse pathway begins with contamination of a phagocyte in the peripheral region. Once disguised, the pathogen may effectively control the phagocyte to advance relocation toward the brain. The contaminated phagocyte arrives at the brain and clings to the luminal side of brain vessels and crosses the BBB, either paracellularly or transcellular. In conditions of decreased invulnerability, the BBB porousness builds, which encourages the entrance of growths into the brain. The pathogens get to the brain parenchyma and multiply causing brain irritation. As the pathogenic variables need to beat the successful barriers encompassing the brain, intrusions are generally connected with immunocompromised states. Consequently, the actuation of nerve cells by fungal cells and the declaration of resistant improving and immunosuppressing cytokines and chemokines assume a deciding job in pathogenesis of FIs-CNS. CNS association happens as the blood-brain barrier, and cerebral and subarachnoid spaces are crossed by the attacking organisms. This procedure is supported by different blood-brain barrier disturbances, for example, injury, medical procedure, or actuation of microglia and cytokines: TNF-α upsets the tight intersections of the barrier. The rate and degree of contamination are affected by the harmfulness of the growth and the movement of the host insusceptible framework. White blood cells, microglia, astrocytes, and endothelial cells assume significant jobs in forestalling disease by repressing fungal development through the creation of cytokines (INFγ, TNF-α, IL-1β, IL-6, and IL-12), chemokines, nitric oxide, and superoxide anion, and by the declaration of MHC I and II particles [111]. TLR-2, 4, and 9 are answerable for the acknowledgment of fungal antigens: polysaccharide case (*C. neoformans*), pseudohyphae (*C. albicans*), or conidia (*Aspergillus* spp.); anyway TLR-2, Dectin-1, and CR-3 are answerable for the acknowledgment of sugars, for example, mannose and β-glucans, present on the outside of *A. fumigatus* and *C. albicans*. Fungal pathogen-related subatomic examples are associated with starches (chitin, mannoproteins, phospholipomannan, and β-glucans) in the cell wall which may permit fungal infections to be constrained by empowering the actuation of microglia yielding master lymphatic and humoral reactions. The enactment of microglia cells relies upon the proximity of opsonins and T cells.

10.3 Treatment of FIs-CNS

Treatment of FIs-CNS Fungal neuroinfections is portrayed by higher death rates and more unfortunate visualization than viral and bacterial infections, and parasitic intrusions. Quick analysis and the utilization of suitable treatment are urgent in forestalling a frequently lethal result. The decision of antifungal treatment relies upon the fungistatic and fungicidal activity of the medication. The fungal cell film or divider segments (ergosterol, chitin, and β-glucans) are significant focuses of the primary gatherings of antifungal specialists in current use, except for flucytosine (antimetabolic impacts). Amphotericin B deoxycholate (AmBd) is profoundly harmful and has poor CNS infiltration, however, it is considered as a potential agent against cryptococcal meningoencephalitis, in combination with flucytosine, and neuroinfections caused by the other fungal agents and possess high BBB penetration (e.g., voriconazole); in these cases, lipid formulations of amphotericin B (L-AmB) ought to be favored [112–114]. Among antifungal medications, voriconazole, fluconazole, and flucytosine promptly enter into the CNS, yet itraconazole and posaconazole just infiltrate to a minor degree [115–117]. Voriconazole is suggested as an essential treatment for CNS aspergillosis, while liposomal amphotericin B (L-AmB) is saved for intolerant patients [118, 119]. Clinical information demonstrates that isavuconazole shows palatable action in obtrusive aspergillosis and scattered mucormycosis in CNS [120]. Notwithstanding pharmacological treatment, careful expulsion of injuries is likewise conceivable. By and large, a blend of careful mediation and antifungal treatment builds the endurance pace of patients with FIs-CNS. It has been demonstrated that neurosurgery is related to an improved result in patients treated with voriconazole for CNS fungal infections [121].

10.4 Conclusion

Every individual on the planet is sustaining commensalism with numerous microorganisms. These microorganisms are varying in diversity including fungi also variable in each individual and depends on the early life, age, dietary and cultural habits and geographical location. These fungal diversity composition sometime imbalance and disrupts the immune system and cause a hidden infection in the body and which leads to fungal diseases. Fungal infection in the mouth to gastrointestinal (GI) tract may occur due to the high load of contaminated consumable. The degree of the disease of an individual body depends on immune power. If individual sufferings from the immunosuppression by the different diseases like diabetes and HIV and wide ranges of diseases affected from colonization of the number of fungi and leads to the fungemia and life threatening.

References

1. Bongomin F, Gago S, Oladele RO, Denning DW (2017) Global and multi-national prevalence of fungal diseases-estimate precision. J Fungi (Basel) 3(4):57. https://doi.org/10.3390/jof3040057
2. Chang CC, Levitz SM (2019) Fungal immunology in clinical practice: magical realism or practical reality? Med Mycol 57(Suppl 3):S294–S306. https://doi.org/10.1093/mmy/myy165. PMCID: PMC7137463
3. Samanta I (2015) Cutaneous, subcutaneous and systemic mycology. Vet Mycol:11–153. https://doi.org/10.1007/978-81-322-2280-4_4
4. Moënne-Loccoz Y, Mavingui P, Combes C, Normand P, Steinberg C (2014) Microorganisms and biotic interactions. In: Environmental microbiology: fundamentals and applications. Springer, Dordrecht, pp 395–444. https://doi.org/10.1007/978-94-017-9118-2_11
5. Ghosh B, Lal H, Srivastava A (2015) Review of bioaerosols in indoor environment with special reference to sampling, analysis and control mechanisms. Environ Int 85:254–272. https://doi.org/10.1016/j.envint.2015.09.018
6. Lee PP, Lau YL (2017) Cellular and molecular defects underlying invasive fungal infections-revelations from endemic mycoses. Front Immunol 8:735. https://doi.org/10.3389/fimmu.2017.00735
7. Lanternier F, Cypowyj S, Picard C et al (2013) Primary immunodeficiencies underlying fungal infections. Curr Opin Pediatr 25(6):736–747. https://doi.org/10.1097/MOP.0000000000000031
8. Miller JM, Binnicker MJ, Campbell S et al (2018) A guide to utilization of the microbiology laboratory for diagnosis of infectious diseases: 2018 update by the Infectious Diseases Society of America and the American Society for Microbiology. Clin Infect Dis 67(6):e1–e94. https://doi.org/10.1093/cid/ciy381
9. Li Z, Lu G, Meng G (2019) Pathogenic fungal infection in the lung. Front Immunol 10:1524. https://doi.org/10.3389/fimmu.2019.01524
10. Tanaka RJ, Boon NJ, Vrcelj K et al (2015) In silico modeling of spore inhalation reveals fungal persistence following low dose exposure. Sci Rep 5:13958. https://doi.org/10.1038/srep13958
11. Paterson RRM, Lima N (2017) Filamentous fungal human pathogens from food emphasising Aspergillus, Fusarium and Mucor. Microorganisms 5(3):44. https://doi.org/10.3390/microorganisms5030044
12. Nag PK (2018) Sick building syndrome and other building-related illnesses. Office Buildings:53–103. https://doi.org/10.1007/978-981-13-2577-9_3
13. Paulussen C, Hallsworth JE, Álvarez-Pérez S et al (2017) Ecology of aspergillosis: insights into the pathogenic potency of Aspergillus fumigatus and some other Aspergillus species. Microb Biotechnol 10(2):296–322. https://doi.org/10.1111/1751-7915.12367
14. Dagenais TR, Keller NP (2009) Pathogenesis of *Aspergillus fumigatus* in invasive aspergillosis. Clin Microbiol Rev 22(3):447–465. https://doi.org/10.1128/CMR.00055-08
15. Azoulay E, Russell L, Van de Louw A et al (2020) Diagnosis of severe respiratory infections in immunocompromised patients. Intensive Care Med 46(2):298–314. https://doi.org/10.1007/s00134-019-05906-5
16. Schett G, Casati B, Willinger B et al (1998) Endocarditis and aortal embolization caused by *Aspergillus terreus* in a patient with acute lymphoblastic leukemia in remission: diagnosis by peripheral-blood culture. J Clin Microbiol 36(11):3347–3351

17. Gupta V, Rajagopalan N, Patil M, Shivaprasad C (2014) Aspergillus and mucormycosis presenting with normal chest X-ray in an immunocompromised host. BMJ Case Rep 2014:bcr2014204022. https://doi.org/10.1136/bcr-2014-204022
18. Blackwell M (2011) The fungi: 1, 2, 3 ... 5.1 million species? Am J Bot 98(3):426–438. https://doi.org/10.3732/ajb.1000298
19. Köhler JR, Casadevall A, Perfect J (2014) The spectrum of fungi that infects humans. Cold Spring Harb Perspect Med 5(1):a019273. https://doi.org/10.1101/cshperspect.a019273
20. Góralska K, Blaszkowska J, Dzikowiec M (2018) Neuroinfections caused by fungi. Infection 46(4):443–459. https://doi.org/10.1007/s15010-018-1152-2
21. Revankar SG, Sutton DA (2010) Melanized fungi in human disease [published correction appears in Clin Microbiol Rev. 2012 Oct;25(4):720]. Clin Microbiol Rev 23(4):884–928. https://doi.org/10.1128/CMR.00019-10
22. Zupančič J, Novak Babič M, Zalar P, Gunde-Cimerman N (2016) The black yeast *Exophiala dermatitidis* and other selected opportunistic human fungal pathogens spread from dishwashers to kitchens. PLoS One 11(2):e0148166. https://doi.org/10.1371/journal.pone.0148166
23. Sil A, Andrianopoulos A (2014) Thermally dimorphic human fungal pathogens—polyphyletic pathogens with a convergent pathogenicity trait. Cold Spring Harb Perspect Med 5(8):a019794. https://doi.org/10.1101/cshperspect.a019794
24. Cleare LG, Zamith-Miranda D, Nosanchuk JD (2017) Heat shock proteins in histoplasma and paracoccidioides. Clin Vaccine Immunol 24(11):e00221–e00217. https://doi.org/10.1128/CVI.00221-17
25. Li Z, Nielsen K (2017) Morphology changes in human fungal pathogens upon interaction with the host. J Fungi (Basel) 3(4):66. https://doi.org/10.3390/jof3040066
26. Lee SC, Billmyre RB, Li A et al (2014) Analysis of a food-borne fungal pathogen outbreak: virulence and genome of a *Mucor circinelloides* isolate from yogurt. *mBio* 5(4):e01390–e01314. https://doi.org/10.1128/mBio.01390-14
27. Geramizadeh B, Heidari M, Shekarkhar G (2015) Gastrointestinal basidiobolomycosis, a rare and under-diagnosed fungal infection in immunocompetent hosts: a review article. Iran J Med Sci 40(2):90–97
28. Vargas KG, Joly S (2002) Carriage frequency, intensity of carriage, and strains of oral yeast species vary in the progression to oral candidiasis in human immunodeficiency virus-positive individuals. J Clin Microbiol 40(2):341–350. https://doi.org/10.1128/jcm.40.2.341-350.2002
29. Iliev ID, Leonardi I (2017) Fungal dysbiosis: immunity and interactions at mucosal barriers. Nat Rev Immunol 17(10):635–646. https://doi.org/10.1038/nri.2017.55
30. Bertolini M, Ranjan A, Thompson A et al (2019) *Candida albicans* induces mucosal bacterial dysbiosis that promotes invasive infection. PLoS Pathog 15(4):e1007717. https://doi.org/10.1371/journal.ppat.1007717
31. Salvatori O, Puri S, Tati S, Edgerton M (2016) Innate immunity and saliva in *Candida albicans*-mediated oral diseases. J Dent Res 95(4):365–371. https://doi.org/10.1177/0022034515625222
32. Liu F, Fan X, Auclair S et al (2016) Sequential dysfunction and progressive depletion of *Candida albicans*-specific CD4 T cell response in HIV-1 infection. PLoS Pathog 12(6):e1005663. https://doi.org/10.1371/journal.ppat.1005663
33. de Oliveira Santos GC, Vasconcelos CC, Lopes AJO et al (2018) *Candida* infections and therapeutic strategies: mechanisms of action for traditional and alternative agents. Front Microbiol 9:1351. https://doi.org/10.3389/fmicb.2018.01351
34. (2015) Abstracts from the 38th annual meeting of the society of general internal medicine. J Gen Intern Med 30(Suppl 2):45–551. https://doi.org/10.1007/s11606-015-3271-0
35. Jabra-Rizk MA, Kong EF, Tsui C et al (2016) *Candida albicans* pathogenesis: fitting within the host-microbe damage response framework. Infect Immun 84(10):2724–2739. https://doi.org/10.1128/IAI.00469-16
36. Williams D, Lewis M (2011) Pathogenesis and treatment of oral candidosis. J Oral Microbiol 3. https://doi.org/10.3402/jom.v3i0.5771

37. Garcia-Cuesta C, Sarrion-Pérez MG, Bagán JV (2014) Current treatment of oral candidiasis: a literature review. J Clin Exp Dent 6(5):e576–e582. https://doi.org/10.4317/jced.51798
38. Hallen-Adams HE, Suhr MJ (2017) Fungi in the healthy human gastrointestinal tract. Virulence 8(3):352–358. https://doi.org/10.1080/21505594.2016.1247140
39. Guarner J, Brandt ME (2011) Histopathologic diagnosis of fungal infections in the 21st century. Clin Microbiol Rev 24(2):247–280. https://doi.org/10.1128/CMR.00053-10
40. Davies SF, Sarosi GA (1983) Fungal infection of the lung. The big 3—histoplasmosis, blastomycosis, coccidioidomycosis. Postgrad Med 73(6):242–251
41. Dieterich W, Schink M, Zopf Y (2018) Microbiota in the gastrointestinal tract. Med Sci (Basel) 6(4):116. https://doi.org/10.3390/medsci6040116
42. Li J, Jiang H, Li L, Zhang X, Chen J (2019) The effect of disease and season to hepatopancreas and intestinal mycobiota of *Litopenaeus vannamei*. Front Microbiol 10:889. https://doi.org/10.3389/fmicb.2019.00889
43. Underhill DM, Iliev ID (2014) The mycobiota: interactions between commensal fungi and the host immune system. Nat Rev Immunol 14(6):405–416. https://doi.org/10.1038/nri3684
44. Tamboli CP, Neut C, Desreumaux P, Colombel JF (2004) Dysbiosis in inflammatory bowel disease. Gut 53(1):1–4. https://doi.org/10.1136/gut.53.1.1
45. Qiu X, Zhang F, Yang X et al (2015) Changes in the composition of intestinal fungi and their role in mice with dextran sulfate sodium-induced colitis. Sci Rep 5:10416. https://doi.org/10.1038/srep10416
46. Leonardi I, Li X, Iliev ID (2018) Macrophage interactions with fungi and bacteria in inflammatory bowel disease. Curr Opin Gastroenterol 34(6):392–397. https://doi.org/10.1097/MOG.0000000000000479
47. Sokol H, Leducq V, Aschard H et al (2017) Fungal microbiota dysbiosis in IBD. Gut 66(6):1039–1048. https://doi.org/10.1136/gutjnl-2015-310746
48. Klaile E, Müller MM, Zubiría-Barrera C et al (2019) Unaltered fungal burden and lethality in human CEACAM1-transgenic mice during *Candida albicans* dissemination and systemic infection. Front Microbiol 10:2703. https://doi.org/10.3389/fmicb.2019.02703
49. Kumamoto CA (2011) Inflammation and gastrointestinal Candida colonization. Curr Opin Microbiol 14(4):386–391. https://doi.org/10.1016/j.mib.2011.07.015
50. Sonoyama K, Miki A, Sugita R, Goto H, Nakata M, Yamaguchi N (2011) Gut colonization by *Candida albicans* aggravates inflammation in the gut and extra-gut tissues in mice. Med Mycol 49(3):237–247. https://doi.org/10.3109/13693786.2010.511284
51. Schmidt-Dannert C (2016) Biocatalytic portfolio of Basidiomycota. Curr Opin Chem Biol 31:40–49. https://doi.org/10.1016/j.cbpa.2016.01.002
52. Díez B, Pedrós-Alió C, Marsh TL, Massana R (2001) Application of denaturing gradient gel electrophoresis (DGGE) to study the diversity of marine picoeukaryotic assemblages and comparison of DGGE with other molecular techniques. Appl Environ Microbiol 67(7):2942–2951
53. Chehoud C, Albenberg LG, Judge C et al (2015) Fungal signature in the gut microbiota of pediatric patients with inflammatory bowel disease. Inflamm Bowel Dis 21(8):1948–1956. https://doi.org/10.1097/MIB.0000000000000454
54. Praneenararat S (2014) Fungal infection of the colon. Clin Exp Gastroenterol 7:415–426. https://doi.org/10.2147/CEG.S67776
55. Garcia-Rubio R, de Oliveira HC, Rivera J, Trevijano-Contador N (2020) The fungal cell wall: *Candida*, *Cryptococcus*, and *Aspergillus* species. Front Microbiol 10:2993. https://doi.org/10.3389/fmicb.2019.02993
56. Andrutis KA, Riggle PJ, Kumamoto CA, Tzipori S (2000) Intestinal lesions associated with disseminated candidiasis in an experimental animal model. J Clin Microbiol 38(6):2317–2323
57. Lamps LW, Lai KK, Milner DA Jr (2014) Fungal infections of the gastrointestinal tract in the immunocompromised host: an update. Adv Anat Pathol 21(4):217–227. https://doi.org/10.1097/PAP.0000000000000016

58. Coker OO, Nakatsu G, Dai RZ et al (2019) Enteric fungal microbiota dysbiosis and ecological alterations in colorectal cancer. Gut 68(4):654–662. https://doi.org/10.1136/gutjnl-2018-317178
59. Lin L, Zhao CH, Yin XY et al (2017) *Aspergillus niger* bloodstream infection in gastric cancer after common hepatic artery embolization: a case report. Exp Ther Med 14(2):1427–1432. https://doi.org/10.3892/etm.2017.4693
60. https://www.adiclair.com/manifestations-of-candida-mycoses/fungal-infections-of-the-gastrointestinal-tract.html
61. Johnson MD, MacDougall C, Ostrosky-Zeichner L, Perfect JR, Rex JH (2004) Combination antifungal therapy. Antimicrob Agents Chemother 48(3):693–715. https://doi.org/10.1128/AAC.48.3.693-715.2004
62. Gunsalus KT, Tornberg-Belanger SN, Matthan NR, Lichtenstein AH, Kumamoto CA (2015) Manipulation of host diet to reduce gastrointestinal colonization by the opportunistic pathogen *Candida albicans*. mSphere 1(1):e00020–e00015. https://doi.org/10.1128/mSphere.00020-15
63. Latgé JP (1999) *Aspergillus fumigatus* and aspergillosis. Clin Microbiol Rev 12(2):310–350
64. Schlesinger RB (1988) Biological disposition of airborne particles: basic principles and application to vehicular emissions. In: Watson AY, Bates RR, Kennedy D (eds) Air pollution, the automobile, and public health. National Academies Press (US), Washington, DC. Available from: https://www.ncbi.nlm.nih.gov/books/NBK218161/
65. Kuhn DM, Ghannoum MA (2003) Indoor mold, toxigenic fungi, and *Stachybotrys chartarum*: infectious disease perspective. Clin Microbiol Rev 16(1):144–172. https://doi.org/10.1128/cmr.16.1.144-172.2003
66. Denning DW, Pashley C, Hartl D et al (2014) Fungal allergy in asthma-state of the art and research needs. Clin Transl Allergy 4:14. https://doi.org/10.1186/2045-7022-4-14
67. Kwon-Chung KJ, Fraser JA, Doering TL et al (2014) *Cryptococcus neoformans* and *Cryptococcus gattii*, the etiologic agents of cryptococcosis. Cold Spring Harb Perspect Med 4(7):a019760. https://doi.org/10.1101/cshperspect.a019760
68. Chang YC, Stins MF, McCaffery MJ et al (2004) Cryptococcal yeast cells invade the central nervous system via transcellular penetration of the blood-brain barrier [published correction appears in Infect Immun. 2004 Nov;72(11):6753. Paul-Satyasee, Maneesh [corrected to Paul-Satyaseela, Maneesh]]. Infect Immun 72(9):4985–4995. https://doi.org/10.1128/IAI.72.9.4985-4995.2004
69. Morris A, Norris KA (2012) Colonization by *Pneumocystis jirovecii* and its role in disease. Clin Microbiol Rev 25(2):297–317. https://doi.org/10.1128/CMR.00013-12
70. Gigliotti F, Limper AH, Wright T (2014) Pneumocystis. Cold Spring Harb Perspect Med 4(12):a019828. https://doi.org/10.1101/cshperspect.a019828
71. https://www.mayoclinic.org/diseases-conditions/histoplasmosis/symptoms-causes/syc-20373495
72. Ross AA, Müller KM, Weese JS, Neufeld JD (2018) Comprehensive skin microbiome analysis reveals the uniqueness of human skin and evidence for phylosymbiosis within the class Mammalia. Proc Natl Acad Sci U S A 115(25):E5786–E5795. https://doi.org/10.1073/pnas.1801302115
73. Richard ML, Sokol H (2019) The gut mycobiota: insights into analysis, environmental interactions and role in gastrointestinal diseases. Nat Rev Gastroenterol Hepatol 16:331–345. https://doi.org/10.1038/s41575-019-0121-2
74. Strati F, Di Paola M, Stefanini I et al (2016) Age and gender affect the composition of fungal population of the human gastrointestinal tract. Front Microbiol 7:1227. https://doi.org/10.3389/fmicb.2016.01227
75. Liu XZ, Wang QM, Göker M et al (2015) Towards an integrated phylogenetic classification of the Tremellomycetes. Stud Mycol 81:85–147. https://doi.org/10.1016/j.simyco.2015.12.001
76. Limon JJ, Skalski JH, Underhill DM (2017) Commensal fungi in health and disease. Cell Host Microbe 22(2):156–165. https://doi.org/10.1016/j.chom.2017.07.002

77. Gupta VK, Paul S, Dutta C (2017) Geography, ethnicity or subsistence-specific variations in human microbiome composition and diversity. Front Microbiol 8:1162. https://doi.org/10.3389/fmicb.2017.01162
78. Naranjo-Ortiz MA, Gabaldón T (2019) Fungal evolution: major ecological adaptations and evolutionary transitions. Biol Rev Camb Philos Soc 94(4):1443–1476. https://doi.org/10.1111/brv.12510
79. Auchtung TA, Fofanova TY, Stewart CJ et al (2018) Investigating colonization of the healthy adult gastrointestinal tract by fungi. mSphere 3(2):e00092–e00018. https://doi.org/10.1128/mSphere.00092-18
80. Tomova A, Bukovsky I, Rembert E et al (2019) The effects of vegetarian and vegan diets on gut microbiota. Front Nutr 6:47. https://doi.org/10.3389/fnut.2019.00047
81. Rinninella E, Raoul P, Cintoni M et al (2019) What is the healthy gut microbiota composition? A changing ecosystem across age, environment, diet, and diseases. Microorganisms 7(1):14. https://doi.org/10.3390/microorganisms7010014
82. Van Ende M, Wijnants S, Van Dijck P (2019) Sugar sensing and signaling in *Candida albicans* and *Candida glabrata*. Front Microbiol 10:99. https://doi.org/10.3389/fmicb.2019.00099
83. Viswanatha B, Naseeruddin K (2011) Fungal infections of the ear in immunocompromised host: a review. Mediterr J Hematol Infect Dis 3(1):e2011003. https://doi.org/10.4084/MJHID.2011.003
84. Kazemi A, Majidinia M, Jaafari A, Ayatollahi Mousavi SA, Zarei Mahmoudabadi A, Alikhah H (2015) Etiologic agents of otomycosis in the North-Western area of Iran. Jundishapur J Microbiol 8(9):e21776. https://doi.org/10.5812/jjm.21776
85. Ismail MT, Al-Kafri A, Ismail M (2017) Otomycosis in Damascus, Syria: etiology and clinical features. Curr Med Mycol 3(3):27–30. https://doi.org/10.29252/cmm.3.3.27
86. Sousa, Neto AL d, de Aquino RL, Vargas LS, Lopes AFA, Maganhoto AMS, Teixeira NF, de Paula Silva SF, Marra MD (2019) Fungal and bacterial infections in hospitalized HIV carriers. J Nurs UFPE/Revista de Enfermagem UFPE 13
87. Nadkarni T, Goel A (2005) Aspergilloma of the brain: an overview. J Postgrad Med 51(5):37
88. Lowes DJ, Hevener KE, Peters BM (2020) Second-generation antidiabetic sulfonylureas inhibit *Candida albicans* and Candidalysin-mediated activation of the NLRP3 inflammasome. Antimicrob Agents Chemother 64(2)
89. Kang SW, Tran VG, Nguyen NZN, Lee S, Kim J, Kim HJ, Lee JS, Cho HR, Kwon B (2019) CCR5-mediated recruitment of NK cells to the kidney is a critical step for host defense to systemic *Candida albicans* infection. Am Assoc Immnol 202(1 Suppl):190.55
90. Whitehead W, McNeil JC (2019) Infections complicating neurosurgical procedures/devices. In: Healthcare-associated infections in children. Springer, New York, pp 153–175
91. Sanches MD'A, Mimura LAN, Oliveira LRC, Ishikawa LLW, Garces HG, Bagagli E, Sartori A, Kurokawa CS, Fraga-Silva TFC (2019) Differential behavior of non-Albicans Candida species in the central nervous system of immunocompetent and immunosuppressed mice. Front Microbiol 9:2968
92. Brieland J, Essig D, Jackson C, Frank D, Loebenberg D, Menzel F, Arnold B, DiDomenico B, Hare R (2001) Comparison of pathogenesis and host immune responses to *Candida glabrata* and *Candida albicans* in systemically infected immunocompetent mice. Infect Immun 69(8):5046–5055
93. Bodensteiner DC, Skikne B (1982) Central nervous system involvement in mycosis fungoides. diagnosis, treatment and literature review. Cancer 50(6):1181–1184
94. Chakrabarti A (2007) Epidemiology of central nervous system mycoses. Neurol India 55(3):191
95. Shukla A, Bansal M, Husain M, Chhabra DK (2014) Central nervous system mycosis: analysis of 10 cases. Indian J Pathol Microbiol 57(4):591
96. Kloss S, Schuster A, Schroten H, Lamprecht J, Wahn V (1991) Control of proven pulmonary and suspected CNS Aspergillus infection with itraconazole in a patient with chronic granulomatous disease. Eur J Pediatr 150(7):483–485

97. Shah A, Dar NJ, Hassan QP, Ahmad M (2016) Endophytes and neurodegenerative diseases: a hope in desperation. CNS Neurol Disord Drug Targets 15(10):1231–1239
98. Nadell J, Sanders CV, Sardenga L (1976) Brain abscess caused by *Cladosporium trichoides* (Bantianum): a case with paranasal sinus involvement. South Med J 69(11):1519–1521
99. Sorrell TC, Juillard P-G, Djordjevic JT, Kaufman-Francis K, Dietmann A, Milonig A, Combes V, Grau GER (2016) Cryptococcal transmigration across a model brain blood-barrier: evidence of the Trojan horse mechanism and differences between *Cryptococcus neoformans* var. *grubii* strain H99 and *Cryptococcus gattii* strain R265. Microbes Infect 18(1):57–67
100. de Lange ECM (2012) The physiological characteristics and transcytosis mechanisms of the blood-brain barrier (BBB). Curr Pharm Biotechnol 13(12):2319–2327
101. Chang YC, Stins MF, McCaffery MJ, Miller GF, Pare DR, Dam T, Paul-Satyasee M, Kim KS, Kwon-Chung KJ (2004) Cryptococcal yeast cells invade the central nervous system via transcellular penetration of the blood-brain barrier. Infect Immun 72(9):4985–4995
102. Jong A, Wu C-H, Chen H-M, Luo F, Kwon-Chung KJ, Chang YC, LaMunyon CW, Plaas A, Huang S-H (2007) Identification and characterization of CPS1 as a hyaluronic acid synthase contributing to the pathogenesis of *Cryptococcus neoformans* infection. Eukaryot Cell 6(8):1486–1496
103. Chang YC, Jong A, Huang S, Zerfas P, Kwon-Chung KJ (2006) CPS1, a homolog of the *Streptococcus pneumoniae* type 3 polysaccharide synthase gene, is important for the pathobiology of *Cryptococcus neoformans*. Infect Immun 74(7):3930–3938
104. Huang S-H, Long M, Wu C-H, Kwon-Chung KJ, Chang YC, Chi F, Lee S, Jong A (2011) Invasion of *Cryptococcus neoformans* into human brain microvascular endothelial cells is mediated through the lipid rafts-endocytic pathway via the dual specificity tyrosine phosphorylation-regulated kinase 3 (DYRK3). J Biol Chem 286(40):34761–34769
105. Jong A, Wu C-H, Prasadarao NV, Kwon-Chung KJ, Chang YC, Ouyang Y, Shackleford GM, Huang S-H (2008) Invasion of *Cryptococcus neoformans* into human brain microvascular endothelial cells requires protein kinase C-α activation. Cell Microbiol 10(9):1854–1865
106. Denaro FJ, Lopez-Ribot JL, Chaffin WLJ (1995) Adhesion of *Candida albicans* to brain tissue of *Macaca mulata* in an ex vivo assay. Infect Immun 63(9):3438–3441
107. Zhang J-R, Tuomanen E (1999) Molecular and cellular mechanisms for microbial entry into the CNS. J Neurovirol 5(6):591–603
108. Liu Y, Mittal R, Solis NV, Prasadarao NV, Filler SG (2011) Mechanisms of *Candida albicans* trafficking to the brain. PLoS Pathog 7(10):e1002305
109. Fu Y, Phan QT, Luo G, Solis NV, Liu Y, Cormack BP, Edwards JE, Ibrahim AS, Filler SG (2013) Investigation of the function of *Candida albicans* Als3 by heterologous expression in *Candida glabrata*. Infect Immun 81(7):2528–2535
110. Filler SG (2013) Can host receptors for fungi be targeted for treatment of fungal infections? Trends Microbiol 21(8):389–396
111. Pan W, Kastin AJ (1999) Penetration of neurotrophins and cytokines across the blood–brain/blood–spinal cord barrier. Adv Drug Deliv Rev 36(2–3):291–298
112. Banks WA, Kastin AJ, Broadwell RD (1995) Passage of cytokines across the blood-brain barrier. Neuroimmunomodulation 2(4):241–248
113. Baddour LM, Perfect JR, Ostrosky-Zeichner L (2005) Successful use of amphotericin B lipid complex in the treatment of Cryptococcosis. Clin Infect Dis 40(Suppl 6):S409–S413
114. Schwartz S, Ruhnke M, Ribaud P, Reed E, Troke P, Thiel E (2007) Poor efficacy of amphotericin B-based therapy in CNS aspergillosis. Mycoses 50(3):196–200
115. Lopez-Berestein G, Fainstein V, Hopfer R, Mehta K, Sullivan MP, Keating M, Rosenblum MG, Mehta R, Luna M, Hersh EM (1985) Liposomal amphotericin B for the treatment of systemic fungal infections in patients with cancer: a preliminary study. J Infect Dis 151(4):704–710
116. Chiller TM, Sobel RA, Luque JC, Clemons KV, Stevens DA (2003) Efficacy of amphotericin B or itraconazole in a murine model of central nervous system Aspergillus infection. Antimicrob Agents Chemother 47(2):813–815

117. Pitisuttithum P, Negroni R, Graybill JR, Bustamante B, Pappas P, Chapman S, Hare RS, Hardalo CJ (2005) Activity of posaconazole in the treatment of central nervous system fungal infections. J Antimicrob Chemother 56(4):745–755
118. Schwartz S, Ruhnke M, Ribaud P, Corey L, Driscoll T, Cornely OA, Schuler U, Lutsar I, Troke P, Thiel E (2005) Improved outcome in central nervous system aspergillosis, using voriconazole treatment. Blood 106(8):2641–2645
119. Serena C, Javier Pastor F, Marçal M, Mar Rodríguez M, Guarro J (2007) Efficacy of voriconazole in a murine model of cryptococcal central nervous system infection. J Antimicrob Chemother 60(1):162–165
120. Thompson III, George R, Rendon A, dos Santos RR, Queiroz-Telles F, Ostrosky-Zeichner L, Azie N, Maher R et al (2016) Isavuconazole treatment of cryptococcosis and dimorphic mycoses. Clin Infect Dis 63(3):356–362. https://doi.org/10.1093/cid/ciw305
121. Leechawengwongs M, Milindankura S, Liengudom A, Chanakul K, Viranuvatti K, Clongsusuek P (2007) Multiple *Scedosporium apiospermum* brain abscesses after near-drowning successfully treated with surgery and long-term voriconazole: a case report. Mycoses 50(6):512–516. https://doi.org/10.1111/j.1439-0507.2007.01410.x

Diabetic Foot Syndrome: Risk Factors, Clinical Assessment, and Advances in Diagnosis

11

Thomas Antony Thaniyath

11.1 Introduction

Diabetic foot disease (DFD) or syndrome (DFS) is factors' complex array in the macro-vascular (e.g., peripheral arterial disease) and microvascular (e.g., damage in the peripheral nerve) problems which affect diabetic patients and it is estimated one in three of diabetic patients will have the risk of DFD development as well as 10% of them will be developing DFU (Diabetic Foot Ulcer) in their lifetime [1, 2]. WHO defined DFS as "ulceration of the foot (distally from the ankle and including the ankle) associated with neuropathy and different grades of ischemia and infection" [3]. DFU is considered diabetes' serious complication, which may lead to lower extremity amputation, which amounts amid 0.03–1.5% of patients with DFD [4, 5]. Compared to nondiabetic individuals, higher risk for major amputations that is nearly 30–40% has been found in type 2 diabetic patients [6]. Sensation loss due to diabetic peripheral neuropathy, ischemia caused by peripheral arterial diseases or their mixture may contribute to the development of foot ulcers in diabetic patients [7]. In another review, based on epidemiological data, it is estimated that 15% of the cases resulted in peripheral arterial occlusive disease (PAOD), only neuropathy is responsible for diabetic foot syndrome's 50% cases approximately, whereas angiopathy and neuropathy combination results in the development of foot ulcerations which is nearly 35%. The diabetic foot is a distinctive example of diabetic neuropathy's painless complication. The process of nociception-the pain perception developing from encoding's neural processes as well as the noxious stimuli processing is worsening in the diabetic foot. Painless diabetic neuropathy is the underlying main cause for diabetic foot ulcers' development, as it results in painless injuries and inflammation [8]. In addition to the above mentioned etiological factor for the diabetic foot ulcers development, the studies show a clear correlation among incorrectly fitted shoes and foot ulceration in older people with diabetes

T. A. Thaniyath (✉)
Faculty of Medicine, University of Tabuk, Tabuk, Kingdom of Saudi Arabia

M. Zubair et al. (eds.), *Diabetic Foot Ulcer*,
https://doi.org/10.1007/978-981-15-7639-3_11

mellitus. In these studies, the patient with present ulceration, up to five times are likely not to wear correctly fitted shoes in comparison to patients that do not have any foot ulceration [9, 10]. The above evidence is cemented in a review by Andrew and Hylton, stating that the potential for the diabetic foot ulceration occurrence is greater in diabetic patients, who wear incorrectly fitting shoes than those without diabetes [11]. The objective of this chapter is to highlight the diabetic foot syndrome development risk factors, clinical features as well as recent progress in disease's early detection.

11.2 Risk Factors

In a clinical scenario, when diabetic patients are being dealt with them it is of utmost importance that causal pathway must be considered to the foot ulceration as the best method to prevent DFU formation is the risk factors reduction. The four primary components that must be considered are foot deformities, minor trauma, peripheral arterial disease (PAD), and peripheral neuropathy [12].

11.2.1 Diabetes: Duration and Glycemic Control

Long-standing and uncontrolled glycemic profile of the patient influences the peripheral arterial and neuropathy disease complications' development by complicated metabolic pathways. The consequences of these complications lead to loss of sensation and ischemia, which alone or in combination may result in foot ulcers [1, 13]. In a study by Vibha et al. [13] including 620 participants with type 2 diabetes mellitus, 70.5% of 321 patients ($p < 0.001$) with DFS had a history of diagnosed DM for more than 6 years. The duration, as well as high level of glycated hemoglobin, has a strong link with the neuropathy progression and development [1, 14, 15]. It is observed in Diabetes Control and Complications Trials (DCCT) that the HbA1c level's intensive control effectively reduced the neuropathy incidence in 1441 type 1 diabetes mellitus patients by 60% [16]. In another study on type 2 diabetes mellitus, intensive insulin treatment enhanced vibration perception threshold and nerve conduction velocity than those who were under conventional treatment [17]. However, the UK prospective diabetes study (UKPDS) with 3867 type 2 diabetes patients did not show any glycemic control effect on the neuropathy prevalence [18].

11.2.1.1 Peripheral Neuropathy

It is diabetes' common and intractable complication, which causes feeling lost in the lower limb and increases the amputation risk, with the prevalence of 1–2% of diabetic patients [19]. Peripheral sensory neuropathy disrupts the normal protective reflex mechanisms, resulting in a severe trauma or repeated unnoticed mild ones causing wounds. Abnormalities in proprioception cause defective weight support while walking, which also promotes callus or ulcer formation. Sensory and motor neuropathy result in irregular foot mechanism as well as structural alterations and autonomic neuropathy alter sweating and superficial perfusion, which promotes the skin drying and fissure formation [20]. In 2004, van Schie and associates concluded in a case-controlled trial that the neuropathic patients without an ulceration history are at high risk for future ulceration [21].

11.2.1.2 Peripheral Arterial Disease

The risk for PAD (peripheral arterial disease) development is more in diabetic patients as well as it is an estimated two- to fourfold enhancement in risk in comparison to the non-diabetic population. The epidemiological studies observed that the 9.5%PAD prevalence in adult diabetic patients versus 4.5% in the nondiabetic population [22–28]. It is described as a clinical disorder with peripheral arteries' occlusion or stenosis, in which the primary cause is atherosclerosis. Epidemiological studies confirmed the association of diabetes with atherosclerosis. PAD is an important analyst for diabetic foot ulceration development as physicians must evaluate the lower limb vascular status as well as particularly for the ischemia signs, during the patients' examination with diabetes and diabetic foot syndrome [20]. In their cross-sectional study conducted in 2017, Tresierra-Ayala and García Rojas concluded that PAD is among those factors that are associated with type 2 diabetes patients to diabetic foot ulceration and highlights the significance of early assessment as well as peripheral arterial disease treatment.

11.2.1.3 Other Pathological Factors

The other factors, which influence the healing of ulceration in diabetic foot syndrome patients, are the infection and other comorbidities presence [29–31].

11.2.2 Sociodemographic Factors

Several pieces of research suggest the role of sociodemographic factors in diabetes patients with foot ulceration development [32–35]. These studies notify in older patients the high prevalence of DFU, those with low socioeconomic factors, and lower education. Vibha et al. [13], in another community based cross-sectional study observed the high prevalence of DFU among patients with advancing diabetes long duration, sedentary lifestyle, low socioeconomic status, and age.

11.2.3 Foot Deformities

The risk of amputation in patients with DFU rises from 1.7-fold in those with peripheral neuropathy to 12-fold in patients with both foot deformity and sensory loss [36, 37]. Several studies identified that foot deformities as the main contributing element and foot ulceration prediction, possible by skin predisposing to high pressure at foot deformity site [38–40]. Van Schie and associates highlighted the clear relationship between the foot deformities, muscle weakness, and motor nerve conduction deficit in accordance with muscle and individual nerves they innervate [21]. However, they relating conduction deficit of motor nerve with foot deformities, there is no suitable conclusion on the role of abnormal nerve function in the causation of foot deformities.

11.2.4 Incorrectly Fitted Footwear

The modern footwear fulfills three purposes: form, function, and fit [41]. Of these, function intends to protect the feet of the individuals from the risk of injuries and the term fit pertains to how the footwear will maintain the foot's morphology [42]. These statements represent the significant role of footwear in the protection of feet from the risk of injury and to keep the morphology of the foot. The incorrectly fit footwear contributes to pathological alteration in foot morphology, such as hallux valgus and toe deformity [43, 44]. In addition to the above changes, it causes skin lesions like corns and calluses [45], which predispose the foot to ulceration especially in diabetes patients [10].

11.3 Clinical Assessment Guidelines and Advances in the Diagnosis of Diabetic Foot Syndrome

For diabetes as well as diabetic foot syndrome management the significance of foot and footwear evaluation for the deformities existence, gait's abnormalities, and patient's ability to perform physical activities and to determine the risk for the development of ulceration is signified by the clinical practice guidelines [46]. Diabetes patients' screening comprises the individuals' identification who are at high risk of complications development through appropriate screening tests based on appropriate clinical practice guidelines (CPG), which defines standards for health care according to evidence-based interventions [47]. It is proved by several studies, that the patient outcomes are improved when evidence-dependent clinical practice guideline suggestions are used in health care [48]. With appropriate use of reliable clinical practice guidelines, it can be delayed the serious complications of diabetes and diabetic foot syndrome to a certain extend. The international health community and organizations such as WHO and IDF made recommendations with the objective of decreasing the amputations rate by 50% in diabetic foot disease and it suggested that protection program and foot screening implementation for patients at ulceration risk can decrease both health care cost and morbidity [49]. Several internationally accepted CPGs are available for the screening and assessment of diabetes patients and DFS. However, in a systematic review article, Formosa et al., pointed out the inadequacy of these guidelines and recommends the inclusion of current development in science and information technology in accordance with political and ethical issues, competing priorities, assessment tests' specificity, and sensitivity, economic considerations, health system capacity issues, and epidemiological considerations, on revision of guidelines [47].

11.3.1 Highlights of Major Guidelines in Diabetic Foot Disease Prevention and Management

11.3.1.1 National Health and Medical Research Council (NHMRC) Australia; 2011 ("https://www.baker.edu.au/Assets/Files/Foot_FullGuideline_23062011.pdf")

NHMRC clinical guidelines constructed according to evidence-dependent recommendations from literature's systematic review. It recommends temperature perception, vibration, and pinprick's sensory modalities and Achilles reflexes that are dependent on neuropathy disability score [47] to demonstrate the degree of peripheral nerve involvement. Visual inspection of feet and structural deformities and ulceration is an important recommendation of this guideline. For the foot's arterial perfusion the most useful indicators are toe pressure or toe-brachial pressure index, ankle-brachial pressure index, along with peripheral foot pulses' palpation [47]. NHMRC recommends the appropriate footwear and hosiery and the use of therapeutic footwear if indicated. It also considers the use of "Foot Deformity Score" for marking deformation in foot and consists of the following deformities: Charcot's neuro-arthropathy, abnormally wide feet, high-arched, or excessively flat feet, previous amputations, callus, hammer/claw toe, and hallux deformity. The score helps to measure the joint mobility limitation. Foot care education and training provision to all diabetes patients, help to prevent foot complications related to diabetes.

Based on the NHMRC guidelines, it is categorized diabetes patients on the possibility of developing foot complications:

1. Low-risk group: those without risk factors as well as without foot ulcer/amputation history. Yearly evaluation is recommended.
2. Intermediate risk group: those with one risk factor such as foot deformity, PAD, or neuropathy and without foot ulcer/amputation history. Advised to seek expert evaluation every 3–6 months period.
3. High-risk group: those with two or more risk factors as well as/or foot ulceration/amputation history. Recommend for specialized assessment for foot protection programs, including suitable footwear, podiatry review, and foot care education.

In short, NHMRC, 2011 guidelines, provide evidence-based criteria on diabetic foot ulcer management and prevention. It suggests yearly screening of all diabetic patients for prevention and patients with high risk should receive expert and integrated multidisciplinary foot care, comprises wound dressings and debridement, off-loading, and standardized ulcer assessment [50].

11.3.1.2 Canadian Diabetes Association (CDA), Canada; 2013 ("http://guidelines.diabetes.ca/app_themes/cdacpg/resources/cpg_2013_full_en.pdf")

CDA guidelines recommend annual screening (more frequently in patients with higher risk) of diabetic patients for peripheral neuropathy presence with 10 g monofilament over the feet's distal plantar surface. The PAD screening/detection is done with ABPI (ankle-brachial pressure index) with adjunct influence and palpation of foot pulses and systolic toe pressure determination by spectral Doppler waveform analysis, transcutaneous oxygen pressure, and photoplethysmography. Patients' assessment includes determination of bony foot deformities, movement limitation(s) of ankles, and toe joints for the detection of risk for diabetic foot syndrome. It advises the use of expert-designed therapeutic footwear and the foot care education provision for patients with a high risk of foot ulceration. It also recommends the provision of education on foot care for caregivers as well as healthcare professionals for the early detection of signs of DFS, including feet's visual inspection for infection evidence, skin temperature, callus pattern, and skin changes. For the patients who develop foot ulcers, CDA highly recommends the expertise of multidisciplinary healthcare management intending in preventing recurrent foot ulceration as well as amputation.

11.3.1.3 Scottish Intercollegiate Guidelines Network (SIGN), Scotland; 2013 ("https://www.nabcop.org.uk/resources/scottish-intercollegiate-guidelines-network-2013-sign-134/")

SIGN guidelines advise the screening of all diabetic patients by trained health professionals for developing diabetic foot disease's risk. Early assessment for the presence of neuropathy with 10 g monofilament and a neurothesiometer and PAD using Doppler ultrasound detecting ABPI. It recommends arterial reconstruction for all patients with limb ischemia. Simple tests should be used to detect structural abnormalities in these patients and advises preventive footwear and orthoses. Foot care education by a multidisciplinary team is advised for all diabetic patients. SIGN guidelines categorize diabetic patients into:

(a) Low-risk patients with absence of risk factors for diabetic foot: recommends yearly screening by qualified health care expert and provide with verbal and written education, self-management plan, with emergency contact details and suitable access to a podiatrist if needed.
(b) Moderate risk patients with single risk factors: Annual evaluation by a podiatrist, Patient-oriented treatment plan, and provision of written as well as verbal education with emergency contact details.
(c) High-risk patients, having more than one risk factor or amputation/ulceration history: yearly evaluation by a podiatrist with a well-tailored patient-oriented management program with written as well as verbal education with emergency contact details and transfer for expert involvement is needed.
(d) Active diabetic foot disease: a multidisciplinary foot care team's member manages it with a well-tailored patient-oriented management program with written as well as verbal education with emergency contact details and transfer for expert involvement is needed.

11.3.1.4 National Institute for Health and Care Excellence (NICE), England and Wales; 2015 ("https://www.nice.org.uk/guidance/ng19")

NICE guidelines encourage foot's visual inspection and self-monitoring by diabetes patients themselves. It recommends the screening of all diabetic patients for neuropathy and PAD presence by monofilament test or vibration utilizing calibrated tuning fork/bio-thesiometer and palpation respectively. It recommends the provision of adequate training to healthcare professionals as well as those concerned in the diabetic foot assessment. Patient education must be an ongoing basis with different methods until optimal for patients. Specialist footwear and insole should be provided in patients with diabetes and previous ulceration. It also recommends annual review and management plans including diabetic patients' education regarding foot care with low current risk. Patients with elevated neuropathy risk or no pulses or another risk factors should be followed up every 3–6 months for evaluation of foot for enhanced foot care education, footwear, and vascular assessment. High-risk groups with previous ulcers, skin changes, deformity, absent pulse, and neuropathy should be followed up every 1–3 months. The examination includes for nail protection, specialist footwear and skin and insoles, specialized foot care education, vascular assessment, and feet inspection. In case of ulcerated foot and foot care emergency such as new ulceration, swelling, and discoloration, refer the patient with 24 h to a multidisciplinary foot care team. The team must be comprised a diabetologist with expertise in lower limb complications, nurse expert in diabetic wound dressing, and a highly qualified specialist podiatrist as well as orthotist. Revascularization should be considered for the patients of possible benefit. Patients with nonhealing ulcer are suggested with intensive systemic antibiotic therapy.

11.3.1.5 Deutsche Diabetes Gesellschaft (DDG), Germany; 2014 ("https://www.diabetesde.org/system/files/documents/fileadmin/users/Patientenseite/PDFs_und_TEXTE/Infomaterial/Gesundheitsbericht_2014_kl.pdf")

DDG guideline recommends the provision of continuing education programs for diabetic patients and caregivers on foot care intending in preventing diabetic ulcers as well as periodical evaluation of both feet for deformities and limited mobility. It suggests the screening for neuropathy with 10 g monofilament test and/or Rydell-Seiffer tuning fork vibration. The peripheral arterial sufficiency assessment is done with ABPI determination, arterial occlusion pressure over posterior tibial artery, and dorsalis pedis artery measurements, and foot pulses palpation. It advises periodical evaluation of footwear in all diabetics and the provision of footwear as per the diabetic foot risk. Categorizes the diabetic patients in to:

- Risk category 0: no PAD, no sensory neuropathy and recommends annually evaluation.
- Risk category 1: sensory neuropathy with or without deformation: evaluation in each 3–6 months.

- Risk category 2: PAD with or without sensory neuropathy: a specialist examination in each 2–3 months.
- Risk category 3: amputation or ulcer history: specialist evaluation in each 1–2 months.

11.3.1.6 Institute of Clinical Systems Improvement (ICSI), USA; 2014 ("https://www.icsi.org/guideline/diabetes/")

ICSI guideline for diabetic foot prevention as well as management suggests diabetic patients' annual/biannual screening for foot risk assessment as well as foot care counseling to prevent microvascular complications of diabetes. It suggests consideration of foot care specialist if the followings are present: the patient is not able to care their own feet properly, requires suitable footwear, or has conditions like foot deformation(s), the infected lesion(s), or ulcers, thick calluses or deformed nails. Consider vascular surgeon if the patient develops peripheral vascular disease signs and symptoms like claudication and/or peripheral pulses lack. In all patients diagnosed with diabetes, it advises the provision of education/self-management through a healthcare team and feet's daily self-observation for nail problems, redness, and lesions in addition to dermatological changes of color, sweating, infection, ulceration, callus, bleeding, and blistering. The examination of the foot must include the observation for the limitation of joint mobility. It recommends a patient-tailored foot care education based on their individual needs, knowledge as well as the presence of risk factors. It also highlights the importance of physical activities of moderate-intensity exercise at the rate of 150 min per week as well as resistance training three times per week till contraindicated.

11.3.1.7 NZSSD (New Zealand Society for the Study of Diabetes)—Podiatry Special Interest Group; 2014 (www.nzssd.org.nz/healthprofs/pdf)

NZSSD guidelines recommend screening of all diabetic patients by health professionals from the diagnosis time yearly, in case there exists no risk for diabetic foot disease and provision foot care education to each people diagnosed with diabetes as part of multidisciplinary care. In the presence of risk, it advises more frequent assessments every 3–6 months. People with a high diabetic feet risk must consult a multidisciplinary foot care team or a specialist diabetic foot clinic. The screening for neuropathy is done with perception threshold using bio-thesiometer, vibration test using 128 Hz tuning fork, 10 g monofilament. The screening of peripheral arterial disease is done through the rest pain/or symptomatic claudication evaluation and dorsalis pedis artery palpation. The identification of foot deformations and its management is an essential step according to this guideline.

The diabetic foot disease patients are suggested to use cushioned, high-quality sports, or running shoes. It is advised to wear custom made footwear or orthotic insoles in patients who have high-risk feet, deformation, or have previous amputation history with the aim to prevent callus formation or to reduce its severity and to avoid recurrence of ulceration.

11.3.1.8 International Diabetes Federation (IDF); 2015 ("https://www.idf.org/about-diabetes/54-our-activities/222-idf-clinical-practice-recommendations-on-the-diabetic-foot.html")

IDF recommends the provision of a self-management education program which is patient-centered as the main part of therapy for all type 2 diabetes patients from the diagnosis time and ongoing process depending on requirements' regular assessment. An appropriate multidisciplinary team should be assigned to educate the people individually or group-wise considering the suitability of the program and individual and encourages the use of modern technologies as a communication method. Screening of the patients for neuropathy is done with 10 g monofilament or 128 Hz tuning fork. Quantitative measurement is done with bio-thesiometer. It also recommends the use of a non-traumatic pinprick test. The posterior tibial arteries and dorsalis pedis palpation are done for the screening of PAD and quantitative assessment with Doppler measurement of brachial/ankle pressure ratio. Less than 0.9 is considered as the cutoff point for the presence of vascular occlusive disease. The patients are categorized into three groups as per the foot assessment findings;

(a) No added risk: There exist no risk factors such as the previous foot ulceration or amputation history, symptoms of peripheral neuropathy and PAD. Advises the foot care education provision.
(b) At risk: Presence of one risk factor. Review the patient consistently after 6 months by the foot care team. The evaluation processes include the inspection of both feet and ensures the local management provision. Footwear evaluation and suitable advice and enhancement of foot care education.
(c) High risk: There exist two or more risk factors. The foot care team reviews the patient in a more frequent way of 3–6 months gap. The process comprises the inspection of both feet and the local management provision as described. Footwear evaluation and providing specialist insoles as well as shoes if described as well as ensure the suitable intensified foot care education provision.

The patient must be sent to a multidisciplinary foot care team immediately in 24 h after there is of occurrence/presentation of foot ulceration/infection. They should be provided with appropriate wound management. The IDF guidelines classify the infection as;

1. Severe: Accompanied by systemic features of sepsis
2. Moderate: Deeper than skin and more extensive cellulitis
3. Mild: Superficial with minimal cellulitis

Long-term antibiotic therapy should be considered if indicated. In suspected cases of osteomyelitis, appropriate investigations should be considered. Reduction of weight and methods for optimum distribution of pressure should be done such as the use of crutches. The management of vascular insufficiency is the next consideration if needed. The patient should be provided with specialist footwear and orthotic care along with individualized foot care education to prevent recurrence after recovery along with optimal blood glucose regulation.

11.3.1.9 International Working Group on Diabetic Foot (IWGDF); 2015 ("https://iwgdfguidelines.org/")

IWGDF guidelines emphasize the patient education necessity and patient ability assessment to understand the messages, sufficient self-care skills, and motivation to act accordingly. It points to the essentiality of assessment of joint mobility limitation and foot deformation(s). The guideline advises the annual screening of all diabetic patients for peripheral arterial and neuropathy disease presence as well as recommends the suitable footwear to accommodate the modified deformities and biomechanics. IWGDF guidelines raise five key elements for the assessment, screening for the diabetic foot risk: foot at risk's consistent examination and inspection, a foot at risk's identification, education, and family of foot care for prevention and treatment, suitable footwear provision and non-ulcerative pathology treatment such as callus, nail, and skin pathology by specialized podiatrist [49]. This IWGDF 2015 guideline upholds the necessity of three tier foot care management [49]: the different level team includes:

- Level 1—diabetic nurse, podiatrist, and general practitioner
- Level 2—specialized diabetic nurse, podiatrist, surgeon, diabetologist
- Level 3—specialized foot center with multiple disciplines specialized in diabetic foot care

11.3.1.10 American Diabetes Association (ADA), USA; 2019 ("Diabetes Care 2019;42(Suppl 1):S124–S138. https://doi.org/10.2337/dc19-S011")

ADA 2019 guidelines provide a comprehensive criterion for diabetic foot evaluation as well as treatment:

1. ADA recommends for the foot's annual assessment in every diabetic patient for early identification of risk factors for amputation and ulceration and those with signs of prior ulceration/amputation or sensory loss must evaluate their foot on each visit.
2. Check for the nephropathy, retinopathy, cigarette smoking, vascular surgery/angioplasty, Charcot joint, amputation, and ulceration history.
3. Neuropathy's current symptoms were assessed such as vascular occlusions like claudication, and fatigue, numbness, and burning, and pain.
4. The foot examination must consist of skin inspection, foot deformities assessment, and neurological involvement, and peripheral arterial disease assessment.
5. The neurological assessment should be done with 10 g monofilament with a minimum of one other test such as vibration, temperature, or pinprick.
6. The vascular assessment includes pulses palpation in feet and legs. The patients with claudication signs or absent or reduced pedal pulses must be evaluated with ankle-brachial index as well as for other appropriate assessment methods.

7. To all diabetic patients provision of general preventive foot care education.
8. ADA recommends referring the patients with high risks such as smoking habit, history of prior lower extremity amputation, those with peripheral arterial disease, or protective sensation loss, to a foot specialist for ongoing prevention and life-long surveillance.
9. The specialized therapeutic footwear use is suggested for the patients with greater risk for diabetic foot such as severe peripheral neuropathy, amputation history, or foot deformities.
10. Multidisciplinary management is suggested for foot ulceration and high-risk foot patients.

11.3.2 Methods for Peripheral Neuropathy Screening as Well as the Assessment in Diabetic Patients

Painless ulceration of foot as well as/or arthropathy are the cardinal features of diabetic foot. The underlying painless neuropathy is the reason for the masking of the inflammation and the painless repeated foot injuries in diabetic patients. The skin ulcers are completely insensitive to pain and Charcot's joint may reflect with faint dull aching upon load bearing [8]. It is determined that peripheral neuropathy is greatly related to the lower limbs and feet and the most common component for the causation of foot ulceration in diabetic patient [51–53]. The diabetic neuropathy, in most of the patients, affects both the large-fiber nerves of the limbs and in turn, alters the sensations of muscle control, position perception, vibration, and touch, as well as small-fiber nerves for autonomic function, pain, and thermal perception [54]. The diabetic peripheral neuropathy incidence enhances with diabetes duration and age as well as it is common in patients with uncontrolled glycemic profile and obesity [53, 55]. These facts indicate the management and early detection significance of such a condition. Table 11.1 lists important screening tools for peripheral neuropathy's detection. Apart from the abovementioned questionnaire, almost all clinical tools use other confirmatory tests for the confirmation of neuropathy.

11.3.2.1 Touch Sensation Tests

11.3.2.1.1 Semmes-Weinstein Monofilament Test (SWMT)

In every diabetic patient, the test must be done at least once in a year as a part of foot evaluation or the occurrence of a new foot ulcer. During the test, the examiner uses 10 g monofilament, which is calibrated as it requires 10 g of force for bending on touching the foot skin, to know the feel of filament on touch by the patient on closing his/her eyes. The examiner uses the filament on ten different sites randomly on each foot. The maximum score is 10 as the client feels the monofilament at all sites (Fig. 11.1) of touch. Holding the monofilament perpendicular to the skin of the foot and along with a steady, smooth motion, the skin is touched until there is nearly 1 cm bending of filament and after that, for nearly 2 s it is held. On an area, the test is repeated three times, if a patient failed to respond on touch. Mark the positive

Table 11.1 The initial neuropathic pain screening tests

No	Name of instrument	Major components measures	Grading
1	Douleur Neuropathique en 4 (DN4)	Questionnaire for various neuropathic pain, and tactile dynamic allodynia, pin hypothesis and touch's physical examination	Score ≥4/10 specifies the peripheral neuropathy's presence
2	LANSS (Leeds Assessment of Neuropathic Symptoms and Signs) scale	Elicits five symptoms and two clinical signs of diabetic peripheral neuropathy	Maximum score is 24. Patient's score ≥12 indicates diabetic peripheral neuropathy
3	MNSI (Michigan Neuropathy Screening Instrument)	It consists of 15 self-answerable questions and 5 physical assessment criteria, which include monofilament test, great toe's vibration perception, ankle reflexes, ulceration, and feet's appearance	Maximum score is 10. For peripheral neuropathy, a score ≥7 believed to be positive
4	TCNS (Toronto Clinical Neuropathy Score)	Includes assessment of symptoms, sensory loss, and ankle reflexes [56]	Based on the score it classifies into severe neuropathy (≥12), moderate neuropathy (9–11) and mild neuropathy (6–8)
5	NDS (Neuropathy Disability Score)	Assessed by measuring vibration perception, thermal and Achilles tendon reflexes and pinprick sensation	Severity grading: severe (9–10), moderate (6–8), mild (3–5) and none (0–2)
6	UENS (Utah Early Neuropathy Scale)	Measures the pin sensation, allodynia/hyperesthesia, deep tendon reflexes, and motor deficits	Maximum score is 42. 24/42 are devoted to sensory loss's anatomical mapping to pin in lower leg and foot [57]
7	NPQ (Neuropathic Pain Questionnaire)	The questionnaire consists of 32 items: Selected 12 for NPO-SF(short form) 10 related to quality of pain and 2 related to changes in sensitivity [58, 59]	Such tool demonstrated 64.5% sensitivity and 78.6% of specificity with 73% of total forecast accuracy [59]
8	NPSI (Neuropathic Pain Symptoms Inventory)	This neuropathic tool contains 12 questions on the severity of spontaneous pain, severity of painful attacks, the severity of provoked pains, and the severity of abnormal sensations	The grade reaches from 0–10, where 10 represents the worst pain and 0 for no pain
9	NSS (Neurological Symptom Score)	17 item questionnaire, which addresses motor, sensory, and autonomic functions	Specificity as well as sensitivity of 67% and 82% respectively [60]
10	DNE (Diabetic Neuropathy Examination) score	Examine four questions on muscle strength, reflexes, and sensation on index finger and big toe	Maximum score is 16 points. Fast and reliable clinical scoring system for the evaluation of peripheral neuropathy [61]

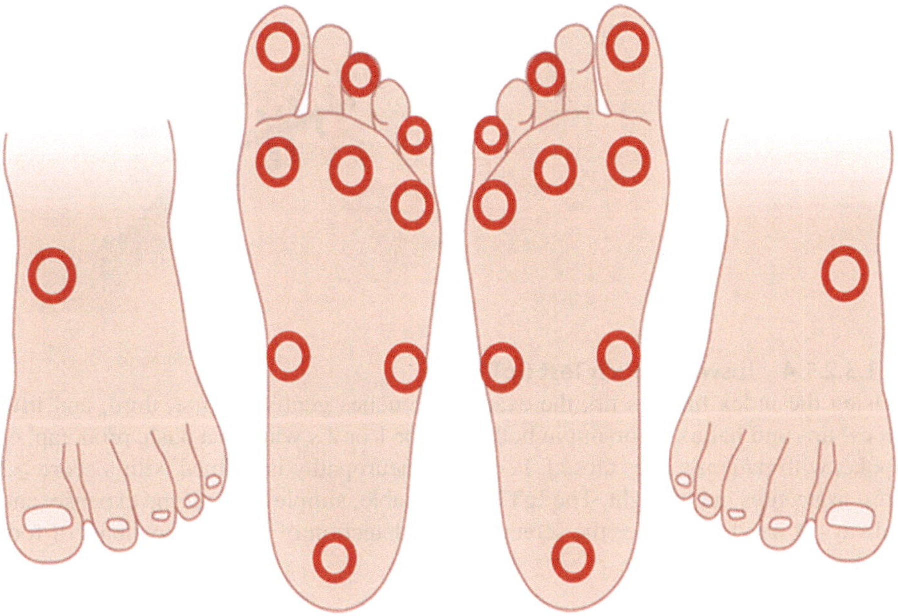

Fig. 11.1 Sites for the monofilament test

result numbers among the total tested sites number. For example, the score 7/9 indicates the seven sites of positive responses, and only nine sites were tested as there is amputation in the patient's right great toe [62].

11.3.2.1.2 Neuropen

This is sensitive as well as an inexpensive alternative approach for evaluating nerve function for identifying moderate to severe neuropathy patients. The sites for tests are restricted to high-pressure areas on the each hallux's plantar surface, and first, second, third, and fifth metatarsal head. The neuropen sensitivity for detecting neuropathy in comparison with the NDS (score $\geq$ 6/10) is higher specificity of the test improves, in a mixture of abnormal Neurotip and abnormal monofilament responses were utilized (68%), instead of the tests of individual (57% and 41%, respectively) [63].

11.3.2.1.3 von Frey Hair Test

The assessment is done with von Frey hair (Fig. 11.2) in five repeated tests at four sites such as leg's lateral part on the dominant lower limb, lateral malleolus, first metatarsal, and interphalangeal joints of the great toe. A positive test is recorded when at least three times out of five hair is felt by the patients. The score of "0" and "1" indicates normal and abnormal, respectively [64].

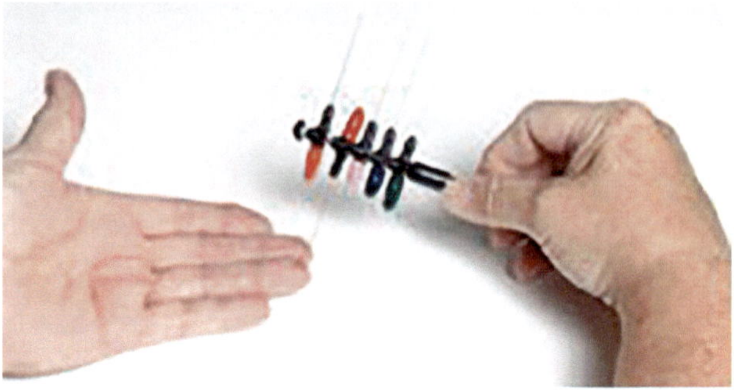

Fig. 11.2 von Frey hair

11.3.2.1.4 Ipswich Touch Test (IpTT)

Using the index finger's tip, the examiner touches gently on first, third, and fifth toes' tips and hallux's dorsum in both feet, for 1 or 2 s without a push, prod, tap, or poke, with patient's eyes closed. Peripheral neuropathy is defined with a score ≥2 insensate sites out of eight. The IpTT is a reliable, simple without the expense, and always at hand, a tool for the screening and detection of high-risk patients of foot ulcers [65].

11.3.2.2 Tests for Vibratory Sensation

11.3.2.2.1 Tuning Fork Test

Vibration sensation is determined by the on–off method placing a vibrating 128-Hz tuning fork at first toe' dorsum to nail bed's proximity on the bony prominence. Patients are requested for reporting the vibration perception's start as well as the cessation. After that, the examiner's thumb distal phalanx dorsal aspect is applied with the tuning fork. Furthermore, a standardized form is used to record the time (in seconds) when according to the perception of the examiner the vibration sensations were faded. On each toe, the test should be repeated twice, and the results should be marked on a standardized form. Also, vibration testing threshold can be described as the total number of times there was no vibrating tuning fork's application as well as vibration's dampening, and the score varies among 0–8. Furthermore, as per the difference in time among perception period signified by the examiner as well as the patient defines the peripheral neuropathy [66].

VibraTip

One of the novel tools is VibraTip used to replace the tuning fork as a source of vibratory stimulus. A vibratory stimulus is produced by it which is the same as 128 Hz tuning fork as well as it is utilized at times of foot examination for DPN detection. Following assessment through the MTEP (Medical technologies Evaluation Program) process, it has been described by the NICE Medical Technology Guidance 22 that VibraTip has a great potential in improving the DPN detection as well as for the NHS cost savings is provided. Although, it cannot be proved against these reasonable doubts due to the available clinical evidence's lack [67].

Bio-Thesiometer

Essentially, the Bio-thesiometer is an "electrical tuning fork" in which a predetermined level of amplitude can be set as well as there will be a gradual increase in amplitude till vibratory sensation's threshold is acquired. On the contrary, the lowering of amplitude is done until there does not exist any vibration. For each case, at a specific level, the determination of amplitudes is done with the greatest accuracy. Being a simple, sensitive, and comfortable method, it is suitable for screening for detection and evaluation of peripheral neuropathy [68].

11.3.2.3 Tactile Circumferential Discriminator

The TCD is a sensory testing device that is portable, which is meant for testing the function of large nerve fibers. TCD is highly sensitive and cost-effective for the community screening for foot ulceration's risk patients identification [69]. The TCD comprises of a handheld disc along with increasing circumferences eight protruding rods, which are meant for assessing the tactile function. In a controlled study by Vileikyte et al. [69], TCD is found a reliable and effective technique for population screening to identify neuronal dysfunction and risk for diabetic foot ulceration.

11.3.2.4 Ball-Bearing Test

A steel ball-bearing with various diameters is used to examine each foot's plantar area over the second metatarsal head. Patients are requested for barefoot walking on flat ground along with the attached plaster of ball-bearing. The contralateral foot is applied with an empty control plaster. The ball-bearing score is defined by the least diameter that can be felt by the patient (range 1–6). The steel ball-bearing test with its high sensitivity and specificity is to be considered for both the evaluation of protective sensory reflexes and screening of patients for risk to neuropathic ulceration [70].

11.3.3 Methods for Peripheral Arterial Disease Screening and Assessment in Diabetic Patients

In diabetic patients, peripheral arterial disease's assessment, as well as early detection, have a significant part in diabetic foot ulcers' prevention as well as management. Even with PAD's high prevalence in diabetic patients, many of them do not report the symptoms of PAD and the symptoms like pain may be blunted by the neuropathic pathology in peripheral nerves [71–74]. The abovementioned facts explain the need for proper screening methods disease in diabetic patients for detecting peripheral arterial.

11.3.3.1 Physical Exam

During the activity, the leg pain (intermittent claudication) and clinical signs like an absent or weak pulse around distal arteries evidence for the peripheral vascular disease's presence and indicates the ulceration risk [75].

11.3.3.2 ABPI Measurement

It is the ratio between the SBP measured on ankles and arms and an effective validated and reproducible screening test for lower limb vascular insufficiency's severity as well as presence's objective assessment. It consists of quantitative methods that are noninvasive to determine the lower limb arteries' patency. It can be easily carried out by any healthcare professional clinic with a Doppler ultrasonic sensor and a BP cuff [76, 77]. The ABPI value of >0.9 is indicative of peripheral arterial disease in both diabetic as well as nondiabetic patients [78].

MESI ABPI MD®, a new device that in clinical settings for PAD screening gives an easy solution along with the ABI's precise, accurate, and fast measurements and depends on an improved oscillometric technology [75].

11.3.3.3 Ultrasound

Doppler ultrasound is useful for identifying narrowed or blocked arteries as well as evaluating the flow of blood in the blood vessels. Arterial duplex ultrasonography demonstrated a 99% specificity and 95% sensitivity for occlusive disease detection, with 92% sensitivity and 97% specificity for hemodynamically significant disease [79].

11.3.3.4 Angiography

Different methodologies for angiography such as DSA (digital subtraction angiography), contrast material-enhanced magnetic resonance (MR) angiography, and CT (computed tomographic) angiography for peripheral arterial disease detection [80].

11.4 Summary

This disease's most usual complication is Diabetic foot disease which causes high morbidity among diabetic patients and leads to high chances for amputation of the lower limb in these patients. The extensive searches in this field identified a number of risk factors which will provoke this complication in diabetic patients, such as comorbidities, peripheral arterial disease presence, peripheral neuropathy disease presence, and glycemic control extension and disease duration. The diabetic foot syndrome development is also influenced by sociodemographic factors such as the age of the patient, financial background, and lifestyle. In addition, the presence of foot deformities and ill-fitting footwear contribute to the causation of this complication of diabetes. Since the diabetic foot syndrome carries a high negative effect on patients' life quality as well as morbidity along with financial burden to the community, risk's early detection for diabetic foot syndrome development and prompt diagnosis and management of the condition has a pivotal role. Different screening tests are described in this chapter for the early evaluation of the peripheral arterial and peripheral neuropathy diseases' presence. There are several guidelines, highlighted above, which suggests various methods and diabetic foot disease management, including multidisciplinary methods and podiatric care.

References

1. Mishra SC, Chhatbar KC, Kshikar A, Mehndiratta A (2017) Diabetic foot. Br Med J 359(Supp 1):1–7. https://doi.org/10.1136/bmj.j5064
2. National Institute for Health and Care Excellence (2016) Diabetic foot problems: prevention and management. https://www.nice.org.uk/guidance/ng19. Accessed 28 Aug 2019
3. Jeffcoate WJ, Macfarlane RM, Fletcher EM (1993) The description and classification of diabetic foot lesions. Diabet Med 10:676–679
4. Parek AK, Goodman RA, Gordon C, Koh HK (2011) HHS interagency workgroup on multiple chronic conditions. Managing multiple chronic conditions: a strategic framework of improving health outcomes and quality of life. Public Health Rep 126(4):460–471. https://doi.org/10.1177/003335491112600403
5. Lazzarini PA, Hurn SE, Fernando ME et al (2015) Prevalence of foot disease and risk factors in general inpatient populations: a systematic review and meta-analysis. BMJ Open 5:e008544. https://doi.org/10.1136/bmjopen-2015-008544. PMID: 26597864
6. Volmer-Thole M, Lobmann R (2016) Neuropathy and diabetic foot syndrome. Int J Mol Sci 17(6):917. https://doi.org/10.3390/ijms17060917
7. Mishra SC, Chhatbar KC, Kashikar A, Mehndiratta A (2017) Diabetic foot. BMJ 359:j5064. https://doi.org/10.1136/bmj.j5064
8. Chantelau EA (2015) Nociception at the diabetic foot, an uncharted territory. World J Diabetes 6(3):391–402. https://doi.org/10.4239/wjd.v6.i3.391
9. Burns S, Leese G, McMurdo M (2002) Older people and ill-fitting shoes. Postgrad Med J 78(920):344–346
10. Nixon BP, Armstrong DG, Wendell C, Vazquez JR, Rabinovich Z, Kimbriel HR, Rosales MA, Boulton AJ (2006) Do US veterans wear appropriately sized shoes? The veterans affairs shoe size selection study. J Am Podiatr Med Assoc 96(4):290–292
11. Andrew KB, Hylton BM (2008) Incorrectly fitted foot wear, foot pain and foot disorders: a systematic search and narrative review of the literature. J Foot Ankle Res 11:43. https://doi.org/10.1186/s13047-018-0284-z
12. Allan J, Munro W, Figgins E (2016) Foot deformities within the diabetic foot and their influence on biomechanics: a review of the literature. Prosthet Orthot Int 40(2):182–192. https://doi.org/10.1177/0309364615592705
13. Vibha SP, Muralidhar MK, Kirthinath ABB, Asha K, Maiya GA (2018) Community based study to assess the prevalence of diabetic foot syndrome and associated risk factor among the pattients with diabetes mellitus. BMC Endocr Disord 18:43. https://doi.org/10.1186/s12902-018-0270-2
14. Sabanayagam C, Liew G, Tai ES et al (2009) Relationship between glycated haemoglobin and microvascular complications: is there a natural cut-off point for the diagnosis of diabetes? Diabetologia 52:1279–1289
15. Pop-Busui R, Lu J, Lopes N et al (2009) Prevalence of diabetic peripheral neuropathy and relation to glycemic control therapies at baseline in the BARI 2D cohort. J Peripher Nerv Syst 14:1–13
16. Diabetes Control and Complications Trial Research Group (1993) The effect of intensive treatment of diabetes on the development and progression of long-term complications in insulin-dependent diabetes mellitus. N Engl J Med 329:977–986

17. Ohkubo Y, Kishikawa H, Araki E et al (1995) Intensive insulin therapy prevents the progression of diabetic microvascular complications in Japanese patients with non-insulin-dependent diabetes mellitus: a randomized prospective 6-year study. Diabetes Res Clin Pract 28:103–117
18. UK Prospective Diabetes Study Group (1998) Intensive blood-glucose control with sulphonylureas or insulin compared with conventional treatment and risk of complications in patients with type 2 diabetes (UKPDS33). Lancet 352:837–853
19. Yagihashi S, Mizukami H, Sugimoto K (2011) Mechanism of diabetic neuropathy: where are we now and where to go? J Diabetes Investig 2(1):18–32. https://doi.org/10.1111/j.2040-1124.2010.00070.x
20. Tresierra-Ayala MÁ, García Rojas A (2017) Association between peripheral arterial disease and diabetic foot ulcers in patients with diabetes mellitus type 2. Med Univ 19(76): 123–126
21. van Schie CH, Vermigli C, Carrington AL, Boulton A (2004) Muscle weakness and foot deformities in diabetes: relationship to neuropathy and foot ulceration in Caucasian diabetic men. Diabetes Care 27(7):1668–1673. https://doi.org/10.2337/diacare.27.7.1668
22. Marso SP, Hiatt WR (2006) Peripheral arterial disease in patients with diabetes. J Am Coll Cardiol 47:921–929
23. Roca MM, Carral F, Baena G, Sánchez Z, Valencia I, Aguilar M (2007) Evaluación de la enfermedad vascular periférica en pacientes con diabetes tipo 2 mediante medición del índice tobillo-brazo. Av Diabetol 23:370–374
24. Rabia K, Khoo EM (2007) Prevalence of peripheral arterial disease in patients with diabetes mellitus in a primary care setting. Med J Malays 62:130–133
25. Poitier L, Halbron M, Bouilloud F et al (2009) Ankle-to-brachial ratio index underestimates the prevalence of peripheral occlusive disease in diabetic patients at high risk for arterial disease [carta]. Diabetes Care 32:e44
26. Mancera J, Paniagua F, Martos I et al (2010) Enfermedad arterial periférica oculta en población diabética seguida en atención primaria. Clin Invest Arterioscl 22:154–161
27. Mukherjee D (2009) Peripheral and cerebrovascular atherosclerotic disease in diabetes mellitus. Best Pract Res Clin Endocrinol Metab 23:335–345
28. Hee YJ, Hwang JY, Mi-Seon S et al (2011) The prevalence of peripheral arterial disease in Korean patients with type 2 diabetes mellitus attending a university hospital. Diabetes Metab J 35:543–550
29. Schaper NC, Andros G, Apelqvist J et al (2012) Specific guidelines for the diagnosis and treatment of peripheral arterial disease in a patient with diabetes and ulceration of the foot 2011. Diabetes Metab Res Rev 28(Suppl 1):236–237
30. Beckert S, Witte M, Wicke C, Königsrainer A, Coerper S (2006) A new wound-based severity scores for diabetic foot ulcers: a prospective analysis of 1000 patients. Diabetes Care 29:988–992
31. Schaper NC, Andros G, Apelqvist J et al (2012) A progress report of the international working group on the diabetic foot. Diagnosis and treatment of peripheral arterial disease in diabetic patients with a foot ulcer. Diabetes Metab Res Rev 28(Suppl 1):218–224
32. Akca AT, Cinar S (2008) Comparison of psychosocial adjustment in people with diabetes with and without diabetic foot ulceration. Aust J Adv Nurs 25(4):87–96
33. DeBerardis G, Pellegrini F, Franciosi M, Belfiglio M, DiNardo B, Greenfield S et al (2005) Are type 2 diabetic patients offered adequate foot care? The role of physician and patient characteristics. J Diabetes Complicat 19(6):319–327
34. Mayfield JA, Reiber GE, Sanders LJ, Janisse D, Pogach LM (1998) Preventive foot care in people with diabetes. Diabetes Care 21(12):2161–2177
35. Bowering CK (2001) Diabetic foot ulcers. Can Fam Physician 47:1007–1016
36. Armstrong DG, Lavery L, Harkless L (1998) Validation of a diabetic wound classification system—the contribution of depth, infection, and ischemia to risk of amputation. Diabetes Care 21:855–859
37. Gooch C, Podwall D (2004) The diabetic neuropathies. Neurologist 10:311–322

38. Boyko EJ, Ahroni JH, Stensel V, Forsberg RC, Davignon DR, Smith DG (1999) A prospective study of risk factors for diabetic foot ulcer: the Seattle Diabetic Foot study. Diabetes Care 22:1036–1042
39. Reiber GE, Vileikyte L, Boyko EJ, del Aguila M, Smith DG, Lavery LA, Boulton AJ (1999) Causal pathways for incident lower-extremity ulcers in patients with diabetes from two settings. Diabetes Care 22:157–162
40. de Sonnaville JJ, Colly LP, Wijkel D, Heine RJ (1997) The prevalence and determinants of foot ulceration in type II diabetic patients in a primary health care setting. Diabetes Res Clin Pract 35:149–156
41. Witana CP, Feng J, Goonetilleke RS (2004) Dimensional differences for evaluating the quality of footwear fit. Ergonomics 47(12):1301–1317. https://doi.org/10.1080/00140130410001712645
42. Goonetilleke RS, Luximon A, Tsui KL (2000) The quality of footwear fit: what we know, don't know and should know. In: Proceedings of the human factors and ergonomics society annual meeting. SAGE Publications, New York, pp 515–518
43. Gorecki G (1978) Shoe related foot problems and public health. J Am Podiatry Assoc 68(4):245. https://doi.org/10.7547/87507315-68-4-245
44. Frey C (2000) Foot health and shoewear for women. Clin Orthop 372:32–44. https://doi.org/10.1097/00003086-200003000-00005
45. Richards R (1991) Calluses, corns, and shoes. Semin Dermatol 10(2):112–114
46. Pérez-Panero A, Ruiz-Muñoz M, Cuesta-Vargas A, Gónzalez-Sánchez M (2019) Prevention, assessment, diagnosis and management of diabetic foot based on clinical practice guidelines: a systematic review. Medicine 98(35):e16877. https://doi.org/10.1097/MD.0000000000016877
47. Formosa C, Gatt A, Chockalingam N (2016) A critical evaluation of existing diabetic foot screening guidelines. Rev Diabet Stud 13(2–3):158–186. https://doi.org/10.1900/RDS.2016.13.158
48. Ryden L, Standl E, Bartnik M, Van den Berghe G, Betteridge J, de Boer MJ, Cosentino F, Jonsson B, Laakso M, Malmberg K et al (2007) Guidelines on diabetes, pre-diabetes, and cardiovascular diseases: executive summary. The Task Force on Diabetes and Cardiovascular Diseases of the European Society of Cardiology (ESC) and of the European Association for the Study of Diabetes (EASD). Eur Heart J 28(1):88–136
49. National Institute for Health and Care Excellence (2014) NICE guideline NG19. Diabetic foot problems: prevention and management. Available from: https://www.nice.org.uk/guidance/ng19
50. https://diabeticfootaustralia.org/wp-content/uploads/DFA-Guides-you-through-guidelines.pdf
51. Reiber GE, Vileikyte L, Boyko EJ, Aguila M, Smith DG, Lavery LA et al (1999) Causal pathways for incident lower-extremity ulcers in patients with diabetes from two settings. Diabetes Care 22:157–162
52. Boulton AJ, Vinik AI, Arezzo JC, Bril V, Feldman EL, Freeman R et al (2005) Diabetic neuropathies: a statement by the American Diabetes Association. Diabetes Care 28(4):956–962
53. Boulton AJM (2005) Management of diabetic peripheral neuropathy. Clin Diabetes 23(1):9–15
54. Vinik AI, Mehrabyan A (2004) Diabetic neuropathies. Med Clin North Am 88(4):947–999
55. Smith AG, Singleton JR (2013) Obesity and hyperlipidemia are risk factors for early diabetic neuropathy. J Diabetes Complications 27(5):436–442
56. Petropoulos IN, Ponirakis G, Khan A, Almuhannadi H, Gad H, Malik RA (2018) Diagnosing diabetic neuropathy: something old, something new. Diabetes Metab J 42:255–269
57. Singleton JR, Bixby B, Russel JW, Feldman EL, Peltier A, Goldstein J, Howard J, Smith G (2008) The Utah Early Neuropathy Scale: a sensitive clinical scale for early sensory predominant neuropathy. J Peripher Nerv Syst 13:21–227
58. May S, Serpell M (2009) Diagnosis and assessment of neuropathic pain. F1000 Med Rep 1:76
59. Eckeli FD, Teixeira RA, Gouvea AL (2016) Neuropathic pain evaluation tools. Rev Dor Sao Paulo 17(Suppl 1):s20–s22

60. Ambreen A, Muhammad AH, Umar AK, Nadeem A, Mujeeb-ur-Rahman AB (2010) Reliability of the neurological scores for assessment of sensorimotor neuropathy in type 2 diabetics. JMPA 60(3) ISSN: 0030-9982
61. Meijer JW, Johen WG, Willem HE, Thera PL, Sounderen EV, Blaauwwiekel EE, Smit AJ (2000) Diabetic neuropathic examination: a hierarchical scoring system to diagnose distal polyneuropathy in diabetes. Diabetes Care 22:75–753
62. https://www.clwk.ca › buddydrive › file › procedure-monofilament-testing
63. Paisley A, Abbott C, van Schie C, Boulton A (2002) A comparison of the Neuropen against standard quantitative sensory-threshold measures for assessing peripheral nerve function. Diabet Med 19(5):400–405
64. Moharić M, Vidmar G, Burger H (2012) Sensitivity and specificity of von Frey's hairs for the diagnosis of peripheral neuropathy in patients with type 2 diabetes mellitus. J Diabetes Complications 26(4):319–322. https://doi.org/10.1016/j.jdiacomp.2012.04.008
65. Rayman G, Vas PR, Baker N, Taylor CG Jr, Gooday C, Alder AI, Donohoe M (2011) Ipswich Touch Test: a simple and novel method to identify inpatients with diabetes at risk of foot ulceration. Diabetes Care 34(7):1517–1518. https://doi.org/10.2337/dc11-0156
66. Perkins BA, Olaleye D, Zinman B, Bril V (2001) Simple screening tests for peripheral neuropathy in the diabetes clinic. Diabetes Care 24(2):250–256. https://doi.org/10.2337/diacare.24.2.250
67. Willits I, Cole H, Jones R, Dimmock P, Arber M, Craig J, Sims A (2015) VibraTip™ for testing vibration perception to detect diabetic peripheral neuropathy: a NICE medical technology guidance. Appl Health Econ Health Policy 13:315–324. https://doi.org/10.1007/s40258-015-0181-6
68. Kasalová Z (2002) Biothesiometry in the diagnosis of peripheral neuropathies. Cas Lek Cesk 141(7):223–225
69. Vileikyte L, Hollis S, Hutchings G, Boulton AJM (1997) The tactile circumferential discriminator—a new, simple screening device to identify diabetic patients at risk of fot ulceration. Diabetes Care 20(4):623–626
70. Papanas N, Gries A, Maltezos E, Zick R (2006) The steel ball-bearing test: a new test for evaluating protective sensation in the diabetic foot. Diabetologia 49(4):739–743
71. Faglia E, Caravaggi C, Marchetti R et al (2005) Screening for peripheral arterial disease by means of the ankle-brachial index in newly diagnosed type 2 diabetic patients. Diabet Med 22:1310–1314
72. Belch J et al (2008) The prevention of progression of arterial disease and diabetes (POPADA) trial. BMJ 337:a1840
73. Bendermacher BL, Teijink JA, Willigendael EM, Bartelink ML, Peters RJ, de Bie RA et al (2007) A clinical prediction model for the presence of peripheral arterial disease—the benefit of screening individuals before initiation of measurement of the ankle-brachial index: an observational study. Vasc Med 12(1):5–11
74. Piarulli F, Sambataro M, Mincuci N, Scarano L, Laverda B, Baiocchi MR et al (2007) Mild peripheral neuropathy prevents both leg muscular ischaemia and activation of exercise induced coagulation in Type 2 diabetic patients with peripheral artery disease. Diabet Med 10:1099–1104
75. Špan M, Geršak G, Millasseau SC, Meža M, Košir A (2016) Detection of peripheral arterial disease with an improved automated device: comparison of a new oscillometric device and the standard Doppler method. Vasc Health Risk Manag 12:305–311. https://doi.org/10.2147/VHRM.S106534
76. Greenland P, Abrams I, Aurigemma GP et al (2000) Prevention conference V: beyond secondary prevention: identifying the high-risk patient for primary prevention: non-invasive tests of atherosclerotic burden: Writing Group III. Circulation 101(1):E16–E22
77. American Diabetes Association (2003) Peripheral arterial dis-ease in people with diabetes. Diabetes Care 26:3333–3341

78. Prompers L, Apelqvist J, Bakker J et al (2007) High prevalence of ischaemia, infection, and serious comorbidity in patients with diabetic foot disease in Europe. Baseline results from the Eurodiale study. Diabetologia 50:18–25
79. Whelan JF, Barry MH, Moir JD (1992) Color flow Doppler ultrasonography: comparison with peripheral arteriography for the investigation of peripheral vascular disease. J Clin Ultrasound 20(6):369–374
80. Philip AH, Ioannis K, Amir HD, Timothy GS, Jeremy DC, John JS, Eugene ED, Navyash G, James CC, Edelman RR (2011) Evaluation of peripheral arterial disease with nonenhanced quiescent-interval single-shot MR angiography. Radiology 260(1):282–293. https://doi.org/10.1148/radiol.11101336

Part III

Developments, Future Prospective, New Possible Treatments

Advances in Prevention and Empirical Treatment of Diabetic Foot Infection

12

Hamid Ashraf, Jamal Ahmad, and Anees Akhtar

12.1 Introduction

Foot-related complications are accountable for up to 50% of all diabetes-related hospital admissions. Lifetime risk of foot ulcer in patients with diabetes is 10–15% and infection complicates over 50% of these ulcerations [1]. Diabetic foot infections (DFIs) are associated with significant morbidity, mortality, reduced quality of life, economic burden, discomfort, need for hospital visits, wound care, antibiotic therapy, and often surgical measures like debridement [1, 2]. More than one-fifth of moderate or severe diabetic foot infections are associated with some level of amputation [3].

Diabetic patients are more prone to infection, secondary to altered immune response, altered circulatory status, and the presence of neuropathy [3]. Sixty percent of lower limb amputation occurs secondary to infections [4–6], making infections the immediate preceding event of this dreaded outcome. Loss of protective sensation predisposes recurrent breach in the skin of diabetic foot, and different kinds of microorganisms colonize and multiply on these ulcers, and this leads to tissue destruction and causes an inflammatory reaction that is regarded as clinical infection [7]. These infections can involve the deeper tissues like bone and leads to osteomyelitis [8]. The presence of ischemia secondary to peripheral arterial disease

H. Ashraf (✉)
Rajiv Gandhi Center for Diabetes & Endocrinology, Faculty of Medicine, J N Medical College & Hospital, Aligarh Muslim University, Aligarh, India

J. Ahmad
Retired Professor & Director Rajiv Gandhi Center for Diabetes & Endocrinology, Faculty of Medicine, J N Medical College & Hospital, Aligarh Muslim University, Aligarh, India

Diabetes & Endocrinology Superspeciality Center, Aligarh, India

A. Akhtar
Department of Microbiology, Faculty of Medicine, J N Medical College & Hospital, Aligarh Muslim University, Aligarh, India

M. Zubair et al. (eds.), *Diabetic Foot Ulcer*,
https://doi.org/10.1007/978-981-15-7639-3_12

(PAD), leads to necrosis and delayed or nonhealing of the ulcer [9]. Infection together with ischemia significantly increases the risk of limb amputation [8].

Management of DFI needs identification and accurate classification of the foot lesion, careful collection of the specimen for culture, timely initiation and careful selection of empirical and definitive antimicrobial therapies, providing timely surgical debridement are needed [9].

Chronic diabetic foot ulcer (DFU) is frequently contaminated with more than one pathogens.

Staphylococcus aureus and *Pseudomonas aeruginosa* are frequently encountered causative pathogens in DFIs. But the distributions of these pathogens vary geographically and they also depend on the duration of the wound, previous use of antimicrobials, and the importance of nosocomial infections [9]. The use of unsuitable antibiotics can lead to drug-resistant bacteria, thereby making the choice of antibiotics difficult [10].

12.2 Etiopathogenesis of Diabetic Foot Infection

Multiple pathological process which gets activated in patients of diabetes mellitus ultimately affects foot. Any structure from the skin, subcutaneous tissue, muscles, nerve fibers, vasculature to bones can be involved. The reasons for the increased incidence of these disorders in patients with diabetes mellitus (DM) involve the interaction of several pathogenic factors: neuropathy, abnormal foot biomechanics, PAD, and poor wound healing. Development of ulceration in diabetics precedes the development of infection [11]. The presence of peripheral sensory neuropathy hinders with normal protective sensations, this leads to sustain major or recurrent minor trauma to the foot, frequently without knowledge of the injury to the patients. After breech in skin continuity because of repeated trauma, microorganism may colonize the site and proliferate. This leads to destruction of the local tissue and initiates the cascade of inflammation, which can have systemic manifestation [12].

12.2.1 Peripheral Neuropathy

Some form of involvement of peripheral nervous system is present in 60% of diabetic patients [10–12]. Loss of protective sensation is an early phenomenon in the development of diabetic neuropathy [13]. All three kinds of nerves (sensory, motor, or autonomic) are usually affected. The involvement of motor nerves leads to imbalances between the flexor and extensor musculatures of foot, leading to deformities in the form of clawing, prominent metatarsals heads, foot drop and equinus deformity. These deformities lead to abnormal distribution of plantar pressure, increasing the risk for ulceration [14].

The involvement of sensory nerves manifests as either positive symptoms such as tingling, burning and pain, or negative symptoms such as numbness. Sensory loss in the form of loss of pain, temperature, touch, and vibration sensation in the feet lead to ill-fitting shoes or early signs of foot abnormality that may go unobserved by the patient and remains uncorrected. The presence of callus is common in neuropathic ulcers and interferes with the healing potential of an ulcer, predisposing to infection [15].

Involvement of the autonomic nervous system manifests as loss of sweat gland function, leading to dry skin, vulnerable to cracking, and infection. Loss of autoregulation leads to increased blood flow. This manifests as edema and osteopenia [16, 17].

12.2.2 Peripheral Arterial Disease

Appearance of atherosclerosis is accelerated in diabetes. Risk of atherosclerosis is two to three times higher in patients with diabetes when compared with nondiabetic population [18]. Risk factors for the development of atherosclerosis are the degree and duration of hyperglycemia, dyslipidemia, obesity, smoking, and a family history of atherosclerosis. Both micro- and macrovessels are involved in diabetic patients. The arteriopathy is also associated with endothelial dysfunction, enhanced arteriovenous shunting, abnormal hyperaemic response to inflammation, enhanced capillary permeability leading to swelling over the lower limb. These changes are associated with delayed and abnormal healing processes in a diabetic foot ulcer [19]. Reduction in the blood supply to the affected limb exacerbates the problems due to neuropathy. Initial features of vascular involvement in the limbs includes atrophic foot, absence of hair on the dorsum, cool temperature of the limb, and thin shiny and atrophic skin [20].

12.2.3 Immune Dysregulation

Patients with diabetes are more susceptible to infections, as hyperglycemia is associated with impaired leukocyte function (chemotaxis, phagocytosis, and killing), structural changes in macrophages, raised inflammatory cytokines, and impairment of polymorphonuclear cell functions [21]. In addition, elevated glucose is a nice medium for the growth of microorganism [18, 19]. Hyperglycemia is also associated with impaired granuloma formation, the protracted occurrence of abscess, compromised production of proteins, fibroblasts, and collagen because of insulin deficiency besides the presence of nutritional inadequacy leading to poor wound healing [22].

12.2.4 Foot Deformity

The involvement of motor nerves leads to imbalances between the flexor and extensor musculatures of foot leading to deformities. These deformities lead to abnormal distribution of plantar pressure, increasing the risk for ulceration. Recurrent trauma from walking and weight bearing or unfitting footwear, leads to augmented plantar pressures, causing the development of callus and break in skin continuity. This causes the formation of blister, tearing of skin and fissuring [23]. Ligament and tendons become inflexible secondary to reduced elasticity and lead to contractures. The presence of these deformities increases the risk of foot ulceration in diabetes.

12.3 Prevention of Diabetic Foot Infection

Awareness of the conjecturers of foot ulcer occurrence, which may be modified by evidence-based interventions, is essential for making a strategy to prevent DFU. Such strategy requires a cohesive approach, education, and awareness of both the patient and treating physicians [24]. Meaningful achievement in the management of diabetic foot-related complications can only be accomplished with a motivated multidisciplinary team approach, with the help of good communication and concerted efforts between the various players. The aim is to provide proper care to the right patient at an appropriate time and in the required amount. Preventive measures are required for both better patient outcomes and cost-effectiveness [25]. A multidisciplinary attitude is suggested for persons with high-risk feet and foot ulcers, particularly those with a previous history of ulcer or amputations [17].

Annual comprehensive examination of foot should be performed, to detect the risk factors for DFU. Foot examination is required at every visit in patients with established loss of protective sensation (LOPS) or previous history of foot ulceration [26]. A careful history regarding foot ulceration, amputation, Charcot foot, any vascular procedure, smoking, retinopathy, nephropathy and intermittent claudication should be obtained. A careful examination of skin integrity and foot deformities should be done. Examination of pedal arteries by palpating the pedal pulses should be done. Neurological examination should focus on detecting LOPS. Use of 10-g monofilament is recommended for detecting LOPS. 10-g monofilament along with any one additional test (pinprick sensation, temperature, or vibration sensation by a 128-Hz tuning fork, or ankle reflexes) should be performed [27].

The negative monofilament test is indicative of LOPS, whereas two normal tests (and no abnormal test) rules out LOPS [27].

Patients with low risk should be examined annually; those with high risk should be examined at each visit. Prevention of foot ulcer occurrence and recurrence entails good glycaemic control, ongoing specialized foot care, and appropriately fitting shoes which has an established effect on the release of plantar pressure [28]. Good education of patient by a dedicated and focussed team may enhance the patients' observance of management recommendations [29]. Management of foot ulcer requires standard protocols for wound care, including off-loading with bed rest, total contact cast, custom-made cast walkers and healing sandals, radical wound debridement. Steps helpful in reducing the foot ulceration and infections are given in Table 12.1.

Table 12.1 Steps helpful in reducing the foot ulceration and infections

• Self-care of foot • Daily examination of feet daily for blisters, scratches, cuts, and inflamed areas • Examination of toe webs • One should always check between the toes • Daily cleaning of feet with mild soap • Dry carefully, especially between the toes • Avoid extreme temperatures • Check the water temperature with hand or elbow prior to bathing. Electric blanket, hot water bottles should be avoided • Avoid barefoot walk • Self-removal of corns should be avoided	• Footwear care • Use properly fitting shoes • Always wear shoes with socks or stockings • Sandals with thongs between the toes should be avoided • Remove shoes during the day to release pressure • People with neuropathy or increased plantar pressure need well-fitted walking shoes or athletic shoes that cushion the feet and redistribute pressure • People with deformities need extra wide or deep shoes • **When to report to doctor** • Cuts, fissures, callus, or breaks in the stem • Alterations in color or discoloration of the foot • Ingrowth of nails • Numbness or loss of sensation • Any apparent deformity

Table 12.2 Summary of IDSA guidelines for obtaining culture form diabetic foot ulcer

Clinically uninfected wounds: Specimen for culture is not recommended
Infected wounds: Properly obtained samples for culture before initial empiric antibiotic therapy
Mild infection in with no history of antibiotic use: Cultures may be unnecessary
Samples should be obtained from deep tissue by biopsy or curettage after cleaning and debridement
Avoid samples collection via swab, especially from inefficiently debrided wounds

12.4 Empirical Management of Diabetic Foot Infection

Empirical antibiotic therapy is needed in the initial management of diabetic foot infections. Many factors may guide to avoid choosing either an unnecessarily broad or inappropriately narrow regimen antibiotic. Before choosing the empirical therapy it is important to document the presence of infection, and if it is present than grade its severity [30, 31]. Since DFU is often chronic, and infected with a number of microorganisms, so proper collection of the microbiological specimen is very important in order to isolate the actual pathogens and their antimicrobial sensitivity. Collection of culture specimen with a swab is not recommended, since they do not provide precise results. Specimen obtained from deep infected tissue or bone should be cultured [32–34]. The culture from superficial swab and deep tissue samples provides discordant results [32, 35]. Culture and sensitivity should be repeated when patients are not responding to the treatment [36]. The Infectious Disease Society of America provided guidelines for the collection of specimen from DFU in 2012 (Table 12.2) [37].

Several basic points need to be considered prior to antibiotic prescription. Initially, the foot infection should be classified clinically. The criteria established by the Infectious Diseases Society of America [37] or the International Working Group on the Diabetic Foot [36] can be used for the same. Those with severe infection, require broad-spectrum parenteral antibiotic therapy, till the culture reports are available. Patients with mild to moderate infection can be often managed with a narrower spectrum antimicrobial agent. Many patients with mild to moderate infections will improve, with the help of proper supportive care, debridement, pressure off-loading, and wound dressing [38]. Antibiotic therapy should always cover aerobic Gram-positive cocci, especially *Staphylococcus aureus*, which is both the most common and virulent pathogen in DFU. Decision to provide coverage for methicillin-resistant *S. aureus* (MRSA), will depend upon the presence or absence of risk factors for MRSA [39]. Risk factors for MRSA include history of recent hospitalization, prior antibiotic intake and renal replacement therapy. Enterococci are often grown on culture, but they rarely cause the infection and are simple colonizer [40]. They require treatment only when patients fail to respond to standard therapy. Up to two-third patients with chronic DFU have infection with aerobic Gram-negative bacilli. Enterobacteriaceae are the commonest Gram-negative isolates from chronic DFU, and these are covered by newer broad-spectrum antibiotics. Once therapy for Gram-negative organism has been decided then the next question is to whether target *Pseudomonas aeruginosa* or not. Findings from a recent study from Korea has identified smoking and previous antibiotic use as a risk factor for *Pseudomonas aeruginosa* [35]. Pseudomonas species is generally found as part of a polymicrobial infection [41]. Another factor that needs especial consideration is the presence of obligate anaerobic microorganism, as they have been found to be present in a significant number of patients [42, 43]. They are commonly found as a part of mixed infection with aerobes, rather than as an only pathogen [44]. Risk factor for anaerobes includes peripheral arterial disease, limb ischaemia and resultant necrosis or gangrene. The presence of foul-smelling discharge from the wound gives clinical clue to the presence of anaerobes. Good debridement leads to removal of necrotic material, and thus eradicating many of the anaerobes and uncovering those remaining to air, could be all that is needed to manage these potential pathogens. Anaerobic coverage is needed only when there is a robust clinical feature of anaerobic infection, i.e., the classical "fetid foot" [45].

Lastly, the route of administration needs some discussion. With the advent of an oral agent with very high bioavailability, results with oral therapy are comparable with parenteral therapy [46]. The result of antibiotic therapy is dependent upon the concentration of antibiotic at local site, rather than on the route of administration. So even though started on parenteral therapy, once they improve, they can be switched to oral therapy [47]. Patients with mild infection can be treated with topical therapy. Table 12.3 summarizes the guidelines for antibiotic treatment for the empirical management of diabetic foot infections.

Table 12.3 Guidelines for antibiotic treatment for the empirical management of diabetic foot infections

Type of infection	Additional characteristic	Likely pathogen	Suggested antibiotic
Acute	No systemic features, no previous antibiotic use, low risk for MRSA	Methicillin sensitive Gram-positive cocci	1st generation cephalosporins, clindamycin
	Penicillin allergy or intolerance	Methicillin sensitive Gram-positive cocci	Clindamycin, fluoroquinolones (FQ)
	High local prevalence of MRSA, previous antibiotic use	Methicillin-resistant *Staphylococcus aureus*	Clindamycin, doxycycline, trimethoprim/sulfamethoxazole, linezolid, daptomycin
Chronic	No systemic feature	Methicillin sensitive Gram-positive cocci Gram-negative bacilli	Second or third generation cephalosporin, aminoglycoside
	Previous antibiotic treatment	Methicillin-resistant staph aureus Gram-negative bacilli ± Anaerobes	b-Lactam, b-lactamase inhibitor; second- or third-generation cephalosporin; group 1 carbapenem; FQ ± aminoglycoside
	Necrotic, gangrenous ischaemic limb; foul odor	Methicillin-resistant *staphylococcus aureus* Gram-negative bacilli	Clindamycin (±FQ); metronidazole (+FQ); b-lactam, b-lactamase inhibitor; carbapenem, cefepime
	Greenish discharge, smoking, macerated ulcer	*Pseudomonas aeruginosa*	Piperacillin/tazobactam, cefepime, imipenem, meropenem, Fluroquinolones
	Risk factors for resistant Gram-negative bacilli	ESBL, MDR Gram-negatives	Piperacillin/ tazobactam + aminoglycoside, imipenem, meropenem

12.5 Recent Advances in Prevention and Empirical Treatment of Diabetic Foot Infection Prevention of Diabetic Foot Infection

Various associations have provided guidelines for the management and prevention of DFU. The International Working Group on the Diabetic Foot has given many evidence-based recommendations to doctors for the prevention of DFU, which can have a substantial influence in decreasing the risk of ulcer recurrence and decreasing the load of this ailment on patients and society [48]. Recent work of the cost-effectiveness of existing integrated and novel methods and of the effectiveness of scientific support and patient response for improving self-management and treatment adherence may foster the development of further effective approaches for averting ulcer recurrence. Adherence to the preventive measures are an important part of management, particular emphasis on behavior and its role in observance to and results of therapy will also be significant [49].

12.5.1 Achieving Optimal Off-Loading

Off-loading is the cornerstone in the management of DFU. The instruments for off-loading in DFU are total contact casts and removable cast walkers, and they are capable to reduce forefoot peak pressure by 90%, compared to barefoot walking [50]. Off-loading devices for the primary or secondary prevention of DFU have a larger margin for improvement in terms of off-loading capacity. Recently, the art of making customized preventative off-loading footwear has benefitted from the availability of advance plantar pressure calculation devices. Two types of modalities have been successfully used. One technique is to incorporate plantar pressure measurement devices into the manufacture of insoles by an electronic milling machine [51]. The second technique is to measure the plantar pressure on users' feet, at the time of wearing conventional footwear, and then the footwear is modified according to the observed pressure values. Many cycles of plantar pressure measurement followed by the footwear adjustment can be done. Both the approaches have been found to be effective in reducing the recurrence of DFU [52, 53]. But to achieve optimal benefit adherence to off-loading is essential.

12.5.2 Thermal Monitoring for DFU Prevention

Another emphasis of current technological developments has been the early identification at risk foot in the pre-ulcerative phase. As the temperature is raised in any inflammation, assessment of temperature multiple times daily over feet, has been found to be effective in the prediction of diabetic foot ulcer [50]. The presence of elevated temperature can be used to counsel persons to reduce their physical activity to reduce their risk of developing a DFU [16]. These suggestions are based on the premise, that an inflammatory response starts in the foot regions, which are exposed to disproportionate physical strain. If two similar sites on two different feet have temperature difference than the warmer site is likely reflective of pre-ulcerative inflammation [50]. In order to reduce the progression to ulcer formation, patients are directed to decrease their physical movement if they notice a "hot spot." Patients can restart their normal physical activities, when temperatures difference normalizes among the 2 feet. Handheld thermometers have been most commonly utilized to assess foot temperatures [50, 52]. Newer version, using a telemedicine system along with a floor mat with embedded temperature sensors has been assessed [49]. This system is easy to use, with individuals need to step on it for 20 seconds. The automated system then analyses the temperature profile of the 2 feet. Using a cut-off of ≥2.22 °C difference between matching sites on opposite feet, the mat identified 97% of DFU with an average time duration of 37 days. Compliance with the mat use was high with 86% of individuals using the mat at least 3 times per week, and average use was 5 times per week. The cut-off of 2.22 °C yielded 97% sensitivity but the specificity was only 43% specificity [50]. The smart socks with the capability of measuring the foot temperature, over one or several times a day, are under development [49]. Because of its ease of use, the temperature-monitoring socks provide the opportunity for continuous temperature assessment. A probable upcoming alternate to instrumented socks is the footwear capable of monitoring the temperature on the plantar surface of the feet. Along with identifying injury to the feet, plantar thermal sensors could deliver the added advantage of monitoring footwear adherence [51].

12.5.3 Molecular Methods for Detection of Pathogens

The diabetic foot infections are variable in character and poses challenge during management. Detecting the variety of microbes colonizing the diabetic ulcer is of paramount importance, and this involves the proper specimens obtained from the wound after debridement [53]. Traditional culture and sensitivity was the only way to detect the causal organism in a DFI for many decades. Frequently fastidious growing microbes are not detected, leading to biased and late results by using traditional bacteriology procedures. Lately, molecular microbiology techniques (direct PCR, 16 ribosomal DNA sequencing, denaturing gradient gel electrophoresis, pyrosequencing, etc.) have confirmed the occurrence of larger numbers and varied varieties of species in various types of wounds than had previously been documented [54]. Techniques of molecular genetics are evolving, and microbial multiplicity of the infected ulcers can be more conveniently and sensitively detected by utilizing the advanced molecular techniques than traditional bacteriological methods [55]. One of the advanced techniques for the detection of microbes depends on PCR amplification method with specifically designed nucleotide primers. PCR has been proposed to be safer, precise, and speedy technique than traditional bacteriological methods for detecting viruses and bacteria [56]. Almost all the studies with molecular microbiological techniques have shown that most DFU has many more bacterial species, than were previously identified based on the results of traditional bacteriological methods [56]. PCR has been found to be sensitive, selective, and specific assay that can detect a smaller number of cultivable as well as non-cultivable organisms. One of the study from our center revealed, that the use of the PCR technique improved the rate of identifying pathogens in pus samples than traditional bacteriological methods. Also, PCR is rapid (4 h) when compared to that of the culture-based methods (48–72 h). The PCR-based technique leads to improvement in the speedy diagnosis of most commonly found bacteria, also yielding greater detection rates of pathogens. PCR has been found to be exceptionally sensitive and dependable being able to detect 100% of culture-confirmed bacterial samples. It also identified few culture-negative, but clinically significant diabetic foot infections, suggesting high level of efficiency [57].

12.6 Summary

There are many difficulties and unmet needs in the management of DFI, comprising a lack of knowledge and awareness of diabetes and its complications, lack of appropriate podiatry services. Management of DFI needs a concerted effort involving a team of health care professionals devoted to the care of diabetes, particularly associated with foot complications. A suitable awareness of the diabetic foot in terms of its biomechanical etiology and the causative risk factors for DFI, availability of newer techniques, involving both clinical and surgical interventions and crucial off-loading strategies to reduce wound pressure is required, among the managing team is needed to efficiently managing DFI in India.

References

1. Singh N, Armstrong DG, Lipsky BA (2005) Preventing foot ulcers in patients with diabetes. JAMA 293:217–228
2. National Diabetes Fact Sheet (2011) US Department of Health and Human Services. Atlanta, GA, Center for Disease Control and Prevention, p 2011
3. Prompers L, Huijberts M, Apelqvist J et al (2007) High prevalence of ischaemia, infection and serious comorbidity in patients with diabetic foot disease in Europe. Baseline results from the Eurodiale study. Diabetologia 50:18–25
4. International Working Group on the Diabetic Foot (1999) International consensus on the diabetic foot. Amsterdam, pp 1–96
5. Pecoraro RE, Ahroni JH, Boyko EJ, Stencil VL (1991) Chronology and determinants of tissue repair in diabetic lower-extremity ulcers. Diabetes 40:1305–1313
6. Reiber GE, Pecoraro RE, Koepsell TD (1992) Risk factors for amputation in patients with diabetes mellitus: a case control study. Ann Intern Med 117:97–105
7. Peters EJ, Lipsky BA (2013) Diagnosis and management of infection in the diabetic foot. Med Clin North Am 97:911–946
8. Nather A, Bee CS, Huak CY, Chew JL, Lin CB, Neo S, Sim EY (2008) Epidemiology of diabetic foot problems and predictive factors for limb loss. J Diabetes Complications 22:77–82
9. Uckay I, Gariani K, Pataky Z, Lipsky BA (2014) Diabetic foot infections: state-of-the-art. Diabetes Obes Metab 16:305–316
10. Miyan Z, Fawwad A, Sabir R, Basit A (2017) Microbiological pattern of diabetic foot infections at a tertiary care center in a developing country. J Pak Med Assoc 67:665–669

11. Armstrong DG, Lavery LA (1998) Diabetic foot ulcers: prevention, diagnosis and classification. Am Fam Physician 57:1325–1332
12. Zubair M, Malik A, Ahmad J (2011) Clinico-microbial study and anti-microbial drug resistance profile of diabetic foot infections in North India. Foot 21:6–14
13. Zubair M, Malik A, Ahmad J (2012) Study of plasmid-mediated extended-spectrum b-lactamase-producing strains of enterobacteriaceae, isolated from diabetic foot infections in a North Indian tertiary-care hospital. Diabetes Technol Ther 14(4):315–324
14. Young MJ, Boulton AJ, Macleod AF et al (1993) A multicentric study of the prevalence of diabetic peripheral neuropathy in the United Kingdom Hospital clinic population. Diabete 36:150–154
15. Reiber GE, Vileikyte L, Boyko EJ, del Aguila M, Smith DG, Lavery LA et al (1999) Causal pathways for incident lower-extremity ulcers in patients with diabetes from two settings. Diabetes Care 22:157–162
16. Noor S, Zubair M, Ahmad J et al (2015) Diabetic foot ulcer—a review on pathophysiology, classification and microbial etiology. Diabetes Metab Syndr 9:192–199
17. Ahmad J (2016) The diabetic foot. Diabetes Metab Syndr 10:48–60
18. The Diabetes Control and Complications Trial Research Group (1993) The effect of intensive treatment of diabetes on the development and progression of long term complications in insulin-dependent diabetes mellitus. N Eng J Med 329(14):977–986
19. Marston WA, Davies SW, Armstrong B et al (2006) Natural history of limbs with arterial insufficiency and chronic ulceration treated with revascularization. J Vasc Surg 44:108–114
20. Bridges RM Jr, Deitch EA (1994) Diabetic foot infections. Path physiology and treatment. Surg Clin North Am 74:537–555
21. Hostetter MK (1990) Perspectives in diabetes. Handicaps to host defense. Effects of hyperglycemia on C3 and *Candida albicans*. Diabetes 39:271–275
22. Geerlings SE, Brouwer EC, Gaastra W, Verhoef J, Hoepelman AIM (1999) The effect of glucose and pH on uropathogenic and non-uropathogenic *Escherichia coli*: studies using urine from diabetics and non-diabetics. J Med Microbiol 48:535–539
23. Schram JC, Dinh T, Vevas A (2006) Microvascular changes in the diabetic foot. Int J Low Extreme Wounds 5:149–159
24. Jaap AJ, Shore AC, Stockman AJ et al (1996) Skin capillary density in subjects with impaired glucose tolerance and patients with type 2 diabetes. Diabet Med 13:160–164
25. Lincoln NB, Radford KA, Game FL, Jeffcoate WJ (2008) Education for secondary prevention of foot ulcers in people with diabetes: a randomised controlled trial. Diabetologia 51:1954–1961
26. Dargis V, Pantelejeva O, Jonushaite A, Vileikyte L, Boulton AJ (1999) Benefits of a multidisciplinary approach in the management of recurrent diabetic foot ulceration in Lithuania: a prospective study. Diabetes Care 22:1428–1431
27. American Diabetes Association (2019) 11. Microvascular complications and foot care: standards of medical care in diabetes—2019. Diabetes Care 42(Suppl 1):S124–S138
28. American Diabetes Association (2003) Peripheral arterial disease in people with diabetes. Diabetes Care 26:3333–3341
29. Hingorani A, LaMuraglia GM, Henke P et al (2016) The management of diabetic foot: a clinical practice guideline by the Society for Vascular Surgery in collaboration with the American Podiatric Medical Association and the Society for Vascular Medicine. J Vasc Surg 63(Suppl):3S–21S
30. Bus SA, van Netten JJ (2016) A shift in priority in diabetic foot care and research: 75% of foot ulcers are preventable. Diabetes Metab Res Rev 32(Suppl 1):195–200
31. Armstrong DG, Bharara M, White M et al (2012) The impact and outcomes of establishing an integrated interdisciplinary surgical team to care for the diabetic foot. Diabetes Metab Res Rev 28:514–518
32. Chakraborti C, Le C, Yanofsky A (2010) Sensitivity of superficial cultures in lower extremity wounds. J Hosp Med 5:415–420

33. Pellizzer G, Strazzabosco M, Presi S, Furlan F, Lora L, Benedetti P, Bonato M, Erle G, de Lalla F (2001) Deep tissue biopsy vs. superficial swab culture monitoring in the microbiological assessment of limb-threatening diabetic foot infection. Diabet Med 18:822–827
34. Nelson EA, Wright-Hughes A, Brown S, Lipsky BA, Backhouse M, Bhogal M, Ndosi M, Reynolds C, Sykes G, Dowson C, Edmonds M, Vowden P, Jude EB, Dickie T, Nixon J (2016) Concordance in diabetic foot ulceration: a cross-sectional study of agreement between wound swabbing and tissue sampling in infected ulcers. Health Technol Assess 20:1–176
35. Rhee SM, Han SK, Kim WK (2010) Difference of microbiology according to tissue sampling in diabetic ulcers. J Korean Soc Plast Reconstr Surg 37:1–6
36. Lipsky BA, Aragon-Sanchez J, Diggle M, Embil J, Kono S, Lavery L, Senneville E, Urbančič-Rovan V, Van Asten S, Peters EJ, International Working Group on the Diabetic Foot (2016) IWGDF guidance on the diagnosis and management of foot infections in persons with diabetes. Diabetes Metab Res Rev 32(Suppl 1):45–74
37. Lipsky BA, Berendt AR, Cornia PB, Pile JC, Peters EJ, Armstrong DG, Deery HG, Embil JM, Joseph WS, Karchmer AW, Pinzur MS, Senneville E, Infectious Diseases Society of America (2012) 2012 Infectious Diseases Society of America clinical practice guideline for the diagnosis and treatment of diabetic foot infections. Clin Infect Dis 54:e132–e173
38. Lipsky BA, Berendt AR, Deery HG et al (2004) IDSA guidelines: diagnosis and treatment of diabetic foot infections. Clin Infect Dis 39:885–910
39. Lipsky BA (2004) A report from the international consensus on diagnosing and treating the infected diabetic foot. Diabetes Metab Res Rev 20(Suppl 1):S68–S77
40. Wagner A, Reike H, Angelkort B (2001) Highly resistant pathogens in patients with diabetic foot syndrome with special reference to methicillin-resistant *Staphylococcus aureus* infections (in German). Dtsch Med Wochenschr 126:1353–1356
41. Tentolouris N, Petrikkos G, Vallianou N et al (2006) Prevalence of methicillin-resistant Staphylococcus aureus in infected and uninfected diabetic foot ulcers. Clin Microbiol Infect 12:186–189
42. Lipsky BA, Armstrong DG, Citron DM, Tice AD, Morgenstern DE, Abramson MA (2005) Ertapenem versus piperacillin/tazobactam for diabetic foot infections (SIDESTEP): prospective, randomised, controlled, double-blinded, multicentre trial. Lancet 366:1695–1703
43. Lipsky BA, Pecoraro RE, Wheat LJ (1990) The diabetic foot. Soft tissue and bone infection. Infect Dis Clin North Am 4:409–432
44. Lee JS, Son ST, Han SK (2017) Risk factors of methicillin-resistant Staphylococcus aureus and Pseudomonas infection in diabetic foot ulcers in Korea. J Wound Manag Res 13:29–34
45. Chung CH, Kim DJ, Kim J, Kim H, Kim H, Min KW, Park SW, Park JH, Baik SH, Son HS, Ahn CW, Oh JY, Lee S, Lee J, Choi KM, Choi I, Park IB (2006) Current status of diabetic foot in Korean patients using national health insurance database. J Korean Diabetes Assoc 30:372–376
46. Korean Society for Diabetic Foot (2014) Korean guideline for management of diabetic foot, 1st edn. Koonja Press, Seoul, pp 49–66
47. Bus SA, Armstrong DG, van Deursen RW, Lewis JE, Caravaggi CF, Cavanagh PR (2016) IWGDF guidance on footwear and offloading interventions to prevent and heal foot ulcers in patients with diabetes. Diabetes Metab Res Rev 32(Suppl 1):25–36
48. Bus SA, Waaijman R, Arts M, de Haart M, Busch-Westbroek T, van Baal J, Nollet F (2013) Effect of custom-made footwear on foot ulcer recurrence in diabetes: a multicenter randomized controlled trial. Diabetes Care 36:4109–4116
49. Frykberg RG, Gordon IL, Reyzelman AM, Cazzell SM, Fitzgerald RH, Rothenberg GM, Bloom JD, Petersen BJ, Linders DR, Nouvong A, Najafi B (2017) Feasibility and efficacy of a smart mat technology to predict development of diabetic plantar ulcers. Diabetes Care 40:973–980
50. Lavery LA, Higgins KR, Lanctot DR, Constantinides GP, Zamorano RG, Athanasiou KA, Armstrong DG, Agrawal CM (2007) Preventing diabetic foot ulcer recurrence in high-risk patients: use of temperature monitoring as a self-assessment tool. Diabetes Care 30:14–20

51. Najafi B, Mohseni H, Grewal GS, Talal TK, Menzies RA, Armstrong DG (2017) An optical-fiber-based smart textile (smart socks) to manage biomechanical risk factors associated with diabetic foot amputation. J Diabetes Sci Technol 11:668–677
52. Baron EJ (2011) Conventional versus molecular methods for pathogen detection and the role of clinical microbiology in infection control. J Clin Microbiol 49(Suppl 9):S43
53. Melendez JH, Frankel YM, An AT, Williams L, Price LB, Wang NY et al (2010) Real-time PCR assays compared to culture-based approaches for identification of aerobic bacteria in chronic wounds. Clin Microbiol Infect 16:1762–1769
54. Lavigne JP, Sotto A, Dunyach-Remy C, Lipsky BA (2014) New molecular techniques to study the skin microbiota of diabetic foot ulcers. Adv Wound Care 4:38–49
55. Babalola O (2003) Molecular techniques: an overview of methods for the detection of bacteria. Africa J Biotechnol 2:710–713
56. Dowd SE, Wolcott RD, Sun Y, McKeehan T, Smith E, Rhoads D (2008) Polymicrobial nature of chronic diabetic foot ulcer biofilm infections determined using bacterial tag encoded FLX amplicon pyrosequencing (bTEFAP). PLoS One 3:e3326
57. Noor S, Raghav A, Parwez I, Ozair M, Ahmad J (2018) Molecular and culture based assessment of bacterial pathogens in subjects with diabetic foot ulcer. Diabetes Metab Syndr 12(3):417–421

Prevention of Diabetic Foot: Indian Experience

13

Vijay Viswanathan and A. Sai Prathiba

13.1 Introduction

Diabetes mellitus, a chronic metabolic disease, is a major risk factor leading to mortality and morbidity due to its potential microvascular and macrovascular complications. The most common cause of hospitalization among diabetics is the diabetic foot infection, apparently, it is the most severe complication and at the same time, the therapy is expensive too. Amputation is 10–20 times more common among diabetic people than non-diabetics, in particular, it is estimated that every 30 s a lower limb or a part of the lower limb is lost somewhere in the world as a consequence of diabetes [1].

13.2 Epidemiology and Problem of Diabetic Foot in India

The global prevalence of the disease is going to be tripled in the next 30 years. The International Diabetic Federation (IDF) states that in 2017, there were 451 million people with diabetes worldwide which is further expected to increase to 693 million in 2045 [2]. The prevalence of this disorder is increasing rapidly among native and migrant Asian populations [3]. ICMR has conducted INDIAB (INDian DIABetes) study in 2011 which has revealed that among all the states in India, Tamil Nadu stands third with 4.8 million patients with diabetes and 3.9 million in prediabetic stage [4]. A study conducted by Murray et al. to identify the Global Burden of the Disease in 2010 had published startling results. He classified diabetes as one of the leading specific causes of Years lived with Disability (YLD) which underscores the burden imposed by diabetes on the individuals. When we refer to the fatal

V. Viswanathan (✉) · A. Sai Prathiba
M. V. Hospital for Diabetes and Prof. M. Viswanathan Diabetes Research Centre (WHO Collaborating Centre for Research, Education and Training in Diabetes), Chennai, India
e-mail: dr_vijay@mvdiabetes.com

M. Zubair et al. (eds.), *Diabetic Foot Ulcer*,
https://doi.org/10.1007/978-981-15-7639-3_13

outcomes, it was estimated that five million deaths all over the world were attributable to people with diabetes in the age group 20–99 years [5]. Systematic and prospective study comparing risk factors for diabetic ulceration and treatment outcomes between centers in industrialized nations and developing countries was carried out in three centers [6] [Southeast Germany (GER), Dar-slaam, Tanzania (TAN) & Chennai, India (IND)] contained 613 consecutive patients with diabetic foot lesions and found that the most important underlying factor of foot ulceration in patients from all three centers was diabetic neuropathy. 368 (60%) of the 613 patients sampled were treated for new diabetic foot lesion. Patients were predominantly male in all three centers and had type 2 diabetes. The average duration of diabetes until the initial foot lesion started was in GER for 14 years and in IND for 12 years, but in TAN for only 5 years. The patient's age was 71, 56, and 51 years. The most common cause of foot lesions in GER was insufficient footwear (19%), although lack of shoes, improper foot care, and burns were the primary precipitating factors among TAN and IND patients. Indicates that there are considerable differences between Western and developing-country diabetic foot patients which should be taken care of while conducting prevention program.

In a developing country like India, the economic boom, the lifestyle changes, migration from rural to urban areas seem to affect diabetes. Contrastingly, this increase in diabetes should have accelerated a large number of studies given the diversity and ethnicity, yet there remains a serious lacuna that needs to be addressed. This can seriously attenuate the proportions of people affected by diabetes in the upcoming years [7]. A multicentric study to estimate the pattern and causes of amputations among diabetics has revealed that infection was the major cause of amputations in India. Among these, a majority (70%) of amputations were minor (involving tarsometatarsal joints, metatarsal bones, toes, or rays). Below-knee amputation was found to be very common among major amputations. Over half of the amputations involved were only toes and rays. Neuropathy was highly prevalent (82%) among the diabetic study population. This study can be generalized to some extent to a national level [8].

13.3 How to Diagnose High-Risk Feet in a Primary Care Center

MNSI: This is Michigan Neuropathy screening instrument which includes 15 item self-answered questionnaires and to assess neuropathy in lower extremity based on vibration sensation and ankle reflex [9]. Diabetic peripheral neuropathy needs to be identified using a simple, inexpensive tool that can screen sensation loss. A graduated tuning fork was used to test vibration perception scores in subjects with sensory neuropathy detected by abnormal biothesiometry. The graduated tuning fork was suitable to detect sensation loss in the feet with high specificity (100%) and fair sensitivity (52%). Furthermore, it was simpler and cheaper to use in outpatient department [10].

Table 13.1 Neuropathy Disability Score (NDS) scoring [12]

Neuropathy Disability Score (NDS)		Right	Left
Vibration perception threshold 128-Hz tuning fork; apex of big toe: normal = can distinguish vibrating/not vibrating	Normal = 0 Abnormal = 1		
Temperature perception on dorsum of the foot Use tuning fork with beaker of ice/warm water			
Pin-prick Apply pin proximal to big toe nail just enough to deform the skin; trial pair = sharp, blunt; normal = can distinguish sharp/not sharp			
Achilles reflex	Present = 0 Present with reinforcement = 1 Absent = 2		
	NDS Total out of 10		

People unable to perceive variations in temperature might have distal symmetric neuropathy. So the need of the hour was to use an instrument that can detect temperature sensitivity. Though the above test was simple and specific, it was not sensitive-enough. Thus, Tip-therm, a pen-like instrument was tested to find if it can be used as an ideal instrument to measure temperature perception in type 2 diabetics. The results were astounding. Tip-therm when compared with monofilament and biothesiometry (established methods of diagnosing diabetic neuropathy) had high specificity (100%) and sensitivity (97.3%) in diagnosing diabetic neuropathy [11]. The NDS score below is used to assess the signs of neuropathy (Table 13.1).

13.4 Development of Footwear in Chennai

Many studies have emphasized the use of specially designed shoes to prevent relapses in diabetics with previous ulceration. Prescription footwear has demonstrated to be a significant factor in preventing ulcer recurrence and amputation [13]. It is for this reason that uniquely designed footwear, in collaboration with the Central Leather Research Institute (CLRI) and Central Footwear Training Institute (CFTI) is available in Chennai. The use of this therapeutic footwear is important especially for Indians as they walk barefoot or wearing improper footwear in extreme heat conditions which can worsen neuropathy.

13.5 Effect of Foot Care Education to Prevent Amputation

The beneficial effects of foot care education cannot be underestimated since there are numerous studies to prove this worthwhile. A study by Vijay et al. has revealed that foot care education and intensive management have proven effective in preventing newer problems and surgeries. There was less frequent recurrence of ulcers and faster healing process in subjects who adhered to foot care advice. Simple advices like examination of feet, how to perform a pedicure, and using proper footwear has reduced foot complications to a larger extent [14]. Another study has proven that foot infections have occurred in 65% of the subjects who did not follow foot care procedures [15]. Amputations rate came down to a considerable extent after the formation of national foot care and health education and prevention in some island populations, such as Fiji and Nauru [16]. In order to reduce the burden of diabetic foot complications, effective foot care advice must be emphasized. The importance of wearing an appropriate footwear and foot care education for all high-risk patients cannot be underscored.

13.6 Use of Modern Technology in India for Wound Care

13.6.1 Hyperbaric Oxygen Therapy (HBOT)

This treatment involves breathing 100% oxygen in a special room under normal atmospheric pressure, thereby making more oxygen available into the bloodstream to promote healing. A systematic review conducted on HBOT in healing foot ulcers was proven to be effective in subjects with concomitant ischemia [17]. The importance of HBOT as adjunctive therapy was proven in a study by Ezhilarasi et al. where it was seen that HBOT has a positive effect in initiating the healing process of ulcer than the standard treatment involving offloading, wound debridement and glucose control [18].

13.6.2 Vacuum-Assisted Closure (VAC) Therapy

This involves using an electronic vacuum pump to apply negative pressure across the wound surface. This is particularly useful in large diabetic wounds where bone, tendon, joint capsule, and fascia are exposed after wound debridement. A clinical trial done among 60 cases with foot ulcers from 3 centers in India for the evaluation of recombinant human epidermal growth factor (REGEN-D™ 150) after administering for a period of 10 weeks found that the trial subjects had reduced wound healing time for the period of 9 weeks compared to the placebo. This trail demonstrated the efficacy of this gel in accelerating the wound healing process [19].

13.7 Conclusion

Diabetic neuropathy which affects the nerves of the feet causes severe damage thereby leading to amputation. With India becoming the diabetic capital of the world, there is a need for more and more people to be aware of the treatment, prevention, and cure of foot ulcers. Educating the patient about maintaining optimum glycemic control, using appropriate footwear at all times, avoiding foot trauma, performing daily examinations of feet, and reporting changes to health care professionals should be insisted.

References

1. International Diabetes Federation. Available from https://www.idf.org/our-activities/care-prevention/diabetic-foot.html
2. Cho NH, Shaw JE, Karuranga S, Huang Y, da Rocha Fernandes JD, Ohlrogge AW, Malanda B (2018) IDF Diabetes Atlas: global estimates of diabetes prevalence for 2017 and projections for 2045. Diabetes Res Clin Pract 138:271–281
3. Ramachandran A, Snehalatha C, Ronald CWM (2010) Diabetes in Asia. Lancet 375(9712):408–418. https://doi.org/10.1016/S0140-6736(09)60937-5
4. Anjana RM et al (2011) Prevalence of diabetes and prediabetes in urban and rural India: Phase I results of Indian Council of Medical Research-INdia DIABetes (ICMR-INDIAB) study. Diabetologia 54(12):3022–3027
5. Murray CJL et al (2012) Disability-adjusted life years (DALYs) for 291 diseases and injuries in 21 regions, 1990–2010: a systematic analysis for the Global Burden of Disease Study 2010. Lancet 380(9859):2197–2223
6. Vijay V, Morbach S, Lutalet JK, Mollenberg J, Ochs HR, Seena R, Ramachandran A, Abbas ZG (2004) Regional differences in risk factors and clinical presentation of diabetic foot lesions. Diabet Med 21:91–95
7. Kaveeshwar SA, Cornwall J (2014) The current state of diabetes mellitus in India. Australas Med J 7(1):45–48
8. Viswanathan V, Kumpatla S (2011) Pattern and causes of amputation in diabetic patients—a multicentric study from India. J Assoc Physicians India 59:148–151
9. MNSI—Michigan Neuropathy Screening Instrument. Michigan Diabetes Research and Training Center. 2010 from http://www.umich.edu/mdrtc/survey/index/html#mnsi
10. Viswanathan V, Snehalatha C, Seena R, Ramachandran A (2001) The Rydel Seiffer tuning fork: an inexpensive device for screening diabetic patients with high-risk foot. Practical Diabetes Int 18(5):155–156
11. Viswanathan V, Snehalatha C, Seena R, Ramachandran A (2002) Early recognition of diabetic neuropathy: evaluation of a simple outpatient procedure using thermal perception. Postgrad Med J 78(923):541–542
12. Boulton AJM (2005) Management of diabetic peripheral neuropathy. Clin Diabetes 23(1):9–15
13. Vijay V, Sivagami M, Saraswathy G, Gautham G, Das BN, Seena R, Ramachandran A (2004) Effectiveness of different types of footwear insoles for the diabetic neuropathic foot. Diabetes Care 27:474–477
14. Viswanathan V et al (2005) Profile of diabetic foot complications and its associated complications – a multicentric study from India. J Assoc Physicians India 53:933–936
15. Amputation Prevention Initiative in South India (2005) Positive impact of foot care education. Diabetes Care 28(5):1019–1021
16. LEA Study Group (1995) Comparing the incidence of lower extremity amputations across the world. The global lower extremity amputation study. Diabet Med 12:14–18
17. Stoekenbroek RM, Santema TB, Legemate DA, Ubbink DT, van den Brink A, Koelemay MJ (2014) Hyperbaric oxygen for the treatment of diabetic foot ulcers: a systematic review. Eur J Vasc Endovasc Surg 47(6):647–655
18. Ezhilarasi K, Palani A, Viswanathan V (2018) Healing effect of hyperbaric oxygen therapy as an adjunctive treatment on diabetic foot ulcer patients in short duration—a brief report. Asian J Sci Tech 9(3):7743–7746
19. Vijay V, Pendsey S, Sekar N, Murthy GSR (2006) A phase III study to evaluate the safety and efficacy of recombinant human epidermal growth factor (REGEN-D™ 150) in healing diabetic foot ulcers. Wounds 18(7):186–196

Low-Cost Management of Diabetic Foot 14

Zulfiqarali G. Abbas

14.1 Introduction and Epidemiology

Diabetes mellitus is a condition with serious outcomes for people with diabetes across the world [1–3]. Diabetes affects all people in the world, has no limitation for age, sex, or status of the person. In 2019 prevalence of diabetes in the world was 463 million [3]. People are living longer, dietary pattern is changing, lifestyle is more of sedentary it is expected that diabetes prevalence rates to increase to 578 million by 2030 and 700 million by 2045 [3].

The continent of Africa is going to suffer and will be hit hard by diabetes and its complications than the rest of the globe. In Africa, people with diabetes are going to increase and will be double every decade we move forward [3]. In 2017 patients with diabetes were 14.2 million, within 2 years in 2019 it increased to 19 million and it is now predicted the way it is increasing to reach 29 million by 2030, and by 2045 to reach 47 million, which is the highest increase in diabetes in Africa than any region of the world of about 143% [3].

Much of the increase in population will happen in Sub-Saharan Africa, which includes many of the poor of the poorest countries. Similar to other parts of the globe as the population will grow, more people in Sub-Saharan Africa will live in cities, consume more processed food, and develop obesity, heart disease, cancer, and type 2 diabetes [4]. People would live longer as life expectancy in undeveloped parts of the region will increase [4]. Diabetes in the world remains one of the leading causes of morbidity and death [5–18]. Complications caused by diabetes, for example, related to eye, kidneys, cardiovascular system, but the most dreadful complications are of diabetic foot ulcers, which are related to highest rates of morbidity and mortality [5–18]. Septic diabetic foot can be extremely serious costly [5–23].

Z. G. Abbas (✉)
Abbas Medical Centre, Dar es Salaam, Tanzania

Muhimbili University of Health and Allied Sciences, Dar es Salaam, Tanzania
e-mail: zabbas@cats-net.co.tz

M. Zubair et al. (eds.), *Diabetic Foot Ulcer*,
https://doi.org/10.1007/978-981-15-7639-3_14

Approximately, 40–60% of all lower limb amputations across the world are performed in patients with diabetes [18, 19]. One million amputations are performed in the world on people with diabetes [18, 19]. The year 2005 was designated to world diabetic foot. It was estimated by the International Working Group of Diabetic Foot (IWGDF) that every 30 s a lower limb is lost due to diabetes somewhere in the world [18, 19]. Today after 15 years in 2020 it was estimated that now every 20 s a lower limb is amputated due to diabetes somewhere in the world [18, 19]. The situation is getting worse rather than improving after all the preventive programmes going on all over the world. With the increase in diabetes-related conferences, diabetic foot conferences, etc., but still instead of improving things are getting worse.

14.2 Diabetic Foot Ulcer Financial Burden

Literature most of them published regarding the cost of treating a diabetic foot ulcer comes from western developed world like USA, Sweden, Holland, and the UK. We are lacking literature on the cost of treating diabetic foot from developing countries. It was important to set up a study to estimate the cost of treating diabetic foot ulcers in the developing world. A study was set up to conduct the cost of treating diabetic foot ulcers in five different countries in the world from three continents [20]. All the countries that participated in this study were given a similar case to estimate the cost in their own country. The cost was estimated to the patient and to the society of treating foot ulcers in five different countries from three continents with completely different health care practices, reimbursement policies, and gross domestic products [20]. It was noted that treating the cost of the same ulcer to the same endpoints in all five countries was estimated at $3060 in Tanzania, which is only 1.6% of the US cost of $188,645 [20].

Medical insurance or reimbursement of medical expenses is not available in the continent of Africa. Management of complicated diabetic foot ulcer can cost more than 2 years of average income for the patient [20]. During the foot ulcer management, the loss of productivity caused by unemployment or sick leave is an added cost to the family, relatives, and community [20–23]. For example, in Senegal the cost of amputation has been estimated to be about 3200 USD not including the orthopaedic equipment [23]. It is devastating and catastrophic if a patient is the only bread earner in an extended family and is very common in Africa [20–23].

14.3 What Is the Reality on the Ground?

14.3.1 Peripheral Neuropathy (PN)

Where ever you are in the world peripheral neuropathy one of the complications of diabetes is the most common. Peripheral neuropathy in the literature ranges from 5–80% of patients with diabetes in the western world [24, 25]. Across Africa, the prevalence rate of peripheral neuropathy is shown the same as seen in the developed world [1, 2, 5–11, 13–16, 26–30]. In the literatures, it has shown that there is no difference in ethnicity or race where ever you are in the world, from Africa being an African, Asia being an Asian or European being Caucasian [14, 15].

14.3.2 Peripheral Arterial Disease (PAD)

Peripheral arterial diseases are one of the important complications of the diabetic foot, which causes high rates of morbidity and mortality. Commonly seen in the western world and used to be not seen in the developing world that is Africa, Asia, and South America. Time is changing and situation across the African continent the rates of PAD are increasing [1–5, 14, 18, 31–34]. As the continent of Africa develop the same time communities in Africa becoming more urbanized, sedentary lifestyle, lack of exercise, change of diet, adopting lifestyle of western people, etc. PAD is increasing in African at the cost of Africa is developing.

14.3.3 Diabetic Foot Ulcers and Amputation

In Africa rates of diabetic foot ulcers are more leading to high morbidity and mortality all over the continent. A study done in Tanzania in 2002 showed 15% of diabetes patients admitted are of foot ulcers, 33% of patients ended up with amputation and 54% of the patients died because of late presentation to the referral hospital are already with extreme pathology (Wagner score ≥ 4) [11]. This is true and seen in most of the parts of the African continent that are with high rates of amputation and death [1, 2, 4, 5, 7, 9, 12, 35–38].

14.4 What Are the Strategies and Challenges?

Developed world has increased research in the past over 20 years on molecular, epidemiology, and genetics. An increase in research of genetics has actually not benefited in patients care and outcome in many countries where basic routine diabetes and diabetic foot care are needed. Increased diabetes burden and limb complications funds allocated in the developed world are most of the time offset for high-tech, medication and antimicrobial are always available. Adequate diabetic foot care delivery in North America is due to the high cost of healthcare insurance rates. The only work that has had any significant impact on patient outcomes in the field of epidemiology carried out in developing nations, including from the African continent, especially for the complication of diabetes is in the diabetic foot, which has been implemented the findings in evidence-based practice. The health systems in the African continent become overwhelmed when there is an increased incidence of PAD [1–5, 14, 18, 31–34].

The major challenges remain that how do we actually achieve successful solutions of the diabetic foot in a poor resource's country, without the high technology and resources available in developed nations? With the existing epidemiological realities and plan in relatively small amounts that could really boost the better outcomes of diabetic foot complications.

14.5 Managing the Diabetic Foot in Low-Cost Setting

In African diabetes patients, almost all foot ulcers are infected on the first presentation as can be seen in the published literature [1, 2, 5–11, 14–16, 18, 35–39]. Patients most of the time present to health centres are already too late with gangrene and infection (Wagner score ≥ 4) or infection has gone to stage of septicaemia and no response to regular antibiotics [11].

Diabetic foot infection is very common in most low resource countries, where no podiatrist facilities, could be several other causes like lesions initially are ignored or noticed relatively late or after unsuccessful home treatment like use of herbal medication, bathroom surgery, soaking in herbal water, application of home remedies, going to faith healer, etc. It is due to these reasons most of the patients with diabetic foot get medical help when serious infection has set in or gangrene of limb has started. It becomes difficult to save foot if presented late to the centre. This can be prevented and can be reduced through proper foot care [18].

Least foot infection is cellulitis, the involvement of deep soft tissue infection is involvement of fascia, muscles, and deep tissue and osteomyelitis when bone is involved [11, 18, 19]. Chronic foot ulcers progress to spread to underlying bone from soft tissue inflammation in an ulcer. Osteomyelitis can be diagnosed by a simple bedside test by probing to the bone beneath an ulcer with a sterile blunt instrument, bone radiography, isotope bone scans, or histology. In Africa, the fact is that most of the centres do not have nuclear medicine services and histology tests routinely available. Abbas and colleagues usually use simple bedside test of probing the bone beneath an ulcer to diagnose the presence or absence of osteomyelitis. When osteomyelitis is detected, the necrotic tissue will be removed until the viable tissue is evident, followed by antibiotic treatment. If the prognosis of foot ulcer looks poor then it is referred for surgical assessment with a view to remove necrotic bone or undergo an amputation if necessary and followed by medical treatment.

The role of microbiology sampling is restricted to the identification of probably pathogens and the sensitivity to antibiotics. Superficial swab specimens for culture and sensitivity are not very useful due to polymicrobial growth, which are largely uninterpretable, but the infection is diagnosed purely on clinical grounds [18, 19, 39].

Deep tissue biopsy gives more useful information. In resources poor countries, microbiology services do not have routine facilities for analysing biopsy specimens [39]. For this reasons, Abbas and colleague had to look for the solution for less developed countries by conducted epidemiologic and microbiology studies and the use of antibiotics.

The use of Gram staining is forgotten as a bedside test and can be done at any place in the world with poor resources. Abbas and colleagues looked at the utility of Gram stains in comparison with culture and sensitivity in the management of limb ulcers in persons with diabetes. We found a sensitivity of more than 90%. In this study, it was concluded that there is no difference in Gram staining and culture for microbiology [39]. Patients with infected foot ulcers empirical broad-spectrum antimicrobials (without microbiology cultures), can be used in conjunction with surgical debridement yielded similar or better outcomes than antimicrobials chosen by antimicrobial susceptibility testing of pathogens isolated from deep tissue cultures [18, 19, 39]. Patients with infected foot ulcers, surgical debridement in conjunction with empirical broad-spectrum antimicrobials (without microbiology cultures), can be used yielded similar or better outcomes than antimicrobials chosen by antimicrobial susceptibility testing of pathogens isolated from deep tissue cultures [18, 19, 39].

Different preparations of antibiotics have limited availability, as well as the cost of some of them, is a major problem in less developed countries, and hence contributes to the relatively poor outcome of infected ulcers and further emphasis the need for early expert assessment. The use of cheap broad-spectrum antibiotics comes from India, as suggested by Abbas and Archibald [6], as there are similar or better than the more expensive western antimicrobials.

14.6 The Surveillance System's Problems and Solutions

Any surveillance system demands first and foremost huge amounts of funding followed by human resources for data collection, statistics analysis of data, etc. Abbas and colleagues had to face challenges in the management of the diabetic foot is to implement and maintenance of this surveillance system. It is important to establish a surveillance system for diabetic limb complications in low and middle-income countries for a number of reasons as follow: (1). To screen high-risk foot (PN and PAD) through this surveillance data; (2) To take proper preventive measures for the selected high-risk diabetes populations and (3) To intervene effectively as needed.

The largest surveillance systems for limb complications in Africa have been instituted by Abbas and colleagues in Tanzania [1–3, 5–11, 13–16]. Due to various reasons surveillance system has been sustained like strict case definition of limb complications, quality questionnaire, the commitment of the staff who are also trained in the collection of data and utilization of these data for evidence-based practice. It has been shown by Abbas and colleagues in Tanzania by maintaining this system it has been seen a good and positive approach on patients, relatives, and friends to know about patient medical condition and how to deal with diabetic foot complications. Patients are more knowledgeable in handling diabetes and its complications. Appointments are maintained and are also reminded by the administrator to attend clinics. In turn involvement of patient's active gives the opportunity to validate further treatment and preventive interventional diabetic foot projects.

14.7 The Importance of Regional/District Hospitals

In developing countries regional or district hospitals are considered large centres with limited resources, but can provide medical, surgical, and basic laboratory services for every region is a way of optimizing resources. This set up is seen mostly in the developing world like in Africa, Southeast Asia, Latin America, and the Caribbean. Regional hospitals are big centres in the region of the country that are the teaching centres for all the disciplines in the medicine. It commonly house medical, surgical, and laboratory facilities including microbiology specialized units. Regional and district are government hospitals and are under the control of the ministry of health. Government agencies from developed countries like World Health Organization, United States Agency for International Development, etc. would generally prefer to maintain collaborative efforts with sentinel centres for reasons such as adequate infrastructure, trained staffs, and access to the ministry of health. The same applies to diabetic foot complications surveillance system and activities in Tanzania.

14.8 Time Is Tissue—The Decision to Seek Medical Help

Time is tissue means the decision to seek medical help in regard to diabetic foot. It is a medical emergency in the field of diabetic foot. As we are all aware that myocardial infarction and cerebral vascular accidents are medical emergencies, in the same way, septic diabetic foot is a medical emergency. What is not known is patients with a diabetic foot ulcer delaying for days, weeks, or a month means a difference in saving a toe, foot, leg, or even saving a life. These patients need to attend the health centre as soon as possible. Abbas and colleagues found in Africa delay presentation was mostly due to cultural traditional and customary behaviour. People with diabetic foot ulcers initially with small lesions on foot, patient, or a relative will try to teat at home by using a razor blade or herbal solution and we call it as bathroom surgery. Next move of the patient will be if this home treatment fails to go to see faith healer or herbal doctor. People in the village and towns usually have very high respect and faith in faith healer. Herbalists are existing in Africa at almost every corner of the cities advertising and claim that cure to all diabetic complications. Patient will decide to move to primary health centre when herbal medications given by herbalist fails. Primary health centres are not trained or equipped to treat diabetic foot ulcers so patient will now go to district or regional hospitals, where we also have no diabetic foot specialist. All these leads to delay in presentation to main specialized referral hospital. By the time patient report at referral hospital it is too late to save foot even prevent death from severe sepsis [11, 18, 35–39]. People with diabetic foot ulcers who strongly beliefs in cultural traditions will prevent getting proper and accurate treatment of diabetic foot and this in turn leads to amputation or death as an outcome [18]. Unfortunately, some patients delay in getting expert opinion because of fear losing a limb as in Africa loss of limb is considered worse thing. At grass root level due to lack of knowledge among healthcare personnel can lead to poor outcomes. It is common practice in the Africa continent soaking diabetic foot, which is a good medium for *pseudomonas* infection and can worsen the condition of the foot. In some centres due to lack of trained personal dealing diabetic foot ulcers management and therefore patients suffer if treated inadequately for a long time [1–3, 5–11, 13–16].

Most of the patients with diabetes are not aware of the need for early reporting to the health centre due to lack of knowledge in the peripheral of the countries in Africa. Lack of knowledge makes things worse by peripheral neuropathy and reduce pain sensations. Patients with loss of protective sensation can sustain unnoticed injuries like rat bite at night [16]. Checking of the feet daily at night to detect injuries or crack due to dry skin is not done due to lack of knowledge on preventive measures of foot care [16]. In contrast, to those with symptomatic (painful) peripheral neuropathy, which is a common complication in both among highly literate and very low literate people with diabetes, but it does not prevent complication even due to education status and not associated with better outcomes [1–3, 5–11, 13–16].

14.9 Sustainable Infrastructure Solution

In Africa education is the most powerful tool for avoiding diabetic foot ulcers. Foot care education is lacking for people with diabetes at the grass root level or district and in some regional health centres [9, 10]. Unfortunately, an ulcer leads to an infected diabetic foot ulcer due to lack of very basic education and hence patient presents severe limb-threatening condition, which leads to amputation in people from 25–50% [19]. The most important thing is the education programme at the primary level to prevent complications of foot ulcer in the developing world [40–47]. In the developing world, the only tool, we have is education, which is free to the patient and can be effective if implemented effectively.

A preventive programme should be targeted health care workers and it should include five main pillars of the preventive diabetic foot as follow: (1). Regular inspection and examination of the feet and footwear, (2). Identification of high-risk patients, (3). Educational of the high-risk patients, relatives, friends, and health care workers, (4). Appropriate footwear for diabetic patients, (5). Treatment of non-ulcerative pathology. By implementing these five pillars limb amputation can be reduced by or more than 50%. Several successful preventive educational programmes have been carried out in developed and developing countries [41–46]. It has been noted, organized, implemented, and published the outcome of the educational programme showed foot complications reduced by more than 50% [41–46].

14.10 *'Step by Step'* Foot Project

It is, for this reason, we had started '*Step by Step*' (*SbS*) *f*oot project to improve educational skills and the management of diabetic foot problems [41, 44–46]. The main goals of the *SbS* foot projects were as follows: (1) Raising awareness among health care workers and patients about diabetic foot problems, (2) Providing effective education in diabetic foot management and to sustain it for health care workers, (3) Cascading the knowledge and skills among health care workers and export ideas to other developing countries, (4) To reduce the risk of complications of the lower limb in people with diabetes, (5) Encourage people with diabetes to take better care of their feet, report earlier, and seek help when problems arise [41, 44–46].

Step by Step foot project showed greater than 50% reduction of amputation rates [41]. Ulceration, infection, and amputation all were prevented through this step by step foot project. It was recorded through this programme which included a preventive and therapeutic approach to save diabetic foot limb [41, 44–46]. It is mandatory that health care workers involved in taking care of patients with diabetes should be able to conduct simple screening of peripheral neuropathy, peripheral arterial, and muscular skeletal system to identify patients with high-risk feet.

It is important that an educational programme should be planned in such a way that people with diabetes should receive maximum information from health care workers. Abbas and colleagues targeted centres at primary health centres who were dealing with the people with diabetes in Tanzania—the first people to see diabetic foot complications. Before we had *SbS* many developing countries, we had a lack of proper management of diabetic foot, lack of trained health care workers, no podiatry services, no specific curriculum of diabetic foot management for the training of health care workers in the country. There is still no concept of a super specialist of diabetic foot. This was the reason *SbS* foot project was designed aimed to educate these health care workers at the primary level and was instituted in several regions across Tanzania [41]. The *SbS* was started in these centres and health workers were largely untrained professionals [41, 44–46].

Step by Step foot project is an educational programme focussing on all the aspects of diabetic foot. It consists of two parts basic and advanced course given a year apart and each course lasts for 3 days. It is very important that eligible centre selected for this course participants should come in pair (doctor and nurse) dealing people with diabetes. All attending health care workers on registration of the first basic course were given educational material and screening, diagnostic and therapeutic basic kit on diabetic foot [41, 44–46].

Educational material directed to diabetic foot ulcers information was given to all the participants, which were in the form of written, posters for the clinics and audio–visual. All these materials either written in the form of booklet or audio–visual were targeted both health care workers (doctors and nurses) and patients [41, 44–46]. Curriculum for step by step foot project was prepared by diabetic foot experts from the developing world on all the aspects of diabetic foot for the health care worker. Step by Step focussed on all aspects of diabetic foot, which includes formal lecture, live workshop with patients, live demonstration on patients and live patients and hands-on experience [41, 44–46]. Once basic and advanced courses are done all the participants are expected to cascade the information knowledge to fellow colleagues and have course at the centre. Basic and advanced foot care educations are given to all health care providers [41, 44–46].

Normal patient with diabetes has no risk can receive normal general education once a year and is enough. Whereas patients with mild to moderate risk foot it means peripheral neuropathy can received education every 6 months. On the other hand, patients with peripheral neuropathy, peripheral arterial diseases and or deformity should receive education every 3 months. Patients with high risk mean all above with a past history an ulcer or previous history of an amputation should receive aggressive foot education every 1–3 months. Patients with a disability who cannot look after themselves special education is given to their assistances and care provider [41, 44–46]. Basic course was conducted in 2004 and advanced course was in 2005 and since the introduction of the *SbS* diabetic foot training programme has improved outcomes of diabetic foot ulcers, as we can see more ulcers are reported at the peripheral health centre at the early stage and more awareness has been created among the patients with diabetes. It has been noticed that a smaller number of patients are referred to tertiary hospital of the country and hence less amputations are registered [41]. Health care workers are now aware of diabetic foot and training is conducted among other health care workers [41, 44–46].

Step by Step foot piolet course conducted in Tanzania was shown to be successful during the period of 2004 and 2005. This leads to recruited further training of 30 private centres which includes 30 teams of medical officers and nurses in total of 60 participants. The same pattern was followed as follow initial with government centres [41, 44–46]. This time cobblers were invited from respected centres in 2010 to extend the approach along with medical workers to make a good training team [41, 44–46].

Centres where physicians and nurses were already trained in government and private health facilities in total of 45 centres, surgeons were invited from the same centres and facility have surgical facilities. In 2009, the first of its kind in the world *SbS* diabetic foot surgical training project specifically aiming surgeons from selected centres in 20 regions was conducted in Tanzania. The main aim was to prevent amputation by salvaging diabetic feet and hence reduce rates of amputation [41].

One of the aims was to export an idea of *SbS* to other developing countries. To date, this original *SbS* diabetic foot project has been conducted in Africa (Democratic Republic of Cong, Guinea, Botswana, Malawi, Kenya, Ethiopia, Egypt and Zimbabwe, Nigeria), and beyond Africa (Pakistan, Saudi Arabia, and Caribbean Barbados, St Lucia, St Maarten, St Kitts and the British Virgin Islands) [41, 44–46].

14.11 'Train the Foot Trainer'

In December 2012, a *SbS* foot care project was transfer to Train the Foot Trainer (*TtFT*) course. Step by Step foot care project could not reach to all the countries in the world. It was decided to conduct *TtFT* course target health workers from different countries in that particular region to come under one roof and then disseminate the knowledge once they go back to their own countries [44–47]. The First *TtFT* course was conducted in Brazil with participants from 14 countries in the continental of South America. In July 2013 course was conducted in Tobago from 22 countries [44–47]. In November 2014 it was exported to Dubai and in February 2015 *TtFT* course was conducted in Slovenia where 17 Eastern European countries participated. In November 2016 it went to the Western Pacific region and trained health care workers from 13 countries. In 2020 it was conducted in the Mena region and trained health care workers from 14 countries.

This is the only unique project which actually started in the developing world (Dar es Salaam, Tanzania) and exported to developing and now developed world and it has touched 110 countries in total [44–47].

In my opinion, to achieve a goal of reducing amputation rates is by focussing only on education. Education is the only powerful tool that can work all over the world. Once we educate the health care worker who would in turn educate other of his colleague in the centre and around his region will have a cascading effect. These healthcare workers in the primary health centre of each country being in the front line of diabetic foot to see would, in turn, educate patients, families of the patients, relatives, and friends.

14.12 Conclusion

In summary, in this manuscript, several reasons of poor diabetic foot care have been discussed in length. While we are waiting for the better technology to improve the situation, the priority at this point and time should be basic principles of training and management in this neglected specialist filed of diabetes. This task can be achieved at a minimal cost. Over the last 20 years, it has shown in developing countries a considerable reduction in the number of major amputations being undertaken for diabetes. The key to improvement is education and to empower health care workers to educate patients with diabetes.

Acknowledgments We would like to acknowledge for the helpful discussion with all our colleagues during the genesis of this manuscript is appreciated. We are grateful to Shabneez Gangji and other staff in Dar es Salaam for their assistance.

References

1. Abbas ZG (2013) Chapter 4: Contemporary management of diabetic foot. In: Pendsey S (ed) The global burden of diabetic foot, 1st edn. JP Medical Ltd, London., www.jpeedigital.com, pp 24–30
2. Abbas ZG, Archibald LK (2006) Chapter 34: The foot in diabetes. In: AJM B, Cavanagh P, Rayman G (eds) Recent international development: Africa, 4th edn. John Wiley & Sons Ltd, Hoboken, NJ., www.wiley.com, pp 379–385
3. International Diabetes Federation, Diabetes Atlas, 9th edition (2019) Available from: https://www.diabetesatlas.org/en/resources/. Accessed 24 June 2020
4. Atun R, Davies JI, Gale EAM et al (2017) Diabetes in sub-Saharan Africa: from clinical care to health policy. Lancet Diabetes Endocrinol 5:622–667
5. Abbas ZG (2016) Diabetic foot—an African perspective. JSM Foot Ankle 1(1):1005

6. Abbas ZG, Archibald LK (2007) Challenges for management of the diabetic foot in Africa: doing more with less. Int Wound J 4:305–313
7. Abbas ZG, Archibald LK (2005) Epidemiology of the diabetic foot in Africa. Med Sci Monit 11:RA262–RRA70
8. Abbas ZG, Viswanathan V (2007) The diabetic foot in Africa and India. Int Diab Monit 19:8–12
9. Abbas ZG, Gill GV, Archibald LK (2002) The epidemiology of diabetic limb sepsis: an African perspective. Diabet Med 19:895–899
10. Abbas ZG, Archibald LK (2007) The diabetic foot in Sub-Saharan Africa: a new management paradigm. Diab Foot J 10:128–136
11. Abbas ZG, Lutale JK, Morbach S, Archibald LK (2002) Clinical outcome of diabetic patients hospitalized with foot ulcers, Dar es Salaam, Tanzania. Diabet Med 19:575–579
12. Tesfaye S, Gill G (2011) Chronic diabetic complications in Africa. African J Diabetes Med 19(1):4–8
13. Abbas ZG, Archibald LK (2000) Foot complications in diabetic patients with symptomatic peripheral neuropathy in Dar es Salaam, Tanzania. Diabetes Int 10:52–56
14. Abbas ZG, Lutale JK, Archibald LK (2009) Diabetic foot ulcers and ethnicity in Tanzania: a contrast between African and Asian populations. Int Wound J 6:124–131
15. Morbach S, Lutale JK, Viswanathan V, Mollenberg J, Ochs HR, Rajashekart S, Ramachandran A, Abbas ZG (2004) Regional difference in risk factors and clinical presentation of diabetic foot lesions. Diabet Med 21:91–95
16. Abbas ZG, Lutale JK, Archibald LK (2005) Rodent bites on the feet of diabetic patients in Tanzania. Diabet Med 22:631–633
17. Hennis AJ, Fraser HS, Jonnalogadda R et al (2004) Explanation for the high risk of diabetes related amputation of black African descent and potential for prevention. Diabetes Care 27:2636–2641
18. Abbas ZG, Bal A (eds) (2019) Pocket Guideline of diabetic foot 2019, 2nd edn. Jaypee Brothers Medical Publishers (P) Ltd, New Delhi
19. International Working group on the Diabetic Foot (IWGDF) (2019) The development of global consensus guidelines on the management and prevention of the Diabetic Foot 2019. www.iwgdf.org
20. Cavanagh P, Attinger C, Abbas ZG, Bal A, Rojas N, Xu ZR (2012) Cost of treating diabetic foot ulcers in five different countries. Diabetes Metab Res Rev 28(Suppl 1):107–111
21. Shobhana R, Rama Rao P, Lavanya A, Vijay V, Ramachandran A (2000) Cost burden to diabetic patients with foot complications—a study from Southern India. JAPI 48(12):1147–1150
22. Ali SM, Fareed A, Humail SM et al (2008) The personal cost of diabetic foot diseases in the developing world—a study from Pakistan. Diabet Med 25:1231–1233
23. Ndour Mbaye M, Sarr A, Diop SN, Diedhiou D, KA-Cisse M, Camara Y, Sidibe EH, Sow AM (2008) Etude descriptive du pied diabétique au Sénégal: à propos de 105 cas. Dakar Médical 53(3):205–212
24. Edmonds M, Boulton A, Buckenham T, Every N, Foster A, Freeman D, Gadsby R, Gibby O, Knowles A, Pooke M, Tovey F, Unwin N, Wolfe J (1996) Report of the diabetic foot and amputation group. Diabet Med 13:S27–S42
25. Jeffcoat WJ, Harding KG (2003) Diabetic foot ulcers. Lancet 361:1545–1551
26. Garoushi S, Johnson MI, Tashani OA (2019) A cross-sectional study to estimate the point prevalence of painful diabetic neuropathy in Eastern Libya. BMC Public Health 19(1):78
27. Khalifa WA (2018) Risk factors for diabetic foot ulcer recurrence: a prospective 2-year follow-up study in Egypt. Foot (Edinb) 35:11–15. https://doi.org/10.1016/j.foot.2017.12.004
28. Awadalla H, Noor SK, Elmadhoun WM, Almobarak AO, Elmak NE, Abdelaziz SI, Sulaiman AA, Ahmed MH (2017) Diabetes complications in Sudanese individuals with type 2 diabetes: overlooked problems in sub-Saharan Africa? Diabetes Metab Syndr 11(Suppl 2):S1047–S1051
29. Olamoyegun M, Ibraheem W, Iwuala S, Audu M, Kolawole B (2015) Burden and pattern of micro vascular complications in type 2 diabetes in a tertiary health institution in Nigeria. Afr Health Sci 15(4):1136–1141

30. Kuate-Tegueu C, Temfack E, Ngankou S et al (2015) Prevalence and determinants of diabetic polyneuropathy in a Sub-Saharan African referral hospital. J Neurol Sci 355:108–112
31. Khalil SA, Megallaa MH, Rohoma KH, Guindy MA, Zaki A, Hassanein M, Malaty AH, Ismael HM, Kharboush IF, El Kafash DN, Sallam HN, Desouky IA (2019) Prevalence of chronic diabetic complications in newly diagnosed versus known type 2 diabetic subjects in a sample of Alexandria population, Egypt. Curr Diabetes Rev 15(1):74–83
32. Ogbera AO, Adeleye O, Solagberu B et al (2015) Screening for peripheral neuropathy and peripheral arterial disease in persons with diabetes mellitus in a Nigerian University Teaching Hospital. BMC Res Notes 8:533
33. Codjo HL, Adoukonou TA, Wanvoegbe A et al (2016) Prevalence of peripheral artery disease among diabetics in Parakou in 2013. Ann Cardiol Angeiol 65:260–264
34. Mwebaze RM, Kibirige D (2014) Peripheral arterial disease among adult diabetic patients attending a large outpatient diabetic clinic at a national referral hospital in Uganda: a descriptive cross sectional study. PLoS One 9(8):e105211
35. Isiguzo CM, Jac-Okereke C (2015) Diabetic foot ulcer—12 months prospective review of pattern of presentation at Enugu State university of technology teaching hospital, Parklane, Enugu: a basis for diabetic foot clinic? Niger J Med 24:125–130
36. Ngim NE, Ndifon WO, Udosen AM et al (2012) Lower limb amputation in diabetic foot disease: experience in a tertiary hospital in southern Nigeria. African J Diabetes Med 1:13–15
37. Enweluzo GO, Giwa SO, Adekoya-Cole TO et al (2010) Profile of amputations in Lagos University Teaching Hospital, Lagos, Nigeria. Nig Q J Hosp Med 20:205–208
38. Sié Essoh JB, Kodo M, Djè Bi Djè V et al (2009) Limb amputations in adults in an Ivorian teaching hospital. Niger J Clin Pract 12:245–247
39. Abbas ZG, Lutale JK, Ilondo MM, Archibald LK (2012) The utility of Gram stains and culture in the management of limb ulcers in persons with diabetes. Int Wound J 9(6):677–682
40. Abbas Z, Morbach S (2005) Diabetes foot damage in developing countries: the urgent need for education. Diabetes Voice 50:15–17
41. Abbas ZG, Lutale JK, Bakker K, Baker N, Archibald LK (2011) The 'Step by Step' Diabetic Foot Project in Tanzania: a model for improving patient outcomes in less-developed countries. Int Wound J 8:169–175
42. Bakker K, Abbas ZG, Pendsey S (2006) Step by step, improving diabetic foot care in the developing world. A pilot study for India, Bangladesh, The "Step by Step" Diabetic Foot Project in Tanzania, 2004–2010 Sri Lanka and Tanzania. Pract Diab Intern 23:365–369
43. Pendsey S, Abbas ZG (2007) The step-by-step program for reducing diabetic foot problems: a model for the developing world. Curr Diab Rep 7(6):425–428
44. Abbas ZG (2013) Preventing foot care and reducing amputation: a step in right direction for diabetes care. Diabetes Manag 3(5):427–435
45. Abbas ZG (2015) Reducing diabetic limb amputations in developing countries. Expert Rev Endocrinol Metabol 10(4):425–434
46. Abbas ZG (2014) Chapter 39: Preventive foot care programs. In: Hinchliffe RJ, Schaper NC, Thompson MM, Tripathi RK, Timaran CH (eds) The diabetic foot, 1st edn. JP Medical Ltd, London., www.jpeedigital.com, pp 24–30
47. Baker N, Van Acker K, Urbancic-Rovan V, Abbas ZG, Morbach S (2017) The worldwide implementation of the 'Train the Foot Trainer' programme. Diabet Foot J 20(2):71–76

Role of Growth Factors in the Treatment of Diabetic Foot Ulceration

15

Deepti Singh and Hifzur R. Siddique

Abbreviation

ECM	Extracellular matrix
rhEGF	Recombinant human epidermal growth factor
rhPDGF	Recombinant human platelet-derived growth factor
S4PL	Syndecan-4 proteo liposomes

15.1 Introduction

Growth factors are the naturally occurring polypeptides promoting growth and differentiation of cells in the body and also the repair of tissue [1, 2]. Growth factors such as Platelet-Derived Growth Factor (PDGF), Vascular Endothelial Growth Factor (VEGF), Fibroblast Growth Factor (FGF), Insulin-like Growth Factor (IGF), Hypoxia-inducible factor (HIFs), Transforming Growth Factor beta-1 (TGF-β-1) have also been implicated in playing role in the process of diabetic foot ulceration (DFU) [3]. Growth factors have been implicated to play a role in both normal and impaired wound healing. The growth factors are responsible for the rapid increase in the cell number and therefore can be used in enhancing the process of wound healing in the case of DFU. Recently, various clinical interventions have been reported emphasizing the role of growth factors for the healing of the wound [4].

Diabetes mellitus is one of the common metabolic diseases, which is due to the failure of the machinery to maintain the normal blood glucose level and includes defects such as failure of insulin secretion, insulin action, or both. There are three

D. Singh · H. R. Siddique (✉)
Molecular Cancer Genetics and Translational Research Lab, Section of Genetics, Department of Zoology, Aligarh Muslim University, Aligarh, India
e-mail: hifzur.zo@amu.ac.in

M. Zubair et al. (eds.), *Diabetic Foot Ulcer*,
https://doi.org/10.1007/978-981-15-7639-3_15

main types of diabetes viz. Type-1 diabetes resulting from the loss of the insulin-secreting β cells of the pancreas; Type-2 diabetes resulting from the peripheral resistance of insulin and the third one, gestational diabetes mellitus resulting from deterioration of glucose tolerance occurring particularly in third trimester [5–7]. Diabetes mellitus has been reported to have a high incidence rate in the adult population [8]. The various symptoms that are associated with diabetes mellitus include polyuria, polyphagia, polydipsia, hyperglycemia, retinopathy, nephropathy, risk of foot ulceration, etc. Further, patients are at a very high risk of lower extremity amputation and the main reason leading to amputation includes peripheral neuropathy, infection, peripheral vascular disease, and foot ulceration.

Diabetic ulcers are mainly lesions in which a loss of the epithelium is involved. These abrasions may also expand to the deeper layers, dermis, and sometimes to the muscles and bone. DFU is one of the most common predisposing factors which leads to lower extremity amputation. About 4–10% of the population suffering from diabetes is estimated to have foot ulceration [9–11]. The various risk factors which are responsible for the increased incidence of ulceration in the foot include gender (male has more risk), having diabetes for more than 10 years, high body mass index (BMI), diabetic neuropathy, peripheral arterial disease, poor glycemic control, and the structural abnormalities and deformities in the foot such as claw toes, flat foot, hallux valgus, etc. [12–15]. The diabetic foot has been classified into two categories viz. (1) the neuropathic foot in which the factor responsible for the disease is the neuropathies and (2) neuroischemic foot in which apart from neuropathy, occlusive vascular disease is the primary risk factor [16].

Wound healing is a process that involves the activation of cellular machinery such as fibroblasts, platelets, endothelial cells, macrophages, and keratinocytes. Wound healing involves four phases, i.e., hemostasis, inflammation, fibroplasia, and maturation. The phases of wound healing are summarized in Fig. 15.1.

Induction of hypoxia is a necessary requisite for wound healing, which is followed by the release of Vascular Endothelial Growth Factor (VEGF) by the fibroblast, macrophages, and epithelial cells of the body leading to the phosphorylation

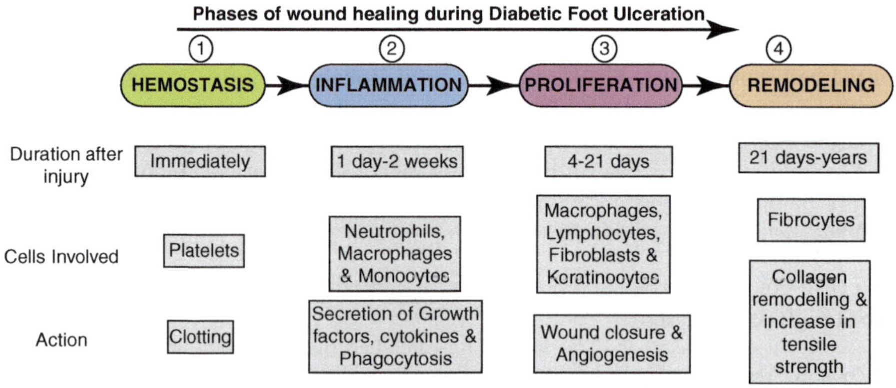

Fig. 15.1 Phases of wound healing during diabetic foot ulceration

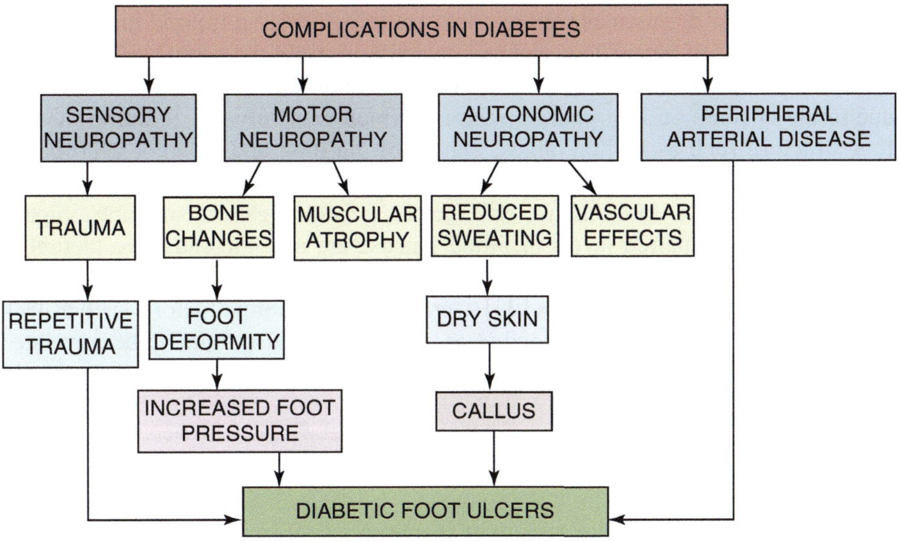

Fig. 15.2 Risk factors associated with diabetic foot ulceration

and ultimate activation of nitric oxide synthase. These series of events are decelerated in the patients of diabetes due to the blood glucose level [17]. In this chapter, we will be focusing on the various growth factors that play a major role in the treatment of DFU.

15.2 Factors Responsible for Diabetic Foot Ulceration

DFU is a common complication related to diabetes. Many risk factors (Fig. 15.2) are responsible for the pathogenesis of diabetic foot ulcers. In most of the cases, it results from the synchronous action of these multiple causes. However, the factors that have been implicated to be the major cause of DFU are ischemia resulting from peripheral vascular diseases and peripheral neuropathy. In approximately 90% of the cases of DFU, damage to the nerve affecting the motor, sensory, and autonomic fibers has been observed. This condition is referred to as diabetic neuropathy [18, 19]. Damage to the nerves innervating intrinsic foot muscles results in an imbalance in the flexion and extension of the affected foot. This results in anatomical foot deformations thereby leading to the breakdown of skin and ulceration.

Peripheral diabetic neuropathy is a condition in which sensation is lost in the feet as a result of repetitive injuries. Due to the loss of sensation, wounds go unnoticed and undetected and keep on worsening leading to foot ulceration. The condition is further worsened by an infection in the ulcer leading to foot amputation particularly in patients with peripheral arterial disease. Peripheral arterial disease is another cause of foot ulceration. It is a dysfunction of the circulatory system in which the supply of blood to the limbs is reduced by narrowed arteries. This increases the risk of cardiovascular diseases as well as foot ulceration [20]. An injured limb requires an increased rate of blood flow, and any decrease in the blood supply results in foot ulceration, which further progresses to limb amputation [21, 22]. DFU also results due to the uncommon foot plantar pressure, which is mainly due to deformities in foot structure such as hallux valgus, claw toes, flatfoot, and Charcot neuropathy, which is a condition causing bone and joint architecture destruction and loss of function. In addition to the above risk factors, gender, cigarette smoking, impairment of vision, impaired levels of blood glucose are also the causative factors of ulceration [22, 23]. Studies have shown the prevalence of foot ulceration more common in males rather than females [23]. Certain socioeconomic factors, such as lack of access to health care facilities and poor education, are also found to be correlated to frequent foot ulceration [22, 23].

15.3 Development of Ulcer in Diabetes

Ulcers in diabetic patients are a result of synchronous effects of motor, sensory, and autonomic neuropathy. Motor neuropathies result in foot deformities and biochemical abnormalities in the foot. Sensory neuropathy is a loss of protective sensation in the foot. Furthermore, autonomic neuropathy leads to decreased sweating in the foot thereby resulting in dry skin [24]. The combined effect of these neuropathies is the formation of callus which is the initial stage of diabetic ulcer formation. After callus formation, continuous trauma, stress, and repetitive injuries lead to skin breakdown thereby resulting in the formation of foot ulcers [24].

15.4 Therapeutic Role of Various Growth Factors in the Lesioning of Ulcers

Growth factors are the molecules that regulate the growth of cells and repair of tissues by modulating various cell signaling pathways. They are involved not only in case of healthy wound healing but also in the impaired wound healing process. Growth factors play a role in wound healing by inducing cellular proliferation, migration, chemotaxis, the formation of the extracellular matrix, establishment of cell integrity, and angiogenesis. The effect of growth factors in strengthening the process of wound healing has been demonstrated by various *in vitro* and *in vivo* studies. Among the growth factors playing role in the process of healing of diabetic foot ulcers, the most frequently studied are PDGF, FGF, EGF, VEGF, and TGF-β1 [25–27]. The sequential process of wound healing requires several growth factors and cells resulting in the appropriate closure of the wound. A decrease in the level of growth factor secretion, as well as an increase in the destruction of growth factors, may lead to a delay in the process of wound healing. Therefore, growth factors may serve as an effective therapeutic agent in the treatment of DFU. Various growth factors along with their source of origin and mechanism of action have been summarized in Table 15.1.

Table 15.1 Summary of the various growth factors with their source of origin and mechanism

Growth factor	Description	Source	Mechanism
PDGF	Represent a family of four closely related peptides encoded by four genes (A, B, C, and D). These four peptides get activated by the formation of homo- or heterodimer (AA, AB, BB, CC, and DD)	Platelets, fibroblasts, macrophages, and vascular endothelial cells	Chemoattractant for fibroblast, neutrophils, monocytes Promotes the proliferation of fibroblasts and the production of ECM
FGF	Binds to heparin and heparin sulfate. FGF family includes 22 members and 5 distinct receptors	Fibroblasts, macrophages, and endothelial cells	Increased cellular proliferation, migration, epithelialization, restoring, and remodeling of ECM
EGF	Founding member of the EGF family proteins	Platelets, fibroblasts, and macrophages	Reduction in the healing duration
VEGF	A subfamily of PDGF family of growth factors. Five isoforms include VEGF-A, placental growth factor, VEGF-B, VEGF-C, and VEGF-D	Platelets, fibroblasts, macrophages, and keratinocytes	Increased proliferation and migration of keratinocytes and upregulation in the VEGFR2 mRNA expression level
KGF	A signaling molecule which is also known as FGF-7	Fibroblasts	Enhanced healing by re-epithelialization and formation of granular tissue, mitogen for epithelial cells
TGF-α	Encoded by the TGFA gene. Binds to EGFR	Platelets, macrophages, and keratinocytes	Stimulates angiogenesis
TGF-β1–3	Member of the EGF family of proteins. Functions by interacting with EGFR	Platelets, fibroblasts, macrophages, and keratinocytes	Chemoattractant for macrophages, mitogen for fibroblasts, stimulates granulation tissue formation
IGF	Related to proinsulin	Fibroblasts, macrophages, neutrophils, and hepatocytes	Enhances the re-epithelialization and fibroblast proliferation

15.4.1 Platelet-Derived Growth Factor (PDGF)

PDGF is released and delivered to the wound by the platelets and the local fibroblasts of the injured capillary vessels [28]. It is a 30 kDa dimer formed of two chains A and B. Two additional chains C and D were later identified. Each chain is encoded by the gene present on chromosomes 7, 22, 4, and 11, respectively [29–31]. PDGF exists as a family of homo-heterodimeric growth factors, including PDGF-AA, PDGF-AB, PDGF-BB, PDGF-CC, and PDGF-DD [32]. The four isoforms of PDGF (A, B, C, and D) form dimers and activate the downstream tyrosine kinase receptors resulting in the reorganization of actin filament and proliferation of the fibroblast cells inducing the formation of myofibroblasts [33]. PDGF plays a role in various phases of diabetic wound healing. PDGF based topical interventions are used for the treatment and induction of healing in case of neuropathic diabetic foot ulcers. Administration of PDGF to wounds has been found to significantly increase the influx of fibroblasts and the cells involved in inflammation.

PDGF is also known to enhance the deposition of extracellular matrix protein and the formation of collagen [34]. Further, PDGF acts as a cellular chemoattractant and promotes the migration of various cells such as fibroblasts, neutrophils, and monocytes to the site of injuries. Besides, PDGF is also responsible for the differentiation of fibroblast cells into myofibroblast thereby supporting the contraction of collagen fibers and the wound [35]. The effectiveness of the topical application of recombinant human PDGF (rhPDGF) in the healing of chronic lower extremity neurotropic ulcers has been reported by Steed [36]. Another study by Bennett et al. [37] reported the benefit of topical application of PDGF in the treatment of non-healing, well-perfused ulcers [37]. According to a report by Mandial et al. [38], exogenous daily application of PDGF is effective and safe in the healing of lower extremity non-healing diabetic ulcers. Further, the topical application of PDGF increases the rate of ulcer closure and also enhances the formation of granulation tissue at the site of the ulcer. The approach of co-delivering PDGF-BB with an enhancer such as Syndecan-4 Proteoliposomes (S4PLs) has been found to significantly increase the wound healing activity of PDGF-BB. This shows that the delivery of syndecan-4 is an effective and beneficial method to enhance the wound healing activity of PDGF-BB [39]. A similar study by Rangaswamy et al. [40] showed that the wounds of the patients treated with rhPDGF contracted more than the non-treated control cohort. The above studies indicate that the PDGF dressings are more effective and can be used for the healing of diabetic wounds and ulcers. PDGF is sold as Regranex/Becaplermin and has also been approved for clinical use by the US Food and Drug Administration (FDA) [41–44]. The treatment of DFU with Becaplermin along with good care of the wound has been found to be more effective in treating the foot ulcer [45, 46].

15.4.2 Epidermal Growth Factor (EGF)

EGF family includes members such as EGF, TGF-α, and Heparin-binding EGF. EGF acts by binding to its receptor EGFR and stimulating cell growth, proliferation, and differentiation. EGF is produced by platelets, macrophages, monocytes and stimulates the growth of epithelial cells around the wound. It also acts on smooth muscle cells and fibroblasts [47–49]. The role of EGF in the treatment of DFU has been determined by various clinical studies. In case of early human wound repair, EGF stimulates epithelialization and has also been reported to stimulate the healing process in chronic wounds such as the DFU [48, 50, 51]. The role of rhEGF in diabetic foot ulcers on Wagner's Grade 1 and 2 (the most commonly used classification system for diabetic foot ulcers) ulcers has been reported by Singla et al. [52]. This study involved 50 patients and concluded that the administration of rhEGF could reduce the length of healing time of the ulcer. Another study involved a double-blinded controlled trial with 50 patients in which rhEGF was applied intra-lesionally. The study demonstrated that rhEGF increases the rate of healing of ulcers and also improves the epithelialization of the wound [53]. In the case of chronic diabetic foot ulcers, the effectiveness of rhEGF has also been reported [54]. A recent study involving 294 patients and four randomized controlled trials have shown the potential of rhEGF in increasing the rate of diabetic ulcer healing and found a fourfold increase in the healing process [55]. According to another study, the treatment of diabetic patients with EGF resulted in complete healing of 76% of patients [56]. As compared to the conventional povidone-iodine dressing group, the group that has been treated with EGF topically has a 100% probability of wound healing in 7 weeks. The result of this study also suggests that EGF, when applied topically, causes a reduction in the number of non-healing ulcers [57]. A genetically engineered form of EGF is Regen-D™ which has been expressed in *E. coli* before being purified. Regen-D™ is a topical gel used at a dose of 150 μg/g and is applied two times a day until the wound is completely healed. The clinical trial carried out with Regen-D™ showed a healing rate of about 9 weeks and a success rate of about 86% [58]. Another form of EGF is Easyef, which is a dermal spray solution (50 mg/mL). It is a recombinant human EGF which comes with a generic name of Nepidermin and recommended to apply two times a day until the wound is fully closed. The clinical trial of Easyef in South Korea and Vietnam has shown more than 50% complete healing [54, 59]. The results of the above studies suggest the potential role of EGF in the treatment of diabetic foot ulcers.

15.4.3 Transforming Growth Factor (TGF-β)

TGF-β is a member of a group of cytokines collectively referred to as TGF-β superfamily. TGF-β regulates the growth, differentiation, organization, apoptosis of epithelial cells. TGF-β1, TGF-β2, and TGF-β3 are the forms found in mammals. Out of them, the predominating form is TGF-β1. The cells producing TGF-β include macrophages, fibroblasts, keratinocytes, lymphocytes, and platelets [49, 60, 61]. In the process of wound healing, TGF-β1 is produced early, and an increase in the concentration of TGF-β1 is observed after 5–7 days [62, 63]. TGF-β1 stimulates the chemotaxis of inflammatory cells and the synthesis of extracellular matrix [60]. TGF-β also enhances the production and incorporation of fibronectin and collagen into the extracellular matrix [49]. Another study by Crowe et al. [64] observed that, the absence of TGF-β1 delays the process of wound healing [64]. Topical application of TGF-β1 has been found to stimulate the process of wound repair in young ischemic rabbit skin by increasing the rate of granulation tissue formation [65]. In the healing of partial-thickness and full-thickness wounds like wounds on a distal limb and perforated tympanic membrane in rat, the benefits of local application of TGF-β has been reported [66–68]. Further, TGF-β has also been reported in the healing of hypertrophic scars and chronic ulcers in humans [69, 70].

15.4.4 Fibroblast Growth Factor (FGF)

FGF is a family of closely related polypeptides, including acidic FGF (aFGF/FGF-1), basic FGF (bFGF/FGF-2), few oncogenic proteins (int-2, hst/K-FGF) and KGF. Among them, aFGF, bFGF, and KGF are the most important regulators of wound healing [71–74]. Both aFGF and bFGF have a strong affinity for heparin sulfate making them insoluble molecules that are always associated with the extracellular matrix. Basic FGF has a lot of cells as its target including most of the cells involved in the process of wound healing [75]. FGF is produced by endothelial cells, neural cells, keratinocytes, and smooth muscle cells [61]. FGF stimulates the proliferation and migration of a number of cells (endothelial cells, chondrocytes, myoblasts, and epithelial cells) involved in wound healing both *in vitro* and *in vivo* [60, 73, 76, 77]. Acidic and basic FGF are also angiogenic factors and play a role in the process of angiogenesis. Since angiogenesis mainly occurs during the healing of wounds and fractures, FGF is evaluated mostly in the healing tissues [76, 78]. An upregulation of bFGF is observed which is followed by an increase in the phosphorylation of ERK 1/2 proteins [79] thereby suggesting that FGF regulates wound healing by ERK 1/2 signaling cascade. Despite being accepted as an important factor in the healing of the diabetic wound, the use of FGF in the treatment of diabetic foot ulcers is not much reported. A recent study on the use of recombinant human bFGF in the treatment of periodontal intra-bony defects has shown that recombinant bFGF can promote wound regeneration but its efficacy is not satisfactory on clinical level [80]. Some clinical studies have reported the use of bFGF in wound healing [81], but later it was shown that the exogenous application of bFGF failed to support wound closure and bFGF gets washed away by other molecules in the areas of wound thus failing to stay in the areas of the wound [82]. The use of a form of recombinant human bFGF namely Fiblast® spray has been reported by Uchi et al. [83]. It is a lyophilized powdered form and has a generic name Trafermin and is supplied in a spray like formulation. The formulation is applied 5 cm away from the site of ulcer with an approximate dose of 30 μg per day. It binds to the ECM of several tissues and has been shown to improve the process of healing [83]. Further, if bFGF is combined with other drugs, its efficacy could be improved for treating diabetic ulcers.

15.4.5 Vascular Endothelial Growth Factor (VEGF)

VEGF is similar in structure to PDGF and placental growth factor [84] and was discovered mainly as playing a role in increasing the permeability of blood vessels to the circulating molecules in tumor cells. VEGF is produced mainly by tumor cells, endothelial cells, macrophages, pericytes, smooth muscle cells, lymphocytes, monocytes, granulocytes, and megakaryocytes [85, 86]. VEGF is a cell-specific mitogen with potential angiogenic activity. Angiogenesis mainly occurs during the healing of wounds and fractures. During the repair of the wound, angiogenesis provides the essential nutrients required for wound healing and helps in the formation of granulation tissue [87]. An increase in the expression of VEGF mRNA/protein within a day of wounding has been reported [88–91]. In case of rabbit tracheal reconstruction [92] and dermal ulcer of the ear [93], an increase in the healing process has been reported through the application of VEGF. Further, gene therapy with VEGF has also increased the deposition of granular tissue in case of rabbit ear wounds [94] and increased the healing of the wound in the skin of rat [95]. The above studies suggest the great potential of VEGF in the treatment of wounds by the delivery of VEGF via the gene transfection method. Further, a decrease in the level of VEGF-A has been observed in patients with DFU as compared to the patients without DFU. This further leads to a decrease in the level of VEGF receptor-2 [96] which was supposed to be the cause of poor healing of wound [97]. A study by Amoli et al. [98] further confirmed the role of VEGF in DFU. The study reported that a low frequency of AA genotypes and A alleles of the VEGF gene is associated with the incidence of ulcers in the foot of diabetic patients [98]. Recombinant human VEGF (Telbermin) has undergone a phase I trial in 2008 [99] on chronic neuropathic DFU. The trial was done on 55 patients with type 1 and 2 diabetes. They were divided into two groups of 29 and 26 patients. The first group received Telbermin whereas the second group received a placebo. It was reported that Telbermin has a tendency of increasing the rate of healing of ulcer and also reduces the duration of ulcer healing [99]. Lois et al. [100] reported that the use of FGF-2 loaded nanoparticles and fibrin-based scaffold with VEGF could promote the healing of the wound in diabetic mouse models [100]. The above studies suggest the role of VEGF in the treatment of diabetic ulcers and further suggests that rhVEGF combined with other components might be used as an innovative therapeutic approach to the treatment of DFU.

15.4.6 Keratinocyte Growth Factor (KGF)

KGF is a heparin-binding growth factor promoting the growth, proliferation, migration, and morphogenesis of epithelial cells thus encouraging the repair of injured tissue and skin. Keratinocytes form epithelium over the wound in the epithelialization phase of wound healing and also induces the deposition of collagen in the wound [101]. A truncated form of rhKGF-2 is Repifermin. It has been reported to be used in the healing of chronic venous stasis ulcers [102, 103]. The study reported that Repifermin accelerated the process of wound healing significantly and 75% of patients treated with Repifermin achieved wound closure as compared with placebo.

15.4.7 Insulin-Like Growth Factor (IGF)

IGF, previously known as somatomedin is produced in the liver and exists in two forms IGF-1 and IGF-2 which produce glycogen and glycosaminoglycans, respectively. It is present in high concentrations in the platelets and is released by platelets during the clotting of the wound. It has been reported that in the case of diabetic mice and humans, the level of IGF-1 is reduced and IGF-2 is increased in the epidermal basal layer. Also, after wounding, the expression of both IGF-1 and IGF-2 is delayed. All these results in a delay in the healing of wounds [104, 105]. During the healing of the wound, IGF participates in cellular granulation in patients of DFU. IGF-1 expression is lowered in patients with diabetes which leads to a failure in cell granulation. IGF is a potent mitogen for fibroblasts and keratinocytes and enhances the production of ECM [106].

15.5 Molecular Targets in DFU and Their Delivery Systems

The management of DFU is based on the molecular targets which are directly or indirectly involved in the modulation of DFU. The molecular targets of DFU as discussed in the previous sections of this chapter include growth factors such as PDGF, EGF, VEGF, FGF, IGF, KGF, and TGF. Several agents can directly or indirectly influence these molecular targets by suppressing or enhancing the expression of growth factors and factors stimulating angiogenesis. Several approaches such as the use of growth factors, dual growth factors, cytokines modulators, anti-inflammatory drugs, MMP inhibitors, ECM stimulators have been evaluated in the treatment of DFU but have shown little achievement.

For the use of growth factors in the treatment of DFU, two points need to be considered. First, the use of growth factors effectively for therapeutic purposes depends on the delivery system. This area has been covered by the use of specialized delivery platforms like the use of polymer gels, coated dressings, chamber devices, and nanoparticles [107–110]. Micro and nanospheres are synthesized using natural and synthetic materials such as Poly Lactic-Co-Glycolic Acid (PLGA), Gelatin, and Chitosan [111–113]. For entrapping growth factors, PLGA is the most commonly used polymer due to its biocompatibility and biodegradability. It is also less hydrophilic, absorbs less water, and degrades slowly allowing the sustainable release of the drug [114, 115]. Also, the degradation of PLGA produces lactate which stimulates angiogenesis, activates the pro-collagen factors, and also recruits endothelial cells at the site of the wound. Human recombinant EGF-loaded PLGA microspheres have been developed by Dong et al. [114], which demonstrated an 85.6% encapsulation efficiency. Preclinical and clinical studies have reported that EGF-PLGA-MS when applied topically to wounds resulted in an increased fibroblast proliferation rate and also improved wound healing as compared to using human recombinant EGF alone. Another study reported that the use of bioinspired hydrogels, which are based on the nanomorphology of algal adhesive along with gum Arabic, calcium, pectin when combined with bFGF serves as a promising treatment for wound healing and enhance the cell proliferation, wound epithelialization and deposition of collagen [116].

The second key point that needs to be considered in growth factor therapy is that complex microenvironments are generated at the sites of chronic inflammation, making them difficult to be treated by a single growth factor [117]. The strategy for this is the sustained delivery of growth factors such that they can resist the proteases in the wound microenvironment. Further, the secretion of growth factor at the appropriate time and in appropriate concentration is necessary to achieve positive outcomes. Appropriate wound care is done with the combined action of several cell types such as fibroblasts, platelets, etc. [118]. Recently, one exciting study related to surgical sutures reported that standard surgical threads can be bioactivated with a genetically modified form of microalgae to release both oxygen and recombinant growth factor at the site of the wound [119]. Gene therapy is another new option for wound treatment. Shi et al. [120] reported the transfer of genes of VEGF-A and PDGF-B for DFU in rats for the treatment of wounds [120] and observed positive results. However, this field further requires thorough investigation. Therefore, Research is still going to assess more beneficial treatment options for DFU.

15.6 Conclusions

Impaired wound healing is a common diabetes-related complication in diabetic patients. Several studies have reported the importance of growth factors in the treatment of DFU. The molecular steps involved in the healing of ulcers in diabetic patients have also been critically studied to contribute to DFU management. Significant improvements have been made to develop newer approaches such as the use of dual growth factors, cytokine modulators, anti-inflammatory drugs, MMP inhibitors, and angiogenesis stimulators. Although several compounds for the treatment of DFU have been reported, the concern remains in their efficiency, side effects, and cost-effectiveness. Further, the integrity, stability, and the release efficiency of these compounds is a major concern and needs thorough preclinical and clinical studies. Several recent studies generate hope for the researchers in designing novel delivery systems for the growth factors (single or in combination). Drug delivery systems based on the use of combination pharmaceutical products appear as one of the future innovative approaches for treating DFU. A combination of materials such as a combination of growth factors, dressings, and scaffolds can be used to improve the efficiency of the treatment. The release efficiency of each of the biomaterials used in the treatment needs to be regularly checked to attain desirable results, and the degradation of the growth factors in the area of the wound should be minimized. The efficacy of these approaches needs further studies and exploration in the future.

Acknowledgments D.S. expresses her sincere gratitude to CSIR, India for Fellowship. H.R.S. is thankful to the UGC [Grant no. F.30-377/2017(BSR)] and DST-SERB (Grant no. EMR/2017/001758), New Delhi, for providing financial help.

References

1. McGrath MH (1990) Peptide growth factors and wound healing. Clin Plast Surg 17:421–432
2. Rothe MJ, Falanga V (1992) Growth factors and wound healing. Clin Dermatol 9:553–559

3. Papanas N, Maltezos E (2008) Becaplermin gel in the treatment of diabetic neuropathic foot ulcers. Clin Interv Aging 3:233–240
4. Park JW, Hwang SR, Yoon IS (2017) Advanced growth factor delivery systems in wound management and skin regeneration. Molecules 22(8):1259
5. Craig ME, Hattersley A, Donaghue KC (2009) Definition, epidemiology and classification of diabetes in children and adolescents. Pediatr Diabetes 10:3–12
6. Galtier F (2010) Definition, epidemiology, risk factors. Diabetes Metab 36:628–651
7. American Diabetes Association (2014) Diagnosis and classification of diabetes mellitus. Diabetes Care 37:S81–S90
8. Kharroubi AT, Darwish HM (2015) Diabetes mellitus: the epidemic of the century. World J Diabetes 6:850–867
9. Abbott CA, Carrington AL, Ashe H, North-West Diabetes Foot Care Study et al (2002) The North-West Diabetes Foot Care Study: incidence of, and risk factors for, new DFU in a community-based patient cohort. Diabet Med 19:377–384
10. Centers for Disease Control and Prevention (2005) Lower extremity disease among persons aged ≥40 years with and without diabetes—United States, 1999–2002. MMWR Morb Mortal Wkly Rep 54:1158–1160
11. Lauterbach S, Kostev K, Kohlmann T (2010) Prevalence of diabetic foot syndrome and its risk factors in the UK. J Wound Care 19:333–337
12. Iraj B, Khorvash F, Ebneshahidi A, Askari G (2013) Prevention of diabetic foot ulcer. Int J Prev Med 4:373–376
13. McEwen LN, Ylitalo KR, Herman WH, Wrobel JS (2013) Prevalence and risk factors for diabetes-related foot complications in Translating Research Into Action for Diabetes (TRIAD). J Diabetes Complicat 27:588–592
14. Shahbazian H, Yazdanpanah L, Latifi SM (2013) Risk assessment of patients with diabetes for foot ulcers according to risk classification consensus of International Working Group on Diabetic Foot (IWGDF). Pak J Med Sci 29:730–734
15. Waaijman R, de Haart M, Arts ML, Wever D, Verlouw AJ, Nollet F et al (2014) Risk factors for plantar foot ulcer recurrence in neuropathic diabetic patients. Diabetes Care 37:1697–1705
16. Edmonds ME, Foster AV (2006) Diabetic foot ulcers. BMJ 332:407–410. Review
17. Omanakuttan A, Nambiar J, Harris RM, Bose C, Pandurangan N, Varghese RK et al (2012) Anacardic acid inhibits the catalytic activity of matrix metalloproteinase-2 and matrix metalloproteinase-9. Mol Pharmacol 82:614–622
18. Kumar S, Ashe HA, Parnell LN, Fernando DJ, Tsigos C, Young RJ et al (1994) The prevalence of foot ulceration and its correlates in type 2 diabetic patients: a population-based study. Diabet Med 11:480–484
19. Tesfaye S, Stevens LK, Stephenson JM, Fuller JH, Plater M, Ionescu-Tirgoviste C et al (1996) Prevalence of diabetic peripheral neuropathy and its relation to glycaemic control and potential risk factors: the EURODIAB IDDM Complications Study. Diabetologia 39:1377–1384
20. Pendsey S (2003) Diabetic foot: a clinical atlas. Jaypee Brothers Medical Publishers, New Delhi
21. Management of peripheral arterial disease (PAD). TransAtlantic Inter-Society Consensus (TASC) (2000) Eur J Vasc Endovasc Surg 19:S1–250
22. Prompers L, Huijberts M, Apelqvist J, Jude E, Piaggesi A, Bakker K et al (2007) High prevalence of ischaemia, infection and serious comorbidity in patients with diabetic foot disease in Europe. Baseline results from the Eurodiale study. Diabetologia 50:18–25
23. Benotmane A, Mohammedi F, Ayad F, Kadi K, Azzouz A (2000) Diabetic foot lesions: etiologic and prognostic factors. Diabetes Metab 26:113–117
24. Armstrong DG, Boulton AJM, Bus SA (2017) Diabetic foot ulcers and their recurrence. N Engl J Med 376:2367–2375
25. Grotendorst GR, Martin GR, Pencev D, Sodek J, Harvey AK (1985) Stimulation of granulation tissue formation by platelet-derived growth factor in normal and diabetic rats. J Clin Invest 76:2323–2329

26. Buckley A, Davidson JM, Kamerath CD, Woodward SC (1987) Epidermal growth factor increases granulation tissue formation dose dependently. J Surg Res 43:322–328
27. Broadley KN, Aquino AM, Hicks B, Ditesheim JA, McGee GS, Demetriou AA et al (1988) Growth factors bFGF and TGF beta accelerate the rate of wound repair in normal and in diabetic rats. Int J Tissue React 10:345–353
28. Trojanowska M (2008) Role of PDGF in fibrotic diseases and systemic sclerosis. Rheumatology (Oxford) 47:v2–v4
29. Li X, Pontén A, Aase K, Karlsson L, Abramsson A, Uutela M et al (2000) PDGF-C is a new protease-activated ligand for the PDGF alpha-receptor. Nat Cell Biol 2:302–309
30. Bergsten E, Uutela M, Li X, Pietras K, Ostman A, Heldin CH et al (2001) PDGF-D is a specific, protease-activated ligand for the PDGF beta-receptor. Nat Cell Biol 3:512–516
31. Frederiksson L, Li H, Eriksson U (2004) The PDGF family: four gene products form five dimeric isoforms. Cytokine Growth Factor Rev 15:197–204
32. Heldin CH, Eriksson U, Ostman A (2002) New members of the platelet derived growth factor family of mitogens. Arch Biochem Biophys 398:284–290
33. Werner S, Grose R (2003) Regulation of wound healing by growth factors and cytokines. Physiol Rev 83:835–870
34. Pierce GF, Mustoe TA, Altrock BW, Deuel TF, Thomason A (1991) Role of platelet-derived growth factor in wound healing. J Cell Biochem 45:319–326. Review
35. Heldin CH, Rönnstrand L (1988) The platelet-derived growth factor receptor. In: Moudgil VK (ed) Receptor phosphorylation. CRC Press, Boca Raton, pp 149–162
36. Steed DL (1994) Clinical evaluation of recombinant human platelet derived growth factor for the treatment of lower extremity diabetic ulcers. J Vasc Surg 21:71–81
37. Bennett SP, Griffiths GD, Schor AM, Leese GP, Schor SL (2003) Growth factors in the treatment of diabetic foot ulcers. Br J Surg 90:133–146. Review
38. Mandial V, Gupta M, Sharma R (2017) Evaluation of recombinant human platelet derived growth factor-BB in healing of chronic diabetic foot ulcers. Int J Contemp Med Res 4:1607–1610
39. Das S, Majid M, Baker AB (2016) Syndecan-4 enhances PDGF-BB activity in diabetic wound healing. Acta Biomater 42:56–65
40. Rangaswamy P, Rubby SA, Prasanth K (2017) Prospective study if platelet derived growth factor in wound healing of diabetic foot ulcers in Indian population. Int Surg J. https://doi.org/10.18203/2349-2902.isj20164428
41. Robson MC, Mustoe TA, Hunt TK (1998) The future of recombinant growth factors in wound healing. Am J Surg 176:80S–82S
42. Kunimoto BT (1999) Growth factors in wound healing: the next great innovation? Ostomy Wound Manage 45:56–64
43. Ladin D (2000) Becaplermin gel (PDGF-BB) as topical wound therapy. Plastic Surgery Educational Foundation DATA Committee. Plast Reconstr Surg 105:1230–1231
44. Nagai MK, Embil JM (2002) Becaplermin: recombinant platelet derived growth factor, a new treatment for healing diabetic foot ulcers. Expert Opin Biol Ther 2:211–218
45. Ghatnekar O, Persson U, Willis M, Odegaard K (2001) Cost effectiveness of Becaplermin in the treatment of diabetic foot ulcers in four European countries. PharmacoEconomics 19:767–778
46. Kantor J, Margolis DJ (2001) Treatment options for diabetic neuropathic foot ulcers: a cost-effectiveness analysis. Dermatol Surg 27:347–351
47. Brown GL, Curtsinger L, Brightwell GR, Ackerman DM, Tobin GR, Polk HC Jr et al (1986) Enhancement of epidermal regeneration by biosynthetic epidermal growth factor. J Exp Med 163:1319–1324
48. Nanney LB (1990) Epidermal and dermal effect of epidermal growth factor during wound repair. J Invest Dermatol 94:624–629
49. Servold SA (1991) Growth factor impact on wound healing. Clin Podiatr Med Surg 8:937–953
50. Brown GL, Curtsinger L, Jurkiewics MJ, Nahai F, Schultz G (1991) Stimulation of healing of chronic wounds by epidermal growth factor. Plast Reconstr Surg 88:189–196

51. Tsang MW, Wong WK, Hung CS, Lai KM, Tang W, Cheung EY et al (2003) Human epidermal growth factor enhances healing of diabetic foot ulcers. Diabetes Care 26:1856–1861
52. Singla S, Garg R, Kumar A, Gill C (2014) Efficacy of topical application of beta urogastrone (recombinant human epidermal growth factor) in Wagner's Grade 1 and 2 diabetic foot ulcers: comparative analysis of 50 patients. J Natl Sci Biol Med 5:273–277
53. Gomez-Villa R, Aguilar-Rebolledo F, Lozano-Platonoff A, Teran-Soto JM, Fabian Victoriano MR, Kresch-Tronik NS et al (2014) Efficacy of intralesional recombinant human epidermal growth factor in diabetic foot ulcers in Mexican patients: a randomized double-blinded controlled trial. Wound Repair Regen 22:497–503
54. Dumantepe M, Fazliogullari O, Seren M, Uyar I, Basar F (2015) Efficacy of intralesional recombinant human epidermal growth factor in chronic diabetic foot ulcers. Growth Factors 33:128–132
55. Yang S, Geng Z, Ma K, Sun X, Fu X (2016) Efficacy of topical recombinant human growth factors in diabetic foot ulcers 315 © 1996–2018 epidermal growth factor for treatment of diabetic foot ulcer: a systematic review and meta-analysis. Int J Low Extrem Wounds 15:120–125
56. Hong JP, Jung HD, Yun W (2006) Recombinant human epidermal growth factor (EGF) to enhance healing for diabetic foot ulcers. Ann Plast Surg 56:394–398
57. Manoharan GV, Venkatesh G, Shanmugam S (2016) A comparative study on wound healing with topical application of human epidermal growth factor verses application of povidone-iodine in diabetic wounds. Sch J App Med Sci 4:2302–2306
58. Mohan VK (2007) Recombinant human epidermal growth factor (REGEN-D™ 150): effect on healing of diabetic foot ulcers. Diabetes Res Clin Pract 78:405–411
59. Tuyet HL, Quynh N, Tran T, Minh H, Bich DN, Dinh T et al (2009) The efficacy and safety of epidermal growth factor in treatment of diabetic foot ulcers: the preliminary results. Int Wound J 6:159–166
60. Bennett NT, Schultz GS (1993) Growth factors and wound healing: biochemical properties of growth factors and their receptors. Am J Surg 165:728–737
61. Lawrence WT, Diegelman RF (1994) Growth factors in wound healing. Clin Dermatol 12:157–169
62. Yang L, Qiu CX, Ludlow A, Fergusson MWJ, Brunner G (1999) Active transforming growth factor-β in wound repair. Determination using a new assay. Am J Pathol 154:105–111
63. Breuing K, Andree C, Helo G, Slama J, Liu PY, Eriksson E (1997) Growth factors in the repair of partial thickness porcine skin wounds. Plast Reconstr Surg 100:657–664
64. Crowe MJ, Doetschman T, Greenhalgh DG (2000) Delayed wound healing in immunodeficient TGF-β1 knockout mice. J Invest Dermatol 115:3–11
65. Wu L, Xia YP, Roth SI, Grushkin E, Mustoe TA (1999) Transforming growth factor-β1 fails to stimulate wound healing and impairs its signal transduction in an aged ischaemic ulcer model. Am J Pathol 154:301–309
66. Graham A (1998) The use of growth factors in clinical practice. J Wound Care 7:536–540
67. Ishimoto S, Ishibashi T, Bottaro DP, Kaga K (2002) Direct application of keratinocyte growth factor, basic fibroblast growth factor and transforming growth factor-alpha during healing of tympanic membrane perforation in glucocorticoid-treated rats. Acta Otolaryngol 122:468–473
68. Van Der Boom R, Wilmink JM, O'Kane S, Wood J, Ferguson MW (2002) Transforming growth factor-beta levels during second-intention healing are related to the different course of wound contraction in horses and ponies. Wound Repair Regen 10:188–194
69. Fu X, Shen Z, Chen Y et al (2000) Recombinant bovine basic fibroblast growth factor accelerates wound healing in patients with burns, donor sites and chronic dermal ulcers. Chin Med J 113:367–371
70. Beck PL, Rosenberg IM, Xavier RJ, Koh T, Wong JF, Podolsky DK (2003) Transforming growth factor-beta mediates intestinal healing and susceptibility to injury in vitro and in vivo through epithelial cells. Am J Pathol 162:597–608
71. Redmer DA, Reynolds LP (1996) Angiogenesis in the ovary. Rev Reprod 1:182–192

72. Reynolds LP, Redmer DA (1998) Expression of the angiogenic factors, basic fibroblast growth factor and vascular endothelial growth factor, in the ovary. J Anim Sci 76:1671–1681
73. Zimmerman MA, Selzman GH, Harken AH (1999) Surgical implications of therapeutic angiogenesis. Surgery 125:243–249
74. Gerwins P, Skoldenberg E, Claesson-Welsh L (2000) Function of fibroblast growth factors and vascular endothelial growth factors and their receptors in angiogenesis. Crit Rev Oncol/Hematol 34:185–194. 796
75. Kibe Y, Takenaka H, Kishimoto S (2000) Spatial and temporal expression of basic fibroblast growth factor protein during wound healing of rat skin. Br J Dermatol 43:720–727
76. Limat A, French LE (1999) Therapy with growth factors. Curr Probl Dermatol 27:49–56
77. Takehara K (2000) Growth regulation of skin fibroblasts. J Dermatol Sci 24:70–77
78. Greenhalgh DG (1996) The role of growth factors in wound healing. J Trauma 41:159–167
79. Yang SL, Han R, Liu Y, Hu LY, Li XL, Zhu LY (2014) Negative pressure wound therapy is associated with up-regulation of bFGF and ERK1/2 in human diabetic foot wounds. Wound Repair Regen 22:548–554
80. Khoshkam V, Chan HL, Lin GH, Mailoa J, Giannobile WV, Wang HL et al (2015) Outcomes of regenerative treatment with rhPDGF-BB and rhFGF-2 for periodontal intra-bony defects: a systematic review and meta-analysis. J Clin Periodontol 42:272–280
81. Robson MC, Phillips LG, Lawrence WT, Bishop JB, Youngerman JS, Hayward PG et al (1992) The safety and effect of topically applied recombinant basic fibroblast growth factor on the healing of chronic pressure sores. Ann Surg 216:401
82. Richard JL, Parer-Richard C, Daures JP, Clouet S, Vannereau D, Bringer J et al (1995) Effect of topical basic fibroblast growth factor on the healing of chronic diabetic neuropathic ulcer of the foot: a pilot, randomized, double-blind, placebo-controlled study. Diabetes Care 18:64–69
83. Uchi H, Igarashi A, Urabe K, Koga T, Nakayama J, Kawamori R et al (2009) Clinical efficacy of basic fibroblast growth factor (bFGF) for diabetic ulcer. Eur J Dermatol 19:461–468
84. Ferrara N (1999) Molecular and biological properties of vascular endothelial growth factor. J Mol Med 77:527–543
85. Redmer DA, Doraiswamy V, Bortnem BJ, Fisher K, Jablonka-Shariff A, Grazul-Bilska AT et al (2001) Evidence for a role of capillary pericytes in vascular growth of the developing ovine corpus luteum. Biol Reprod 65:979–989
86. Svendsen MN, Werther K, Nielsen HJ, Kristjansen PE (2002) VEGF and tumour angiogenesis. Impact of surgery, wound healing, inflammation and blood transfusion. Scand J Gastroenterol 37:373–379
87. Nissen NN, DiPietro LA (2000) Angiogenic mediators in healing wounds. In: Angiogenesis in health and disease. Springer, Boston, MA, pp 417–427
88. Nissen NN, Polverini PJ, Koch AE, Volin MV, Gamelli RL, DiPietro LA (1998) Vascular endothelial growth factor mediates angiogenic activity during the proliferative phase of wound healing. Am J Pathol 152:1445–1452
89. Sheikh AY, Gibson JJ, Rollins MD, Hopf HW, Hussain Z, Hunt TK (2000) Effect of hyperoxia on vascular endothelial growth factor levels in a wound model. Arch Surg 135:1293–1297
90. Taub PJ, Silver L, Weinberg H (2000) Plastic surgical perspectives on vascular endothelial growth factor as gene therapy for angiogenesis. Plast Reconstr Surg 105:1034–1042
91. Howdieshell TR, Callaway D, Webb WL, Gaines MD, Procter CD Jr, Sathyanarayana et al (2001) Antibody neutralization of vascular endothelial growth factor inhibits wound granulation tissue formation. J Surg Res 96:173–182
92. Dodge-Khatami A, Backer CL, Holinger LD, Mavroudis C, Cook KE, Crawford SE (2001) Healing of a free tracheal autograft is enhanced by topical vascular endothelial growth factor in an experimental rabbit model. J Thorac Cardiovasc Surg 122:554–561
93. Corral CJ, Siddiqui A, Wu L, Farrell CL, Lyons D, Mustoe TA (1999) Vascular endothelial growth factor is more important than basic fibroblastic growth factor during ischemic wound healing. Arch Surg 134:200–205

94. Breitbart AS, Grande DA, Laser J, Barcia M, Porti D, Malhotra S et al (2001) Treatment of ischemic wounds using cultured dermal fibroblasts transduced retrovirally with 798 wound healing: the role of growth factors PDGF-B and VEGF121 genes. Ann Plast Surg 46:555–561
95. Deodato B, Arsic N, Zentilin L, Galeano M, Santoro D, Torre V et al (2002) Recombinant AAV vector encoding human VEGF165 enhances wound healing. Gene Ther 9:777–785
96. Kulwas A, Drela E, Jundziłł W, Góralczyk B, Ruszkowska-Ciastek B, Rość D (2015) Circulating endothelial progenitor cells and angiogenic factors in diabetes complicated diabetic foot and without foot complications. J Diabetes Complicat 29:686–690
97. Zhou K, Ma Y, Brogan MS (2015) Chronic and non-healing wounds: the story of vascular endothelial growth factor. Med Hypotheses 85:399–404
98. Amoli MM, Hasani-Ranjbar S, Roohipour N, Sayahpour FA, Amiri P, Zahedi P et al (2011) VEGF gene polymorphism association with diabetic foot ulcer. Diabetes Res Clin Pract 93:215–219
99. Hanft JR, Pollak RA, Barbul A, van Gils C, Kwon PS, Gray SM et al (2008) Phase I trial on the safety of topical rhVEGF on chronic neuropathic diabetic foot ulcers. J Wound Care 17(30–2):34–37
100. Losi P, Briganti E, Errico C, Lisella A, Sanguinetti E, Chiellini F et al (2013) Fibrin-based scaffold incorporating VEGF- and bFGF-loaded nanoparticles stimulates wound healing in diabetic mice. Acta Biomater 9:7814–7821
101. Gardner JC, Wu H, Noel JG (2016) Keratinocyte growth factor supports pulmonary innate immune defense through the maintenance of alveolar antimicrobial protein levels and macrophage function. Am J Phys Lung Cell Mol Phys 310:L868–L879
102. Fricker J (1998) Keratinocyte growth factor on trial for wound repair. Mol Med Today 4:229
103. Robson MC, Phillips TJ, Falanga V, Odenheimer DJ, Parish LC, Jensen JL et al (2001) Randomized trial of topically applied repifermin (recombinant human keratinocyte growth factor-2) to accelerate wound healing in venous ulcers. Wound Repair Regen 9:347–352
104. Brown DL, Kane CD, Chernausek SD, Greenhalgh DG (1997) Differential expression and localization of insulin-like growth factors I and II in cutaneous wounds of diabetic and non-diabetic mice. Am J Pathol 151:715–724
105. Blakytny R, Jude EB, Martin Gibson J, Boulton AJ, Ferguson MW (2000) Lack of insulin-like growth factor 1 (IGF1) in the basal keratinocyte layer of diabetic skin and diabetic foot ulcers. J Pathol 190:589–594
106. Mason RM, Wahab NA (2003) Extracellular matrix metabolism in diabetic nephropathy. J Am Soc Nephrol 14:1358–1373
107. Vranckx JJ, Hoeller D, Velander PE, Theopold CF, Petrie N, Takedo A et al (2007) Cell suspension cultures of allogenic keratinocytes are efficient carriers for ex vivo gene transfer and accelerate the healing of full-thickness skin wounds by overexpression of human epidermal growth factor. Wound Repair Regen 15:657–664
108. Demidova-Rice TN, Hamblin MR, Herman IM (2012) Acute and impaired wound healing: pathophysiology and current methods for drug delivery, Part 2: Role of growth factors in normal and pathological wound healing: therapeutic potential and methods of delivery. Adv Skin Wound Care 25:349–370
109. Moura LI, Dias AM, Carvalho E, de Sousa HC (2013) Recent advances on the development of wound dressings for diabetic foot ulcer treatment—a review. Acta Biomater 9:7093–7114
110. Smith DM, Simon JK, Baker JR (2013) Applications of nanotechnology for immunology. Nat Rev Immunol 13:592–605
111. Degim Z (2008) Use of microparticulate systems to accelerate skin wound healing. J Drug Target 16:437–448
112. Ye M, Kim S, Park K (2010) Issues in long-term protein delivery using biodegradable microparticles. J Control Release 146:241–260
113. Gainza G, Villullas S, Pedraz JL, Hernandez RM, Igartua M (2015) Advances in drug delivery systems (DDSs) to release growth factors for wound healing and skin regeneration. Nanomedicine 11:1551–1573

114. Dong X, Xu J, Wang W, Luo H, Liang X, Zhang L et al (2008) Repair effect of diabetic ulcers with recombinant human epidermal growth factor loaded by sustained-release microspheres. Sci China C Life Sci 51:1039–1044
115. Porporato PE, Payen VL, De Saedeleer CJ, Preat V, Thissen JP, Feron O et al (2012) Lactate stimulates angiogenesis and accelerates the healing of superficial and ischemic wounds in mice. Angiogenesis 15:581–592
116. Zhang X, Kang X, Jin L, Bai J, Liu W, Wang Z (2018) Stimulation of wound healing using bioinspired hydrogels with basic fibroblast growth factor (bFGF). Int J Nanomedicine 13:3897–3906
117. Dwivedi C, Pandey I, Pandey H, Patil S, Mishra SB, Pandey AC et al (2018) In vivo diabetic wound healing with nanofibrous scaffolds modified with gentamicin and recombinant human epidermal growth factor. J Biomed Mater Res A 106:641–651
118. Akita S, Hayashida K, Takaki S, Kawakami Y, Oyama T, Ohjimi H (2017) The neck burn scar contracture: a concept of effective treatment. Burns Trauma 5:22
119. Centeno-Cerdas C, Jarquin-Cordero M, Chavez MN, Hopfner U, Holmes C, Schmauss D et al (2018) Development of photosynthetic sutures for the local delivery of oxygen and recombinant growth factors in wounds. Acta Biomater 81:184–194
120. Shi R, Lian W, Han S, Cao C, Jin Y, Yuan Y et al (2018) Nanosphere-mediated co-delivery of VEGF-A and PDGF-B genes for accelerating diabetic foot ulcers healing in rats. Gene Ther 25:425–438

Stem Cells in the Treatment of Diabetic Foot Ulcers

16

Rashid Mir, Imadeldin Elfaki, Ajaz Ahmad Waza, and Faisel M. AbuDuhier

16.1 Introduction

Diabetic foot ulcer is a major clinical complication of type 2 diabetes mellitus and remained an important clinical challenge to global health. The prevalence of Diabetic foot ulcers is 16–25% among type 2 diabetes mellitus patients in the Americans. Diabetic foot ulcers (DFU) are an economic burden on our health care system and society. Diabetic (DFUs) are the leading cause of lower limb amputation and is the most common chronic complication from T2D (Type 2 diabetes) and affecting 4–10% of patients. More than 85% of amputations are preceded by an active foot ulcer. Clinical complications of Diabetic foot ulcers are a major cause of hospitalization and amputation in the T2D (Type 2 diabetes) patients. Effective treatment options for curing Diabetic foot ulcers are very far from optimal. Diabetic foot ulcers are a type of wound and its healing is a physiologic response involving the disruption of normal skin architecture therefore requires temporal and spatial coordination of many cell types as well as cytokines.

Diabetic foot ulcer wound healing is the most complex process susceptible to dysregulation secondary to systemic and local factors such as T2D or diabetes and

R. Mir (✉)
Prince Fahd Bin Sultan Research Chair, Division of Molecular Biology, Department of Medical Lab Technology, Faculty of Applied Medical Sciences, University of Tabuk, Tabuk, Kingdom of Saudi Arabia

I. Elfaki
Department of Biochemistry, Faculty of Sciences, University of Tabuk, Tabuk, Kingdom of Saudi Arabia

A. A. Waza
Centre of Research for Development, University of Kashmir, Srinagar, Kashmir, India

F. M. AbuDuhier
Prince Fahd Bin Sultan Research Chair, Department of Medical Lab Technology, Faculty of Applied Medical Sciences, University of Tabuk, Tabuk, Kingdom of Saudi Arabia

M. Zubair et al. (eds.), *Diabetic Foot Ulcer*,
https://doi.org/10.1007/978-981-15-7639-3_16

ischemia which lead to chronic wounds. Diabetic foot ulcer wounds are epidemic as they heal poorly and recur frequently and create a profound impact on the health care system therefore creating an urgent for developing new and advanced therapies. Most of the amputations occurring in the populations with T2D (Type 2 diabetes) reported being due to Diabetic foot ulcer. Several symptoms have been reported of a localized wound infection that indicates Diabetic foot ulcers few of them are as—edema, heat erythema, bad odor from one or both feet and purulent exudate, pain are classic signs of infection linked with wound infection. The various signs specific to secondary symptoms are serous exudate, friable granulation tissue, discolored granulation tissue, pocketing of the wound base, delayed healing, wound breakdown, and foul odor.

Diabetic foot ulcers are vascular disease. It is reported that blood does not flow normally to the tissues and the ulcers do not heal because of poor blood supply. In several cases of Diabetic foot ulcers several foot nerves are damaged that lead to long-term loss of feeling in the foot. In the wounded feet, there is a tingling and painful feeling. The sensitivity to foot pain is reduced because of the nerve damage. Due to nerve damage, poor hygiene painless wounds are formed leading to ulcers besides the use of tobacco which inhibits blood circulation. Diabetic foot ulcers physiology has shown autonomic dysfunction that leads to the drying of the skin. This induces the increased axial and mechanical stress on the patient skin. The drying makes Diabetic foot ulcers more prone to injury.

The gold standard for Diabetic foot ulcer wound management is composed of diagnostic etiology, vascular inflow to reduce ischemia, controlling of infection, off-loading of pressure, and debridement of nonviable tissue. It has been reported that only despite advanced and optimal treatment options still only 51% of Diabetic foot ulcers heal within 15–20 weeks however more than 50% under *recurrence* within 19 months. Therefore improved, novel, and modern methods of Diabetic foot ulcer wound healing are required.

Current treatment options are reported to recover about 31% of Diabetic foot ulcers and even the most modern and advanced therapies like cell-based therapies composed of skin-derived fibroblasts and keratinocytes however only 50% cure rate has been reported, therefore leaving a void and a tremendous scope for developing new effective therapeutic options for Diabetic foot ulcers. It has been established that mesenchymal stem cell therapy (Stem cell) holding a great promise as an advanced therapy for Diabetic foot ulcers. Stem cell therapy has been reported to have a great potential in accelerating the healing of Diabetic foot ulcer wounds.

Mesenchymal stem cells proved to high curative potential as they secrete stimulatory molecules and provide base for collagen scaffolding that can generate a template on which new tissue can be rebuilt and regenerate. Several studies established that mesenchymal stem cell—scaffold device is a pre-conditioned and its regenerative and reparative properties can be maximized. Mesenchymal stem cell therapy (Stem cell) therapy has limited scope because of the requirement for invasive harvesting techniques, having short cell survival in vivo and immunogenicity.

Several studies established that embryonic stem cell-derived mesenchymal stem cells are more advantageous and superior to adult-derived mesenchymal stem cell because they have high potency, display a consistent phenotype and have the proliferative ability. Because of the ethical issues, the utilization of Adult-derived mesenchymal stem cell has become limited by the ethical issues. The limited use of embryonic stem cells is due to invasive harvesting techniques, limited cell survival in vivo, and high immunogenicity with the use of embryonic stem cells. Similarly, the Induced pluripotent stem cells (iPSC) have a high potential for self-renewal, are pluripotent, and can differentiate into any adult cell type. They can be used in wound healing as well as regenerative medicine. Induced pluripotent stem cells (iPSC) have translational potential and enhanced therapeutics. Induced pluripotent stem cells (iPSC) can be harvested non-invasively and can be transplanted autonomously and reducing immune rejection. Induced pluripotent stem cells (iPSC) iPSC are capable of differentiation into all cell types in the human skin.

16.1.1 Role of Induced Pluripotent Stem Cells (iPSC) in Diabetic Foot Wound Healing

16.1.1.1 Pluripotent Stem Cells

Pluripotent stem cells are commonly called as master cells, which are able to produce any type of cell and are able to self-renew, i.e., can produce more copies of them. iPSCs are pluripotent stem cells derived from adult somatic cells through reprogramming strategy. Such cells have the capability to differentiate into any type of adult cell and therefore have emerged as a novel strategy for wound healing therapy [1]. IPSC have the capability to augment diabetic wound healing via direct and paracrine signaling [2]. They are a source of autologous and allogeneic cell types and therefore can improve the outcome in DFU wound healing. Although iPSCs can differentiate into various cell types essential for DFU healing, but have not been exploited yet for the repair of chronic wounds [3, 4]. Till date, iPSC have not yet been used to treat recalcitrant DFUs.

16.1.1.2 Current Methods for Generating Induced Pluripotent Stem Cells

Induced pluripotent stem cells (iPSCs) are produced by artificial reprogramming/manipulation of adult cell. Currently, different strategies are followed to achieve reprogramming and are discussed in Table 16.1.

Although different strategies like nuclear transfer, cell extracts, forced expression of defined factors, synthetic molecules, and miRNA are adapted to produce iPSCs, but the optimal method is yet to be explored. Out of all these, the forced expression technique is well defined and the most studied one.

16.1.2 Dysregulation of Wound Healing in Diabetic Wounds

Long-standing diabetes is associated with numerous complications like cardiovascular diseases, cerebrovascular diseases, neuropathy, retinopathy, nephropathy, and

Table 16.1 Techniques adopted for iPSC production

Method	Technique	Refernces
Nuclear transfer	In this technique, the nucleus of a somatic cell is allowed to fuse with a mature enucleated oocyte.	[5, 6]
Cell extracts	This technique involves incubation of differentiated cells with ES cells extracts, so to induce them to express profiles of ES cells.	[7, 8]
Forced expression of defined factors	This technique involves the transfection of embryonic cells with a known combination of different genes like Oct4, Sox2, c-Myc, Klf4, Lin28, Stat3, Nanog, UTF-1, Esrrb SV40LT, Wnt3a, hTERT, Nr5a2, and p53 siRNA.	[9, 10]
Synthetic molecules	This technique involves the use of low molecular weight compounds for reprogramming purposes. For example, Reversina is used to produce cells with adipogenic and osteogenic differentiation potential from myoblasts. Other compounds used for this purpose include valproic acid (VPA), Suberoylanilide hydroxamic acid (SAHA), valproic acid (VPA), trichostatin A (TSA), BIX-01294, 5′ azaC, dexamethasone, and BayK8644.	[11, 12]
miRNA	This technique involves the use of microRNAs to alter the protein profile of the target cell.	[13, 14]

poor wound healing. Out of these complications, poor wound healing also called DFU is devastating and can even lead to amputation. A normal healing process is not followed during diabetic wound healing but a dysregulation in proliferation, deposition of extracellular matrix, and cell migration has been observed [15, 16]. Role of hypoxia and hypoxia inducible factor-1 (HIF-1) in wound healing and extracellular matrix deposition is well established in fibroblasts essential for wound healing [17]. HIF-1 activates wound repair associated genes like GLUT-1 (transporter -1) and VEGF (vascular endothelial growth factor) [17]. Duscher and his colleagues found that the deletion of HIF-1 in fibroblasts resulted in delaying wound healing with poor vascularization [18]. Similarly, insulin is considered to be a key factor in the wound healing process and selective insulin resistance (insulin unresponsiveness) has been found in fibroblasts and endothelial cells. As a result, insulin-associated endogenous signaling mediated through the IRS/PI3K/AKT pathway is not activated in these wound healing essential cells [19, 20].

16.1.3 Human-Induced Pluripotent Stem Cells in Ischemic Wounds

Ischemia is a condition resulted from a decreased blood flow to some tissue/organs and occurs due to obstruction of the arteries. Insufficient blood flow to brain and heart can lead to heart attack and stroke respectively, while decreased blood flow to skin can lead to wound formation. Currently, iPSC are being studied in various ischemia disease models, which includes myocardial infarction, retinopathy, osteonecrosis, and peripheral arterial disease. As evident from skin-related wound healing studies, it has been observed that iPSC healing potential is mainly attributed to their pro-angiogenic property [21]. Till date, iPSCs have been investigated with respect to peripheral arterial disease models but research has not been carried out yet regarding wound healing in severe ischemic limbs. In peripheral arterial disease models, iPSC has been found to ameliorate ischemia by decreasing inflammation, enhancing angiogenesis and by reconstitution of viable cells. Use of human-induced pluripotent stem cell-derived endothelial cell (hiPSC-EC) in combination with VEGF in a hind limb ischemia mice model promotes regeneration of muscles and decreases inflammation [22]. Furthermore, hiPSC-EC has been found to increase angiogenesis (increased number of angiogenic related cytokines and growth factors) and therefore resulted in increased blood flow to ischemic limbs [23]. It has been observed that injecting hiPSC-derived pericytes into murine limbs challenges with ischemia is associated with increased limb reperfusion by fourfold [24].

16.1.4 Limitations of Induced Pluripotent Stem Cells to Achieve Wound Healing

Although the use of iPSC has emerged as an exciting and innovative strategy in the field of regenerative medicine and holds the potentials to enhance wound healing. Before using in clinical settings, their role must be fully understood with respect to their tumorigenic potential [1]. HiPSC derived from chronic disease patients can be reprogrammed into the cells identical to those derived from a healthy individual. But iPSC-EC obtained from mice with induced diabetes are linked with poor healing and therefore, demands further studies to fully understood the nature of hiPSC derived from healthy and diseased donor.

Before using Induced pluripotent stem cells (iPSC) for human use, major hurdles associated with them must be overcome first. Non-integrative methods like the use of small particle and protein transfer for the generation of hiPSC should become speedier and more efficient [25]. Standardized procedures should be developed for teratoma formation assays to confirm pluripotency, so as to derive meaningful conclusions about cell lines. A proper platform for transferring hiPSC into a wound area should be determined. Furthermore, it is important to determine an ideal niche for hiPSC, so as to achieve enhanced intracellular signaling and cell survival.

New strategies/protocols are need of the hour to eliminate undifferentiated hiPSC cells before transplant, as they have tumorigenic tendency. A good number of studies have investigated the tumorigenic tendency of iPSC transferred directly to the murine tissues, but till date no such event has been examined after injection of hiPSC into the cutaneous tissue [26]. Thus it is important to further investigate iPSC in model animals that mimic human skin for their safety and efficacy before their human use.

16.1.5 Induced Pluripotent Stem Cells Reveal Distinct Cellular and Tissue Phenotypes

Diabetic foot ulcers (DFU), have emerged as a major complication associated with diabetes, and to treat these wounds, the use of iPSCs has gained much attention. Recently, it has been reported that iPSC-derived fibroblasts showed enhanced migratory potential in two-dimensional (2D) culture conditions [2]. Interestingly, iPSC-derived fibroblasts (obtained from DFUs) has been found to possess distinct morphology and biochemical composition than parental DFU fibroblasts, when cultured in three-dimensional (3D) conditions [2]. Furthermore, enhanced diabetic wound closure has been reported by using 3D tissues (obtained from iPSC-derived fibroblasts) as compared to primary DFU fibroblasts [2].

16.2 Mesenchymal Stem Cells (MSCS) for Diabetic Foot Wound Healing

Mesenchymal stem cells (MSCs) also called multipotent mesenchymal stromal cells are able to self-renew and have the ability to differentiate into various tissue-forming cell lineages like myocytes, chondrocytes, osteoblasts, tenocytes, and adipocytes [27]. These stem cells can be obtained from different tissues like adipose tissue, bone marrow, and umbilical cord.

16.2.1 Role of Mesenchymal Stem Cells (MSCs)

Various studies have reported that MSCs are able to accelerate wound closure by increasing wound healing [28, 29]. It has been reported that human MSCs (derived from bone marrow) are able to cause wound closure via enhanced migration of keratinocytes and fibroblasts in in vitro conditions [30]. Smith and his colleagues reported an increased wound closure by murine MSCs (derived from bone marrow) via enhanced migration of dermal fibroblasts [31]. Similarly, Jeon and his colleagues reported an increased migratory potential of skin fibroblasts during culturing in umbilical cord blood MSC-conditioned media [32]. The beneficial role of MSCs on skin regeneration and cutaneous wound healing has been well defined and the process is complex. MSCs enhance different processes like wound closure, angiogenesis, re-epithelialization, and formation of tissue granulation, as well as modulate inflammation and regulate extracellular matrix (ECM) remodeling, as shown in Table 16.2. Furthermore, MSCs associated with beneficial effects are mainly attributed to paracrine signaling [33, 34].

16.2.2 Mesenchymal Stem Cells (MSCs): Mechanisms of Action

An intense research had been carried out during the past decade to better understand the molecular mechanism associated with MSCs during regeneration and wound healing. Administrated MSCs promote tissue regeneration and wound healing

Table 16.2 MSCs associated increased cutaneous wound healing

Mesenchymal stem cells	Increased migration of keratinocytes and fibroblasts	Wound closure	Wound healing
	Increased expression of HGF and VEGF	Angiogenesis	
	Increased density of microvessels		
	Decreased inflammatory cells	Inflammation	
	Decreased expression of TNFα and IL-1		
	Decreased expression of ICAM1		
	Increased expression of SOD and GPx		
	Decreased expression of MMP-1	ECM remodeling	
	Increased expression of collagen and elastin		
	Increased proliferation of fibroblasts and HaCaT cells		
	Increased thickness of the regenerated epidermis	Skin regeneration	
	Increased skin appendages		

SOD superoxide dismutase, *GPx* glutathione peroxidase, *TNF-α* tumor necrosis factor-alpha, *HG* hepatocyte growth factor, *HaCaT* immortalized human keratinocyte, *ICAM1* intercellular adhesion molecule 1, *MMP-1* matrix metalloproteinase-1, *IL-1* interleukin-1, *VEGF* vascular endothelial growth factor

through different mechanisms, which include differentiation, migration/homing, paracrine effects, and immunomodulation. Understating the molecular mechanism of each step would be quiet helpful to enhance treatment efficacy, safety, and patient's outcome after administration of MSC.

16.2.3 Differentiation of Mesenchymal Stem Cells

Mesenchymal stem cells (MSCs) have the ability to differentiate into different cell types like epithelial cells, osteocytes, adipocytes, chondrocytes, cardiomyocytes, hepatocytes, vascular endothelial cells, and neurons, and therefore have emerged as a potential cell-based therapy to treat different human diseases [35]. Injection of MSCs (derived from bone marrow) around a cutaneous wound has been found to increase closure of wounds with enhanced angiogenesis, re-epithelialization, and cellularity. Apart from this, MSCs were found to synthesize a keratinocyte-specific protein namely keratin, suggesting differentiation of MSCs into keratinocytes [36]. Furthermore, MSCs have been found to differentiate into epidermal keratinocytes and skin appendages [37].

16.2.4 Migration/Homing of Mesenchymal Stem Cells (MSCs)

The process of delivering MCSs to the site of wound/injury is known as *homing*, and the process is complex. Therapeutic potential of MSCs mainly dependents on paracrine and juxtacrine signaling factors, which are essential for increasing regeneration from endogenous (stem) cells.

In response to injury, certain specific ligands or receptors are upregulated, which not only help in adhesion, infiltration, and trafficking of MSCs, but also provide a feasible niche for marinating pluripotency and self-renewal [38]. Furthermore, MSCs trapped in blood vessels of wound/injured site secretes various cytokines and growth factors that promote wound healing [39].

16.2.5 Paracrine Effects of Mesenchymal Stem Cells (MSCs)

Paracrine signaling associated with MSCs are important for exerting their therapeutic effects [40]. MSCs associated with paracrine signaling promote various beneficial effects on different cell types, which include modulation of proliferation, gene expression, cell survival, and migration [41]. The presence of cytokines and growth factors in MSC-conditioned media promotes wound repair and increases epithelialization, due to the presence of growth factors and cytokines [36]. Conditioned medium obtained from bone marrow-derived MSC has been reported to attract endothelial progenitor cells and macrophages to the wound area [42].

16.2.6 Immunomodulation of Mesenchymal Stem Cells (MSCs)

Suppression of inflammation is considered to be an important event for healing to occur successfully and MSCs possess anti-inflammatory effects. Surface of MSCs possesses low levels of MHC-I (histocompatibility complex-I) and lacks molecules like MHC-II, CD 40, CD 86, and CD 80, thus allowing their successful allogeneic transplantation [43]. Liu et al. observed very low quantity of pro-inflammatory cytokines (like TNF-α and IL-1) and inflammatory cells, when cutaneous rat wounds were transplanted with MSCs (derived from human umbilical cord) [44]. It has been observed that co-culture between human dermal fibroblasts and MSCs (derived from murine bone) resulted in decreased expression of ICAM1 (intercellular adhesion molecule 1) mRNA [45]. Decreased expression of ICAM1 is considered to be essential for suppressing inflammation during wound repair [46].

16.2.7 Optimizing of Mesenchymal Stem Cells (MSCs) Therapeutic Effect

A potential disadvantage associated with the use of MSCs for the treatment of chronic wounds is a variation in cell survival proportion after implantation. On the other hand, MSCs have potential to proliferate fast and therefore does not pose dose-limiting hindrance during MSC therapy. MSCs can be applied in high doses to the wound area or close to the wound, through biomaterials [47]. It has been reported that the use of biomaterials ensures longer MSCs viability, furthermore the use of cell encapsulation technology effectively protects MSCs from mechanical stress, which is a common event during DFU [48]. It is important to better understand the

MSCs niche in diabetic cutaneous wounds, as microenvironment in the niche is essential in controlling MSCs cell fate.

16.2.8 Preclinical Studies on the Stem Cell Usage for Diabetic Foot Ulcers

T2D is resulted from by the genetic and environmental risk factors interaction [49–52]. There are long-term and short-term complications of DM. The long-term complications include the macro vascular complications such as coronary artery disease, peripheral vascular disease, and stroke. Whereas microvascular diabetes complications include neuropathy, nephropathy, and retinopathy [53]. Diabetic foot ulcers (DFU) is a public health concern all over the world. Diabetic foot ulceration and amputation are caused by diabetic cardiovascular and diabetic neuropathy complications. It is considered as a very important cause of illness and deaths among diabetic patients [54]. Every year there are more than one million lower limb amputations because of DFU, and that about 60% of all nontraumatic lower limb amputations are caused by the of diabetes ulcerations [55]. Moreover, DFU costs about 9 billion USD for treatment and care [56]. DFU results from infections, low blood supply, hypoglycemia, and diabetic neuropathy [56].

Stem cells are multipotent cells with the potential of self-renewing and differentiation into multiple tissue-specific daughter cell types with specialized functions [57]. The stem cells are found in all human tissues and play critical roles in growth and homeostasis [58]. The major classes of stem cells include the embryonic (obtained from embryos of human in preimplantation stage), Adult stem cells (derived from tissues of adults), and the induced pluripotent stem cells (iPSCs) which resemble the ESCs and obtained from genetic reprogramming of various somatic cells from many animal species [58]. Due to the ability of the stem cells in self-renewing and differentiation into diverse cell types, they were studied in regenerative medicine for treatment of diabetes mellitus, tumors, and the immunodeficiency virus [49]. The multipotent mesenchymal stem cells (MSCs) represent a good origin for regenerative therapy of inflammation, tissue injuries, tumors, and Diabetic foot wounds [49, 57, 59]. The sources of the MSCs include bone marrows, brain, gingiva, peripheral blood, lungs, heart, and adipose tissues [57, 59].

16.2.9 Source of Mesenchymal Stem Cells

Stem cells can be obtained from the bone marrow. The stem cells obtained from the bone marrow are called the mesenchymal stem cells (BM-MSCs). The BM-MSCs represent an efficient and safe option for DFU therapy [57]. Intramuscular transplantation has been shown to be the most effective way. However, differentiation and numbers of BM-MSCs are reduced with increasing age [60, 61]. The BM-MSCs do not stimulate immune reactions, and they are able to resist the cellular immune response (cytotoxic T and NK lymphocytes) [9] and inhibits the effects of the interferon-gamma (IFN-γ) derived from the T-cells [57, 62]. The BM-MSCs migrate and form the blood vessels in the DFU which would accelerate the wound healing through the protein C-C chemokine receptor type 7, intercellular adhesion molecule 1 (ICAM-1) and the Akt-dependent mechanism cells [49, 63]. The Mesenchymal Stem cells obtained from Umbilical Cord Blood (UCB-MSCs) are able to move like BM-MSCs and have similar multilineage differentiation capacity surface antigen on the cells [49, 61]. The UCB-MSCs have some biological advantages such as increased proliferation capacity, a shorter doubling time, a longer culture time, and a higher anti-inflammation effect [57, 64]. These advantages make the UCB-MSCs more convenient than the BM-MSCs for the application of stem cells in regenerative therapy. Animal and in vitro studies have shown that the UCB-MSCs reduces the neurodegeneration in DFU via the secretion of the neurotrophic factor, the nerve growth factor (NGF) in the femoral nerve that supplies the gastrocnemius muscle of rat diabetic foot. In addition, UCB-MSCs secrete the vascular endothelial (VEGF) and the basic fibroblast (bFGF) growth factors that improve the blood supply for the foot and accelerate diabetic wound healing [57, 64, 65].

16.2.10 The Usage of the BM-MSCs for Diabetic Foot Ulcers in Clinical Studies

The autologous transplantation of BM-MSCs in clinical trials demonstrated decreased pain and size of the wound, in addition to normal liver and kidney functions [66]. The leg perfusion has also improved which decreased the amputation size in critical limb ischemia [57]. The autologous biograft in mixture with BM-MSCs accelerate the ulcer healing and improve the skin angiogenesis and thickness in cases with DFU [57]. The intramuscular injection of BM-MSCs in the quadriceps thigh muscles in patients with DFU resulted in the maintenance of blood sugar and decreased levels of C-reactive protein and tumor necrosis factor alpha levels, in addition to increased vascular endothelial growth factor level [62]. In another study, the intramuscular injection of UCB-MSCs in patients with critical limb ischemia resulted in mild adverse side effects such as diarrhea; mouth wound, and elevated levels of serum creatinine [67, 68]. The body urticaria was treated with antihistamine and the other adverse effects improved without interference [67, 68].

16.2.11 Limitations of the Use of the UCB-MSCs

Limitations of the use of the UCB-MSCs include privacy and ethical issues in addition, to the high costs of the umbilical cord blood preservation. The Mesenchymal stem cells derived from the peripheral blood have been reported to be used frequently in clinical studies. The injection of PB-MSC and angioplasty improved the healing of DFU [49, 56]. In a case-control study, 30 patients with DFU have been treated with stem cells derived adipose tissues (ASCs), and the control group (n = 29) have been treated with polyurethane film for 12 weeks [49]. After the treatment period complete wound healing was achieved in 80% of the group treated with ASCs, and 50% in the control group with no observed side effects [69].

16.3 Administration Route Stem Cell Therapies

One of the most important aspects of the stem cell therapy to improve patient's *treatment* and the outcome is the route of administration of the *stem cells.* Mesenchymal stem cell therapy has been established as a potential, advanced, and effective treatment for Diabetic foot ulcers and can be an alternative treatment to amputation for T2D patients without other treatment options for revascularization. It has been reported that preclinical and clinical studies can be utilized for designing future randomized clinical trials. There are different *routes* of *administration* of *stem cells* used in Diabetic foot ulcers including

1. Nonvascular administration of stem cell therapy
2. Topical administration of stem cell therapy
   (a) Intramuscular
   (b) Subcutaneous
   (c) Intradermal
   (d) Hydrogel and Scaffold
   (e) Spray and Drops
3. Systemic endovascular administration of stem cell therapy
   (a) Endovascular Intraarterial
   (b) Endovascular Intravenous

16.3.1 Nonvascular Injections

Nonvascular injections into tissue have been established as the most utilized route of administration to directly treat Diabetic foot ulcers DFU. More than 28 preclinical studies (52%) have been reported to utilize direct nonvascular injections to directly treat Diabetic foot ulcers [56]. Recently 31 clinical studies (86%) have been conducted with excellent results utilizing direct nonvascular injections to treat Diabetic foot ulcers as depicted in Table 16.3 [56].

Table 16.3 Intramuscular (Nonvascular injections) as administration routes for stem cells its advantages, disadvantages and use in clinical and preclinical studies

Administration route	Injection
Clinical studies	31 (86%)
Preclinical studies	28 (52%)
Administration route subtype	Intramuscular
Disadvantages	Poor engraftment, high cell death, low addressing
Advantages	Low risk, simple and inexpensive
Preclinical studies	2 (3.7%)
Clinical studies	24 (66.7%)

Table 16.4 Topical (Subcutaneous and Intradermal) as administration routes for stem cells its advantages, disadvantages and use in clinical and preclinical studies

Administration route	Topical
Preclinical studies	23 (43%)
Clinical studies	31 (86%)
Administration route subtype	Subcutaneous and intradermal
Advantages	Inexpensive, simple, painless, and low risk
Disadvantages	Low addressing, high cell death, and poor engraftment
Clinical studies	3 (8.3%)
Preclinical studies	6 (11.1%)

16.3.2 Topical Administration of Stem Cell Therapy

Topical administration is also called direct administration stem cells that require a high concentration of stem cells adjacent to the wound as well as at the surface of the wound. It should be kept in mind that the stem cell administration timing is potentially important so that the mesenchymal stem cells undergo functional interaction with the wound cells at critical stages of the healing process. The frequency of direct administration has been performed frequently in 23 (43%) preclinical studies and five clinical studies (14%) [56] as depicted in Table 16.4.

16.3.3 Collagen Hydrogels and Scaffolds Administration of Stem Cell Therapy

Collagen hydrogels are composed of cross-linked hydrophilic polymer networks called extracellular matrix (ECM). The extracellular matrix (ECM) has a property of swelling when coming in contact with water and the extracellular matrix (ECM) is a natural occurring hydrogel which can provide the best microenvironment which provides support to stem cells found resident in tissues, making this polymer desirable for tissue engineering applications using stem cells. It has been established that Collagen hydrogels and scaffolds can be utilized for culturing stem cells in several different tissue engineering applications, including blood, neural tissues [69]. It has been reported that the use of collagen hydrogels or hydrogel scaffolds have attractive characteristics like shape adaptability, ability to access parts of the body that are difficult to reach, and improve the engraftment capacity as well as the survival of the injected Mesenchymal stem cells. These collagen hydrogels or hydrogel scaffolds have the potential to be combined with materials yielding some new or novel hybrid materials that increase cell survival, making it more desirable for drug delivery [69, 70]. Several research studies have reported that collagen hydrogels and scaffolds can be utilized as vehicles to deliver to tissues and cells [71]. It has been reported that hydrogel and scaffold delivery were used in 9 (16.7%) preclinical studies and 0 (0%) clinical studies [56] as depicted in Table 16.5. Similarly, spray and drops administration routes delivery were used in three (8.3%) preclinical studies and clinical studies six (11%) [56] as depicted in Table 16.5.

Table 16.5 Topical (spray and drops and hydrogel and scaffold) as administration routes for stem cells its advantages, disadvantages, and use in clinical and preclinical studies

Administrative route	Topical	
Preclinical research studies	23 (43%)	
Clinical research studies	5 (14%)	
Route subtype	Spray and drops	Hydrogel and scaffold
Advantages	Painless, simple, low risk, and inexpensive	Better retention and engraftment, low risk, high cell density, good spacing control
Disadvantages	Poor engraftment, high cell death, low cell density, and good spacing control	High protocol complexity, expensive and may need debridement
Clinical studies	3 (8.3%)	0 (0.0%)
Preclinical studies	6 (11.1%)	9 (16.7%)

Table 16.6 Systemic Endovascular (Intraarterial and Intravenous) as administration routes for stem cells its advantages, disadvantages, and use in clinical and preclinical studies

Administration route	Systemic endovascular	
Preclinical research studies	5 (9%)	
Clinical research studies	6 (17%)	
Administration route subtype	Intraarterial	Intravenous
Advantages	Can be done during angioplasty, possible	Glucose homeostasis optimizing effect immunomodulation
Disadvantages	Poor engraftment Low addressing High surgical risk	Complex Expensive
Clinical studies	6 (16.7%)	0 (0.0%)
Preclinical studies	1 (1.9%)	4 (7.4%)

16.3.4 Systemic Endovascular Administration of Stem Cell Therapy

Endovascular stem cell administration has been reported in more than five (9%) preclinical and six (17%) clinical studies [56] as depicted in Table 16.6. Intraarterial stem cell delivery has been conducted in one preclinical study (1.9%) and six (16.7%) clinical studies [56] as depicted in Table 16.6. Intravenous stem cell delivery has been conducted four (7.4%) preclinical studies [56] and no clinical studies were conducted till date as depicted in Table 16.6.

Kwon et al. [72] performed a single local injection of allogeneic BM-mesenchymal stem cells that potentially increased the wound healing strength in a rat Diabetic foot ulcers (DFU) model however no significant increase in wound strength was reported by multiple intravenous injections ($P = 0.06$). O'Loughlin et al., [70] in his preclinical studies topically administered stem cells with collagen scaffolds and fibrin spray in a rat Diabetic foot ulcers model, a significant correlation in wound healing was documented similarly Falanga et al., [73] performing preclinical studies delivered stem cells with collagen scaffolds and fibrin spray and reported improved wound healing. In all these three studies, there was a significant correlation in wound healing when at least 1×10^6 stem cells were delivered respectively. Intraarterial stem cell administration proved to be the effective route for immunomodulatory applications in rat kidney transplantation when compared to intravenous administration therefore the reducing the incidence of arteritis, glomerulitis, and tubulitis ($P < 0.01$) [74].

In case of murine diabetic model, multiple intravenous mesenchymal stem cell doses induced high impact on glucose homeostasis, thereby decreasing blood sugar levels after two doses and total remission of T2D within seven doses [75]. It has been reported that the bench-to-bedside approach is the aim of government policies in the globe with collaborations developing between Stem cell Research laboratories, biotechnology industries, pharmaceutical, academia, and clinicians. This bench-to-bedside approach is the focus of government policies throughout the globe with collaborations developing between Stem cell Research laboratories, pharmaceutical, and biotechnology industries, academia, and clinicians. Several research studies have established that mesenchymal Stem Cell therapy that can be utilized to translate technology to a variety of dermatological disorders. Mesenchymal stem cell therapy has increased the attractiveness for industrial investment for further research and development of these products. The most important characteristic for the successful utilization of mesenchymal stem cell treatments is the conducting of rapid and robust randomized controlled clinical trials. It is concluded that stem cell therapy is a potential, advanced, and effective treatment for Diabetic foot ulcers and is utilized as an alternative to amputation for T2D patients for revascularization. This therapy is utilizing tissue engineering as well as regenerative medicine.

References

1. Gorecka J, Kostiuk V, Fereydooni A, Gonzalez L, Luo J, Dash B, Isaji T, Ono S, Liu S, Lee SR et al (2019) The potential and limitations of induced pluripotent stem cells to achieve wound healing. Stem Cell Res Ther 10(1):87
2. Kashpur O, Smith A, Gerami-Naini B, Maione AG, Calabrese R, Tellechea A, Theocharidis G, Liang L, Pastar I, Tomic-Canic M et al (2019) Differentiation of diabetic foot ulcer-derived induced pluripotent stem cells reveals distinct cellular and tissue phenotypes. FASEB J 33(1):1262–1277
3. van Wilgenburg B, Browne C, Vowles J, Cowley SA (2013) Efficient, long term production of monocyte-derived macrophages from human pluripotent stem cells under partly-defined and fully-defined conditions. PLoS One 8(8):e71098

4. Petrova A, Celli A, Jacquet L, Dafou D, Crumrine D, Hupe M, Arno M, Hobbs C, Cvoro A, Karagiannis P et al (2014) 3D In vitro model of a functional epidermal permeability barrier from human embryonic stem cells and induced pluripotent stem cells. Stem Cell Rep 2(5):675–689
5. Kim JS, Choi HW, Choi S, Do JT (2011) Reprogrammed pluripotent stem cells from somatic cells. Int J Stem Cells 4(1):1–8
6. Morgan HD, Santos F, Green K, Dean W, Reik W (2005) Epigenetic reprogramming in mammals. Human Mol Genet 14(Spec No 1):R47–R58
7. Freberg CT, Dahl JA, Timoskainen S, Collas P (2007) Epigenetic reprogramming of OCT4 and NANOG regulatory regions by embryonal carcinoma cell extract. Mol Biol Cell 18(5):1543–1553
8. Hochedlinger K, Jaenisch R (2006) Nuclear reprogramming and pluripotency. Nature 441(7097):1061–1067
9. Kulcenty K, Wroblewska J, Mazurek S, Liszewska E, Jaworski J (2015) Molecular mechanisms of induced pluripotency. Contemp Oncol 19(1A):A22–A29
10. Telpalo-Carpio S, Aguilar-Yanez J, Gonzalez-Garza M, Cruz-Vega D, Moreno-Cuevas J (2013) iPS cells generation: an overview of techniques and methods. J Stem Cells Regenerat Med 9(1):2–8
11. Ma X, Kong L, Zhu S (2017) Reprogramming cell fates by small molecules. Protein Cell 8(5):328–348
12. Zhang Y, Li W, Laurent T, Ding S (2012) Small molecules, big roles—the chemical manipulation of stem cell fate and somatic cell reprogramming. J Cell Sci 125(Pt 23):5609–5620
13. Bhat AA, Younes SN, Raza SS, Zarif L, Nisar S, Ahmed I, Mir R, Kumar S, Sharawat SK, Hashem S et al (2020) Role of non-coding RNA networks in leukemia progression, metastasis and drug resistance. Mol Cancer 19(1):57
14. Zuberi M, Mir R, Khan I, Javid J, Guru SA, Bhat M, Sumi MP, Ahmad I, Masroor M, Yadav P et al (2020) The promising signatures of circulating microRNA-145 in epithelial ovarian cancer patients. MicroRNA 9(1):49–57
15. Garwood CS, Steinberg JS (2016) What's new in wound treatment: a critical appraisal. Diabetes Metab Res Rev 32(Suppl 1):268–274
16. Houreld NN (2014) Shedding light on a new treatment for diabetic wound healing: a review on phototherapy. ScientificWorldJournal 2014:398412
17. Ruthenborg RJ, Ban JJ, Wazir A, Takeda N, Kim JW (2014) Regulation of wound healing and fibrosis by hypoxia and hypoxia-inducible factor-1. Mol Cells 37(9):637–643
18. Duscher D, Maan ZN, Whittam AJ, Sorkin M, Hu MS, Walmsley GG, Baker H, Fischer LH, Januszyk M, Wong VW et al (2015) Fibroblast-specific deletion of hypoxia inducible factor-1 critically impairs murine cutaneous neovascularization and wound healing. Plast Reconstr Surg 136(5):1004–1013
19. Tavakkoly-Bazzaz J, Amoli MM, Pravica V, Chandrasecaran R, Boulton AJ, Larijani B, Hutchinson IV (2010) VEGF gene polymorphism association with diabetic neuropathy. Mol Biol Rep 37(7):3625–3630
20. Elfaki I, Mir R, Abu-Duhier FM, Khan R, Sakran M (2019) Phosphatidylinositol 3-kinase Glu545Lys and His1047Tyr mutations are not associated with T2D. Curr Diabet Rev. https://doi.org/10.2174/1573399815666191015142201
21. Lai WH, Ho JC, Chan YC, Ng JH, Au KW, Wong LY, Siu CW, Tse HF (2013) Attenuation of hind-limb ischemia in mice with endothelial-like cells derived from different sources of human stem cells. PLoS One 8(3):e57876
22. Mulyasasmita W, Cai L, Dewi RE, Jha A, Ullmann SD, Luong RH, Huang NF, Heilshorn SC (2014) Avidity-controlled hydrogels for injectable co-delivery of induced pluripotent stem cell-derived endothelial cells and growth factors. J Controlled Release 191:71–81
23. Rufaihah AJ, Huang NF, Jame S, Lee JC, Nguyen HN, Byers B, De A, Okogbaa J, Rollins M, Reijo-Pera R et al (2011) Endothelial cells derived from human iPSCS increase capillary density and improve perfusion in a mouse model of peripheral arterial disease. Arterioscler Thromb Vasc Biol 31(11):e72–e79

24. Dar A, Domev H, Ben-Yosef O, Tzukerman M, Zeevi-Levin N, Novak A, Germanguz I, Amit M, Itskovitz-Eldor J (2012) Multipotent vasculogenic pericytes from human pluripotent stem cells promote recovery of murine ischemic limb. Circulation 125(1):87–99
25. Brouwer M, Zhou H, Nadif Kasri N (2016) Choices for induction of pluripotency: recent developments in human induced pluripotent stem cell reprogramming strategies. Stem Cell Rev Rep 12(1):54–72
26. Seki T, Fukuda K (2015) Methods of induced pluripotent stem cells for clinical application. World J Stem Cells 7(1):116–125
27. Ding DC, Shyu WC, Lin SZ (2011) Mesenchymal stem cells. Cell Transplant 20(1):5–14
28. Huang Y, Li Q, Zhang K, Hu M, Wang Y, Du L, Lin L, Li S, Sorokin L, Melino G et al (2019) Single cell transcriptomic analysis of human mesenchymal stem cells reveals limited heterogeneity. Cell Death Dis 10(5):368
29. Rodriguez-Menocal L, Shareef S, Salgado M, Shabbir A, Van Badiavas E (2015) Role of whole bone marrow, whole bone marrow cultured cells, and mesenchymal stem cells in chronic wound healing. Stem Cell Res Ther 6:24
30. Walter MN, Wright KT, Fuller HR, MacNeil S, Johnson WE (2010) Mesenchymal stem cell-conditioned medium accelerates skin wound healing: an in vitro study of fibroblast and keratinocyte scratch assays. Exp Cell Res 316(7):1271–1281
31. Smith AN, Willis E, Chan VT, Muffley LA, Isik FF, Gibran NS, Hocking AM (2010) Mesenchymal stem cells induce dermal fibroblast responses to injury. Exp Cell Res 316(1):48–54
32. Jeon YK, Jang YH, Yoo DR, Kim SN, Lee SK, Nam MJ (2010) Mesenchymal stem cells' interaction with skin: wound-healing effect on fibroblast cells and skin tissue. Wound Repair Regenerat 18(6):655–661
33. Lee SH, Jin SY, Song JS, Seo KK, Cho KH (2012) Paracrine effects of adipose-derived stem cells on keratinocytes and dermal fibroblasts. Ann Dermatol 24(2):136–143
34. Schlosser S, Dennler C, Schweizer R, Eberli D, Stein JV, Enzmann V, Giovanoli P, Erni D, Plock JA (2012) Paracrine effects of mesenchymal stem cells enhance vascular regeneration in ischemic murine skin. Microvasc Res 83(3):267–275
35. Volarevic V, Arsenijevic N, Lukic ML, Stojkovic M (2011) Concise review: mesenchymal stem cell treatment of the complications of diabetes mellitus. Stem Cells 29(1):5–10
36. Wu Y, Chen L, Scott PG, Tredget EE (2007) Mesenchymal stem cells enhance wound healing through differentiation and angiogenesis. Stem Cells 25(10):2648–2659
37. Sasaki M, Abe R, Fujita Y, Ando S, Inokuma D, Shimizu H (2008) Mesenchymal stem cells are recruited into wounded skin and contribute to wound repair by transdifferentiation into multiple skin cell type. J Immunol 180(4):2581–2587
38. Si YL, Zhao YL, Hao HJ, Fu XB, Han WD (2011) MSCs: biological characteristics, clinical applications and their outstanding concerns. Ageing Res Rev 10(1):93–103
39. Xu YX, Chen L, Hou WK, Lin P, Sun L, Sun Y, Dong QY, Liu JB, Fu YL (2009) Mesenchymal stem cells treated with rat pancreatic extract secrete cytokines that improve the glycometabolism of diabetic rats. Transplant Proc 41(5):1878–1884
40. Horie M, Choi H, Lee RH, Reger RL, Ylostalo J, Muneta T, Sekiya I, Prockop DJ (2012) Intra-articular injection of human mesenchymal stem cells (MSCs) promote rat meniscal regeneration by being activated to express Indian hedgehog that enhances expression of type II collagen. Osteoarthr Cartil 20(10):1197–1207
41. Hocking AM, Gibran NS (2010) Mesenchymal stem cells: paracrine signaling and differentiation during cutaneous wound repair. Exp Cell Res 316(14):2213–2219
42. Chen L, Tredget EE, Wu PY, Wu Y (2008) Paracrine factors of mesenchymal stem cells recruit macrophages and endothelial lineage cells and enhance wound healing. PLoS One 3(4):e1886
43. Zhang QZ, Su WR, Shi SH, Wilder-Smith P, Xiang AP, Wong A, Nguyen AL, Kwon CW, Le AD (2010) Human gingiva-derived mesenchymal stem cells elicit polarization of m2 macrophages and enhance cutaneous wound healing. Stem Cells 28(10):1856–1868

44. Liu L, Yu Y, Hou Y, Chai J, Duan H, Chu W, Zhang H, Hu Q, Du J (2014) Human umbilical cord mesenchymal stem cells transplantation promotes cutaneous wound healing of severe burned rats. PLoS One 9(2):e88348
45. Hajjar AM, Lewis PF, Endeshaw Y, Ndinya-Achola J, Kreiss JK, Overbaugh J (1998) Efficient isolation of human immunodeficiency virus type 1 RNA from cervical swabs. J Clin Microbiol 36(8):2349–2352
46. Couture P, Paradis-Massie J, Oualha N, Thibault G (2009) Adhesion and transcellular migration of neutrophils and B lymphocytes on fibroblasts. Exp Cell Res 315(13):2192–2206
47. Sorrell JM, Caplan AI (2010) Topical delivery of mesenchymal stem cells and their function in wounds. Stem Cell Res Ther 1(4):30
48. Anderson SB, Lin CC, Kuntzler DV, Anseth KS (2011) The performance of human mesenchymal stem cells encapsulated in cell-degradable polymer-peptide hydrogels. Biomaterials 32(14):3564–3574
49. Steck AK, Rewers MJ (2011) Genetics of type 1 diabetes. Clin Chem 57(2):176–185
50. Almutairi FM, Mir R, Abu-Duhier F, Khan R, Harby K, Elfaki I (2019) SLC2A2 gene (glucose transporter 2) variation is associated with an increased risk of developing T2d in an ethnic population of Saudi Arabia. Indian J Public Health Res Dev 10(1):600–605
51. Elfaki I, Mir R, AbuDuhier FM, Babakr AT, Barnawi J (2019) Potential impact of microRNA gene polymorphisms in the pathogenesis of diabetes and atherosclerotic cardiovascular disease. J Pers Med 9(4):E51
52. Elfaki I, Mir R, Almutairi FM, Duhier FMA (2018) Cytochrome P450: polymorphisms and roles in cancer, diabetes and atherosclerosis. Asian Pac J Cancer Prev 19(8):2057–2070
53. Chawla A, Chawla R, Jaggi S (2016) Microvasular and macrovascular complications in diabetes mellitus: distinct or continuum? Indian J Endocrinol Metab 20(4):546–551
54. American Diabetes Association (2017) 10. Microvascular complications and foot care. Diabetes Care 40(Suppl 1):S88–S98
55. Tindong M, Palle JN, Nebongo D, Aminde LN, Mboue-Djieka Y, Mbarga NTF, Dehayem MY, Choukem SP (2018) Prevalence, clinical presentation, and factors associated with diabetic foot ulcer in two regional hospitals in Cameroon. Int J Low Extrem Wounds 17(1):42–47
56. Lopes L, Setia O, Aurshina A, Liu S, Hu H, Isaji T, Liu H, Wang T, Ono S, Guo X et al (2018) Stem cell therapy for diabetic foot ulcers: a review of preclinical and clinical research. Stem Cell Res Ther 9(1):188
57. Cao Y, Gang X, Sun C, Wang G (2017) Mesenchymal stem cells improve healing of diabetic foot ulcer. J Diabetes Res 2017:9328347
58. Wong VW, Sorkin M, Gurtner GC (2013) Enabling stem cell therapies for tissue repair: current and future challenges. Biotechnol Adv 31(5):744–751
59. Hass R, Kasper C, Bohm S, Jacobs R (2011) Different populations and sources of human mesenchymal stem cells (MSC): a comparison of adult and neonatal tissue-derived MSC. Cell Commun Signal 9:12
60. Wan J, Xia L, Liang W, Liu Y, Cai Q (2013) Transplantation of bone marrow-derived mesenchymal stem cells promotes delayed wound healing in diabetic rats. J Diabetes Res 2013:647107
61. Hua J, Gong J, Meng H, Xu B, Yao L, Qian M, He Z, Zou S, Zhou B, Song Z (2013) Comparison of different methods for the isolation of mesenchymal stem cells from umbilical cord matrix: proliferation and multilineage differentiation as compared to mesenchymal stem cells from umbilical cord blood and bone marrow. Cell Biol Int. https://doi.org/10.1002/cbin.10188
62. Dash NR, Dash SN, Routray P, Mohapatra S, Mohapatra PC (2009) Targeting nonhealing ulcers of lower extremity in human through autologous bone marrow-derived mesenchymal stem cells. Rejuvenation Res 12(5):359–366
63. Amin AH, Abd Elmageed ZY, Nair D, Partyka MI, Kadowitz PJ, Belmadani S, Matrougui K (2010) Modified multipotent stromal cells with epidermal growth factor restore vasculogenesis and blood flow in ischemic hind-limb of type II diabetic mice. Lab Investig 90(7):985–996
64. Jin HJ, Bae YK, Kim M, Kwon SJ, Jeon HB, Choi SJ, Kim SW, Yang YS, Oh W, Chang JW (2013) Comparative analysis of human mesenchymal stem cells from bone marrow, adipose tissue, and umbilical cord blood as sources of cell therapy. Int J Mol Sci 14(9):17986–18001

65. Xia N, Xu JM, Zhao N, Zhao QS, Li M, Cheng ZF (2015) Human mesenchymal stem cells improve the neurodegeneration of femoral nerve in a diabetic foot ulceration rats. Neurosci Lett 597:84–89
66. You HJ, Namgoong S, Han SK, Jeong SH, Dhong ES, Kim WK (2015) Wound-healing potential of human umbilical cord blood-derived mesenchymal stromal cells in vitro—a pilot study. Cytotherapy 17(11):1506–1513
67. Li XY, Zheng ZH, Li XY, Guo J, Zhang Y, Li H, Wang YW, Ren J, Wu ZB (2013) Treatment of foot disease in patients with type 2 diabetes mellitus using human umbilical cord blood mesenchymal stem cells: response and correction of immunological anomalies. Curr Pharm Des 19(27):4893–4899
68. Moon KC, Suh HS, Kim KB, Han SK, Young KW, Lee JW, Kim MH (2019) Potential of allogeneic adipose-derived stem cell-hydrogel complex for treating diabetic foot ulcers. Diabetes 68(4):837–846
69. Ahmed EM (2015) Hydrogel: preparation, characterization, and applications: a review. J Adv Res 6(2):105–121
70. O'Loughlin A, Kulkarni M, Creane M, Vaughan EE, Mooney E, Shaw G, Murphy M, Dockery P, Pandit A, O'Brien T (2013) Topical administration of allogeneic mesenchymal stromal cells seeded in a collagen scaffold augments wound healing and increases angiogenesis in the diabetic rabbit ulcer. Diabetes 62(7):2588–2594
71. Badillo AT, Redden RA, Zhang L, Doolin EJ, Liechty KW (2007) Treatment of diabetic wounds with fetal murine mesenchymal stromal cells enhances wound closure. Cell Tissue Res 329(2):301–311
72. Kwon DS, Gao X, Liu YB, Dulchavsky DS, Danyluk AL, Bansal M, Chopp M, McIntosh K, Arbab AS, Dulchavsky SA et al (2008) Treatment with bone marrow-derived stromal cells accelerates wound healing in diabetic rats. Int Wound J 5(3):453–463
73. Falanga V, Iwamoto S, Chartier M, Yufit T, Butmarc J, Kouttab N, Shrayer D, Carson P (2007) Autologous bone marrow-derived cultured mesenchymal stem cells delivered in a fibrin spray accelerate healing in murine and human cutaneous wounds. Tissue Eng 13(6):1299–1312
74. Zonta S, De Martino M, Bedino G, Piotti G, Rampino T, Gregorini M, Frassoni F, Dal Canton A, Dionigi P, Alessiani M (2010) Which is the most suitable and effective route of administration for mesenchymal stem cell-based immunomodulation therapy in experimental kidney transplantation: endovenous or arterial ? Transplant Proc 42(4):1336–1340
75. Ho JH, Tseng TC, Ma WH, Ong WK, Chen YF, Chen MH, Lin MW, Hong CY, Lee OK (2012) Multiple intravenous transplantations of mesenchymal stem cells effectively restore long-term blood glucose homeostasis by hepatic engraftment and beta-cell differentiation in streptozocin-induced diabetic mice. Cell Transplant 21(5):997–1009

Alternative Medicine in the Management of Diabetic Foot Ulcers/Infections

17

M. Ahmed Mesaik, Hyder O. Mirghani, and Fakhralddin Elfakki

17.1 Introduction

Alternative medicine is nowadays a challenge for healthcare providers and its application remains like to "*separate the pearls from the mud*" [1]. The rising rate of diabetes globally, the search by the patients for better holistic medicine, and the doubt of some patients about the efficacy of current modern medicine made the fitness of the above statement more obvious day by day. We have to admit that segregating efficacious complementary alternative medicine (CAM) treatments from fake treatments will remain a challenging task, and the absence of properly planned and piloted efficacy trials for many treatments further complicates the problem [2]. Nonetheless, to achieve a better collaboration with patients, health care providers must consider the patients' wishes and likeliness in using CAM and provide truthful advice about CAM treatments to those patients. As well both the patient and the health care provider must be well aware of the limitations of the currently available treatments in alternative medicine.

M. A. Mesaik (✉)
Department of Medical Microbiology, Faculty of Medicine, University of Tabuk, Tabuk, Kingdom of Saudi Arabia

H. O. Mirghani
Department of Internal Medicine, Faculty of Medicine, University of Tabuk, Tabuk, Kingdom of Saudi Arabia

F. Elfakki
Department of Family & Community Medicine, Faculty of Medicine, University of Tabuk, Tabuk, Kingdom of Saudi Arabia

M. Zubair et al. (eds.), *Diabetic Foot Ulcer*,
https://doi.org/10.1007/978-981-15-7639-3_17

17.2 What Is Alternative Medicine?

In the beginning, we need to define alternative medicine. In a broader term the complementary and alternative medicine (CAM), are functionally defined as treatments and healthcare practices that are not taught widely in medical schools and are not generally available in the US hospitals [3]. Whereas the National Center for Complementary and Alternative medicine (NCCAM) defines CAM as those healthcare and medical practices that are not currently an integral part of conventional medicine [4]. When describing these approaches, people often use "alternative" and "complementary" interchangeably whoever there are little bit differences in their mean as it is considered complementary when a nonmainstream practice is used *together with* conventional medicine, while considered as an alternative when a nonmainstream practice is used *replacing or in place of the* conventional medicine [5].

17.3 The CAM Included

The different branches of CAM include acupuncture, nutritional advice or lifestyle diets, massage therapy, herbal remedies, biofeedback, meditation, and imagery or relaxation techniques. Other treatments included in this definition of CAM were homeopathic treatment, spiritual healing or prayer, hypnosis, and traditional therapies such as Chinese, Ayurvedic, and Native American medicine. However, not all of them are useful in case of diabetes and the diabetic foot ulcer based on the literature available we are here listing the Alternative and Complementary Practices that are currently in use in case of the diabetic foot ulcer:

17.3.1 Massage

A review based on a meta-analysis that included 27 trials on pharmacological, nonpharmacological, and alternative treatments. Cakici and his co-workers reported *reflexology* and Thai *foot* massage to show beneficial results. They reported signs of progress in *diabetic* peripheral neuropathy symptoms linked with *reflexology* and Thai *foot* massage [6]. Another systematic review based on meta-analyses revealed traditional Chinese medicine *foot* bath while combined with Chinese acupoint massage is more effective for the treatment of DPN alone [7]. Other types of massage like the APIYU massage was proven effective for improving *foot* sensitivity and reducing blood glucose *among diabetic patients* [8]. While the addition of compressed air to the message was found to enhance *ulcer* healing which is thought to act by improving the local tissue oxygenation around the *ulcers* [9]. Additionally, the use of Ozone (O_3) therapy and quick application of the O_3 to an ulcerated foot are rising as new modalities for treating DFUs [10].

17.3.2 Ayurveda Medicine

Ayurveda medicine: Ayurveda is a traditional Indian system of medicine that is more than 3000 years old, consisting mostly of a specific diet, oily infusions, medicinal plants, and yoga. It is based on a naturopathic and anthropological belief in association with the Hinduistic religion. This type of medication has been practiced widely in India but so far it has only been insufficiently appreciated by western medicine, especially psychiatry. An exception is Scharfetter from Zürich who wrote a review article on this topic in 1976. Nevertheless, particularly the immunological mechanisms of psychotic and affective disorders can probably be influenced by the application of ayurvedic methods; however, the empirical data source, particularly concerning randomized controlled trials and meta-analyses regarding psychiatric disorder symptoms is limited. Even if Ayurveda is applied in a highly individualized manner, this should be rapidly improved for further evidential assessment. The first positive experiences in the neuropsychiatric field in Germany are already available.

Use of Ayurveda medicine: Bhandari et al. reported a case of Diabetic Foot Ulcers (DFU) in a 70 years of age patient with a repeated history of Ray's Amputation who was managed by an integrated approach Ayurveda and Allopathy medications and procedures. Several local plant materials have been used, after proper washing and cleaning of the ulcer. The plant used in their trials including Nyagrodha *Ficus benghalensis, Ficus glomerata, Ficus religiosa, Thespesia populnea, Ficus lacor.* Besides the use of special oil where Jasmine is the chief ingredient. This is in addition to maintaining the blood sugar level by the proper food, lifestyle, and medications [11].

The study involved 23 patients of diabetic wounds/ulcers who were treated with a local application of *Securinega leucopyrus* leaf paste with *Sesamum indicum* oil, whereas, in Group B, Betadine ointment was applied on the affected parts, once a day for 30 days. In Group A, diabetic wounds treated with Katupila paste got healed within 28 days with minimal scar formation without any complications, compared to Group B, the wound was healed completely only in two patients within 28 days. In both groups, no patients reported any adverse drug reaction during the entire course of treatment as well as in the follow-up period. The study concluded that the drug Katupila Kalka possesses a wound healing effect with very fine scaring [12]. In another study the local application of *S. leucopyrus* paste once every day resulted in restoration and healing within a month with normal pigmentation and a minimal scar. The case also informed for possible antimicrobial activity of the tested materials [13].

17.3.2.1 *Katupila* Leaves

Katupila leaves have has been found to act as an antiseptic and its paste is used in folklore to extract any extraneous materials from body tissues without surgery [14]. The leaves and the bark are rich with a vast number of important phytochemicals such as alkaloids, terpenoids, steroids, flavonoids, saponins, phenol, and glycosides [15]. The plant was used in the management of wound healing in different forms [16]. Previous clinical studies on this plant in oil form and Kalka (dry powder mixed with sesame oil) also showed encouraging results in the management of nonhealing wounds. The study concluded that *Katupila Kalka* leaves possess cleaning, healing, and depigmentation properties and has a wound healing property.

Securinega leucopyrus as a known herb for the treatment of diabetic foot care was formulated in another study in the name of *Thumari gel* for management non-healing ulcers. In this case, the herb *S. leucopyrus* in the form of a gel applied to the wound and was found very effective in the healing of multiple superficial ulcers [17]. Other cases as well reported its healing potential in a mixer form with *Sesamum indicum* oil where ulcers fully healed within 4 weeks with minor pigmentation [18, 19]. The authors stated that the healing effect could be related to the increase in fibroblast activity, neovascularization, and collagen depositions.

17.3.2.2 Curcumin

Studies evidenced the promotional effect of the natural polyphenol compound curcumin on neovascularization in wound healing of diabetes. Curcumin is known to target multiple signaling molecules. You et al. demonstrated the curative effects of curcumin on ischemic hindlimbs in diabetic mice as it promotes the function of endothelial progenitor cells (EPCs) in the ex-vivo assay. The curcumin application improved the blood reperfusion and increases the capillary density in ischemic hindlimbs. The in vitro studies prove the effect of curcumin on angiogenesis, migration, and proliferation abilities of EPCs. They proposed that curcumin could exert its effect via modulating the functions of EPCs and up-regulation in the VEGF-A and Ang-1 activity [20]. A case report of Brazilian type 2 diabetes mellitus patient, treated for 30 days with photodynamic therapy along with curcumin and blue light-emitting diodes (LEDs), where accelerated wound and complete ulcer healing was noted [21]. Another study conducted to evaluate the efficacy of curcumin nutritional supplements in animal studies. Authors noted the curcumin to exert the most remarkable healing activity beside the L-Arginine, or vitamin E supplements [22].

17.3.2.3 *Commiphora molmol* (Myrrh)

"Jinchuang ointment" is a traditional Chinese herbal medicine complex for the treatment of incised wounds. For more than 10 years, it has been used at China Medical University Hospital (Taichung, Taiwan) for the treatment of diabetic foot Infections and decubitus ulcers. Three different cases are presented in this study. "Jinchuang" ointment is a mixture of natural product complexes from nine different components, the ingredients include myrrh beside dragon's blood, catechu, frankincense, and other different natural components. In vitro cell-based assay was used to test for the biological activities of the ointment the two assays were wound healing and tube formation assay results show that this herbal mixture holds strong activities including stimulation of angiogenesis, cell proliferation, and cell migration, which provides a scientific base for its clinically observed therapeutic effects on nonhealing diabetic wounds [23].

A herbal mixture containing myrrah was reported to modify gene expression markers in the wound in a rat model for type 1 Diabetes. The equal amounts of *Aloe vera*, Henna, *Adiantum capillus-Veneris*, and Myrrha, were mixed with Vaseline and applied as an ointment on wound-induced diabetic and nondiabetic rats. RNA was extracted from the healing region of the wound at different interval days [7, 14, 21] for cDNA extraction. Changes in Tgfb1, Mmp3, Mmp9, Il6, and Tnf α genes expression was monitored by the real-time PCR. The expression of the Mmp3, the Tnf α, and the Tgfb1 genes from wound tissue was significantly different ($p < 0.05$) between the two treated groups [24].

The use of CAM products in the topical treatment of diabetic foot disorders is very common among central Asian Muslim countries patients. Honey is regarded as the most preferable topical preparation alone or in combination with other natural remedies including black seeds and myrrh. The most commonly used CAM product for foot ulcers in Saudi Arabia was Honey (56.6%) followed by *Commiphora molmol* (Myrrh) in (37.4%) [25]. This point will be elaborated later in this chapter.

17.4 Acupuncture and Diabetic Foot, Reporting the Benefits

There is growing evidence that acupuncture is an appealing practice to the general practitioners in the clinical field worldwide especially in the last 25 years [26]. This is more clear in the result of a clinical trial evaluating the application of pestle needle on diabetic foot which reports a significant improvement of the sensory nerve function; besides, it reflects an obvious improvement of the patient-quality of life (QOL) especially patients with high-risk of diabetic foot [27].

Further trials using sham procedures confirms the effectiveness of acupuncture on relieving numbness, spontaneous pain, and alteration in temperature perception in the lower extremities, as well as rigidity in the upper extremities [28]. On the other hand, there is remarkable scientific evidence supporting the quality of reports from acupuncture trials that involve patients with diabetic peripheral neuropathy (DPN); factually, most of these clinical trials have shown noticeable recovery of the clinical symptoms of DPN using acupuncture. Similarly, a systematic review of clinical trials on the effect of electropuncture and diabetic painful neuropathy (DPN) has proven a positive effect and improvement of the DPN and Dpn, as well [29–33].

17.4.1 Acupoint and Appropriate Site for Needle Insertion

A systematic review about the appropriate selection of acupoint for acupuncture revealed that there is common and frequently used foot sites for conducting acupuncture in the treatment of diabetic gastroparesis (DGP); and hence, the compatibility laws for acupoint selection were mainly located in the upper-lower selection, three selection, three regions selection, local selection, and anterior-posterior selection. Further additional study supporting the effectiveness of using both Governor vessel acupoint and local meridian acupoint simultaneously for the greater effect of acupuncture [34, 35].

17.4.2 Herbal Medicine, Placental Extract, and Low Laser Therapy Use on Acupoint

A randomized clinical trial assessing the effect of Chinese Herbal Medicine (CHM) and Tangzhuang Ointment (TYO) for chronic diabetic foot ulcer (DFU) discloses a potential safety and efficacy as well as double healing rate in comparison to the conventional therapy [27, 36, 37]. Unique trials revealed a significant acceleration and regulation of the wound healing process after the application of hominis placenta (HP) and placental extract at the acupuncture points in the middle region of the upper and lower wounds [38–40]. Although it is not yet clinically approved, results from a systematic review revealed that low-level laser therapy has a significant beneficial effect on the treatment of diabetic foot ulcers [41].

17.4.3 The Adverse Effect of Using Acupuncture

Despite a considerable number of published reports on the adverse effect related to acupuncturing techniques in the Chinese literature; however, according to a case study report, most of these unsuccessful clinical experiences are related to lack of cleanliness and sterility before the application of acupuncture on diabetic foot [42, 43].

17.5 Use of Maggot Debridement Therapy

Maggot debridement therapy (MDT) had a significantly positive effect on wound healing when compared to conventional therapies. It does not only shorten the healing period but also enhanced the healing level of chronic ulcers. Therefore, it could be used as an alternative in the treatment of chronic ulcers. It is assumed that these maggots fighting wound infection as the larvae ingest resident bacteria and kill them [44, 45]. Other proposed mechanisms include moistening of the wound by increased exudate, the production stimulated by the larvae ingesting necrotic tissues, or dilution of the wound discharge by the maggots' secretions [46]. currently, doctors consider the use of MDT to be the last option when orthodox treatments failed [47].

17.6 Regenerative Therapy, and the Adipose-Derived Stem Cells (ADSCs)

One therapeutic strategy that rises recently as promising regenerative therapy of chronic diabetic wounds utilizes adipose-derived stem cells (ADSCs). ADSCs can differentiate into multiple cell lineages and are considered an alternative to bone marrow-derived mesenchymal stem cells. They can be easily drawn from the adipose tissue and are expandable in a cell culture system. The studies displayed ADSCs to enhance diabetic wound healing through increasing epithelialization and granulation tissue formation, anti-inflammatory and anti-apoptotic effects, and release of several cytokines needed for the regeneration. Some clinical trials showed that ADSCs treatment in patients with diabetic ulcers caused enhanced ulcer evolution, lower pain scores, and improved claudication walking distances with no reported complications. ADSCs have a promising potential in the regenerative therapy of chronic diabetic wounds. Further studies are required to confirm their efficacy and they are in vivo long-term safety [48]. Furthermore, Dong et al. examined an injectable poly(ethylene glycol) (PEG)-gelatin-based hydrogel system for creating a functional stem cell niche for the transfer of adipose-derived stem cells (ASCs) into diabetic wounds and for effective delivery and engraftment of the stem cells. Significant in vivo improvement in stem cell retention was reached. The decrease in inflammatory cell infiltration enhances neovascularization and remarkably accelerates wound closure in diabetic mice were observed, suggesting a promising potential for the treatment of chronic diabetic wounds [49].

17.7 Honey and Diabetic Septic Foot

Diabetic septic foot remained to be a serious problem despite the advances in the field of antimicrobial therapy. Nearly a quarter of patients with diabetes mellitus had a lifetime risk of developing foot complications. The diabetic septic foot may constitute up to 80% of lower limb amputations. Although the majority of diabetic ulcers involve the toes. However, lower limb amputation is unavoidable if the proper treatment is not provided in due time. Wound healing is complex, so treating wound infections is intensive, and costly. Diabetic foot ulcers precede amputation in 85% limiting physical and social activity and leading to poor quality of life. Due to the emerging of antibiotic-resistant pathogens, attention has been directed to natural products for clinical practice. For these reasons, many forms of therapies have been adopted including topical honey [25, 50].

Honey as a remedy of wound care backdated to ancient times. There are many types of honey [51]. The product may be used alone or in combination with other forms of complementary alternative medicine including herbs and other natural products. It is interesting to note that patients with diabetes may use honey for the treatment of diabetes foot with or without clinical consultation because they thought that it is not important to discuss with the attending physicians [52]. Diabetic foot ulcers are difficult to treat due to poor wound healing of patients with diabetes, chronic inflammation, and colonization of resistant organisms. Honey (ordinary or Manuka) exhibits antibacterial activity mainly due to its osmotic effects leading to bacterial dehydration, also, the acidic nature of honey inhibits bacteria, moreover, methylglyoxal (MGO, one of the phytochemical factors) and other ingredients with antibacterial activity had been identified within honey. The mechanism of the antibacterial of honey is not fully understood, but interruption of cell division, cell lysis, and abnormal protein regulation were observed [50]. The action of Manuka honey on bacteria is high only after 24 h because MGO is low in fresh honey, the concentration of this important ingredient increases when stored at 37 °C [53]. Antioxidants and other ingredients found in Honey act synergistically to reduce both acute and chronic inflammation, also honey activates proinflammatory cytokines and the anti-inflammatory (TNF-α and IL-1β cytokine IL-6, respectively). Importantly, the heat treatment of honey negatively affects the anti-inflammatory actions of honey. Thus supermarket honey is not as effective as a treatment remedy for ulcers [54–56]. When comparing Manuka honey with silver dressing, there is no strong evidence of the superiority of one over the other compound in dressing [50]. A case report showed that honey was effective for an ulcer with tendon exposure [57]. Mohamed et al. [58] reported the treatment of diabetic foot ulcers with commercial honey, offloading, and debridement. A case series (eight diabetic feet ulcers, followed for 3 months) showed that Royal may be an effective dressing measure [59]. A prospective pilot study [60] examined patients with Wagner grade 1–111, and gangrenous ulcers (96 patents, followed for 6 months). The investigators used an ointment containing Royal jelly and panthenol, surgical treatment and saline dressings were applied, but no other specific treatment was given. The research concludes the safety of their ointment and they recommended double-blind randomized controlled trials. A prospective study from Makkah, Saudi Arabia [61] used local honey as a thick layer for dressing the complicated diabetic ulcers (172 patients, followed for 15 months). The authors stated that honey significantly reduced the rate of amputation and improve wound healing. A randomized controlled trial [62] published in the year 2008 (Newcastle Ottawa quality assessment = 7) showed that honey dressing is as effective as povidone-iodine, the study assessed Wagner grade-II ulcers foot ulcers among patients with type 2 diabetes mellitus and followed till healing.

A double-blind placebo-controlled clinical trial [63] included 25 patients with 64 diabetic foot ulcers and followed for 3 months. Offloading, infection control, debridement, and vascular surgery were applied when indicated. The authors found no superiority of topical Royal Jelly over placebo. A randomized controlled trial with a reasonable number (348) and followed for a maximum of 120 days, assessed Beri-honey-impregnated dressing compared to normal saline dressing. The authors showed that honey is more effective in diabetic ulcer healing [64]. A pilot open-labeled randomized controlled trial (31 patients followed for 12 weeks) observed the superiority of Nanocrystalline silver over Manuka honey in terms of ulcer size reduction rate [65]. Eddy et al. [66] reviewed the literature in the year 2008 and stated that honey as a topical therapy for DFUs is cost-effective. However, risks and benefits need to be weighed. A systematic review of five randomized trials and observational studies [67] conducted in the year 2016 showed that honey is safer, however, efficacy cannot be concluded due to quality issues. Zhang et al. [68] conducted a network analysis including 21 randomized control trial and 2159 patients and compared nine dressing including honey, the authors concluded that amniotic membrane and hydrogel dressings are preferred for healing diabetic foot ulcers with no differences between the others including honey.

Because there are many types of honey (e.g., Manuka, Sidr honey, and *Nigella sativa* honey) with various subtypes [51]. Furthermore, honey activity may be dependent on the weather conditions where the bees were raised, grazing grounds, and the natural structure of the blossom nectar. Also, the medical and surgical treatment applied together with topical honed may differ. Thus it is difficult to conclude its effect. The reviewed RCTs showed conflicting results (some showed no superiority over placebo, others showed topical honey is superior to saline dressing), similar to povidone-iodine and inferior to Nanocrystalline and amniotic membrane dressing.

References

1. Jonas WB (1998) Alternative medicine: learning from the past, examining the present, advancing to the future. JAMA 280:1616–1618. https://doi.org/10.1001/jama.280.18.1616
2. Angell M, Kassirer JP (1998) Alternative medicine: the risks of untested and unregulated remedies. N Engl J Med 339:839–841. https://doi.org/10.1056/NEJM199809173391210
3. Eisenberg DM, Kessler RC, Foster C, Norlock FE, Calkins DR, Delbanco TL (1993) Unconventional medicine in the United States: prevalence, costs, and patterns of use. N Engl J Med 328:246–252. https://doi.org/10.1056/NEJM199301283280406
4. National Center for Complementary and Alternative Medicine. Major domains of complementary and alternative medicine [article online]. http://www.nccam.nih.gov/fcp/classify. Accessed 12 Sept 2001
5. From National Center for Complementary and Integrative Health (NCCIH) website. https://nccih.nih.gov/health/integrative-health. Accessed 4 Jan 2020
6. Çakici N, Fakkel TM, van Neck JW, Verhagen AP, Coert JH (2016) Systematic review of treatments for diabetic peripheral neuropathy. Diabet Med 33(11):1466–1476. https://doi.org/10.1111/dme.13083
7. Fu Q, Yang H, Zhang L, Liu Y, Li X, Dai M, Yang Y, Yang S, Xie Y, Liu Y, Fu L, Liu Z, Zhang Q (2019) Traditional Chinese medicine foot bath combined with acupoint massage for the treatment of diabetic peripheral neuropathy: a systematic review and meta-analysis of 31 RCTs. Diabetes Metab Res Rev 36:e3218. https://doi.org/10.1002/dmrr.3218
8. Hasneli Y, Amir Y (2019) Identification and analysis of foot sensitivity and blood glucose levels post Apiyu massage. Enferm Clin 29(Suppl 1):19–22. https://doi.org/10.1016/j.enfcli.2018.11.009
9. Mars M, Desai Y, Gregory MA (2008) Compressed air massage hastens healing of the diabetic foot. Diabetes Technol Ther 10(1):39–45. https://doi.org/10.1089/dia.2007.0240
10. Kushmakov R, Gandhi J, Seyam O, Jiang W, Joshi G, Smith NL, Khan SA (2018) Ozone therapy for diabetic foot. Med Gas Res 8(3):111–115. https://doi.org/10.4103/2045-9912.241076
11. Bhandari M, Rao PN, Gopikrishna BJ, Gudasi D (2019) An integrated approach for the management of diabetic foot ulcer: a case report. Complement Integr Med 16(3) pii: /j/jcim.2019.16.issue-3/jcim-2018-0126/jcim-2018-0126.xml. https://doi.org/10.1515/jcim-2018-0126
12. Ajmeer AS, Dudhamal TS, Gupta SK (2015) Management of Madhumehajanya Vrana (diabetic wound) with Katupila (Securinega leucopyrus [Willd] Muell.) Kalka. Ayu 36(3):351–355. https://doi.org/10.4103/0974-8520.182744
13. Ajmeer AS, Dudhamal TS, Gupta SK, Mahanta V (2014) Katupila (Securinega leucopyrus) as a potential option for diabetic wound management. J Ayurveda Integr Med 5(1):60–63. https://doi.org/10.4103/0975-9476.128872
14. Bakshu LM, Jeevan Ram A, Venkata Raju R (2001) Antimicrobial activity of Securinega leucopyrus. Fitoterapia 72:930–933. https://doi.org/10.1016/s0367-326x(01)00341-0
15. Bulugahapitiya VP, Munasinghe AB, Hettihewa M (2014) Investigation of chemical composition of Flueggea leucopyrus (willd.). World J Pharm Pharmaceut Sci 3(8):79–94
16. Ghodela NK, Kumar V, Dudhamal TS, Naria MK (2016) A wonderful medicinal plant: Securinega leucopyrus (Willd) Muell - a brief review. Int J Sci Innov Today 5(6):472–484

17. Ghodela NK, Dudhamal TS (2017) Clinical efficacy of *Thumari* gel (*Securinega leucopyrus* [Willd.] Muell) in the management of superficial non-healing leg ulcers - a rare case report. Int J Ayush Case Rep 1(1) http://ijacare.in/index.php/ijacare/article/view/3/9
18. Dudhamal TS (2016) Wound healing effect of Humari (Securinega leucopyrus) and supportive Ayurveda therapy in Beurger's ulcer - a case report. Ann Ayurvedic Med 5(1–2):37–43. https://www.aamjournal.in/fulltext/70-1447132744.pdf?1583439012
19. Shah B, Ghodela NK, Dudhamal TS (2017) Healing potency of fresh Katupila Kalka (Securinegaleucopyrus) in Dusta Vrana (nonhealing wound) - a single case report. Ayurlog 5:134–138
20. You J, Sun J, Ma T, Yang Z, Wang X, Zhang Z, Li J, Wang L, Ii M, Yang J, Shen Z (2017) Curcumin induces therapeutic angiogenesis in a diabetic mouse hindlimb ischemia model via modulating the function of endothelial progenitor cells. Stem Cell Res Ther 8(1):182. https://doi.org/10.1186/s13287-017-0636-9
21. Rosa LP, da Silva FC, Vieira RL, Tanajura BR, da Silva Gusmão AG, de Oliveira JM, Dos Santos NAC, Bagnato VS (2017) Application of photodynamic therapy, laser therapy, and a cellulose membrane for calcaneal pressure ulcer treatment in a diabetic patient: a case report. Photodiagn Photodyn Ther 19:235–238. https://doi.org/10.1016/j.pdpdt.2017.06.011
22. Maier HM, Ilich JZ, Kim JS, Spicer MT (2013) Nutrition supplementation for diabetic wound healing: a systematic review of current literature. Skinmed 11(4):217–224; quiz 224–225. https://www.ncbi.nlm.nih.gov/pubmed/24053007
23. Ho TJ, Jiang SJ, Lin GH, Li TS, Yiin LM, Yang JS, Hsieh MC, Wu CC, Lin JG, Chen HP (2014) The in vitro and in vivo wound healing properties of the Chinese herbal medicine "Jinchuang ointment". J Intercult Ethnopharmacol 3(2):56–62. https://doi.org/10.5455/jice.20140130015014
24. Galehdari H, Negahdari S, Kesmati M, Rezaie A, Shariati G (2016) Effect of the herbal mixture composed of Aloe Vera, Henna, Adiantum capillus-veneris, and Myrrha on wound healing in streptozotocin-induced diabetic rats. BMC Complement Altern Med 16:386. https://doi.org/10.1186/s12906-016-1359-7
25. Bakhotmah BA, Alzahrani HA (2010) Self-reported use of complementary and alternative medicine (CAM) products in topical treatment of diabetic foot disorders by diabetic patients in Jeddah, Western Saudi Arabia. BMC Res Notes. 3:254. https://doi.org/10.1186/1756-0500-3-254
26. Ma Y, Dong M, Zhou K, Mita C, Liu J, Wayne PM (2016) Publication trends in acupuncture research: a 20-year bibliometric analysis based on PubMed. PLoS One 11(12). https://doi.org/10.1371/journal.pone.0168123. eCollection 2016
27. Wang Y, Cao HJ, Wang LQ, Lu CL, Yan YQ, Lu H, Liu JP (2019) The effects of Chinese herbal medicines for treating diabetic foot ulcers: a systematic review of 49 randomized controlled trials. Complement Ther Med 44:32–43. https://doi.org/10.1016/j.ctim.2019.03.007
28. Tong Y, Guo H, Han B (2010) Fifteen-day acupuncture treatment relieves diabetic peripheral neuropathy. J Acupunct Meridian Stud 3(2):95–103. https://doi.org/10.1016/S2005-2901(10)60018-0
29. Bailey A, Wingard D, Allison M, Summers P, Calac D (2017) Acupuncture treatment of diabetic peripheral neuropathy in an American Indian community. J Acupunct Meridian Stud 10(2):90–95. https://doi.org/10.1016/j.jams.2016.10.004
30. Xiong W, Feng X, Liu J, Chen W (2016) Electroacupuncture for treatment of diabetic peripheral neuropathy: a systematic review of randomized controlled trials. J Tradit Chin Med Sci 3(1):9–21. https://doi.org/10.1016/j.jtcms.2016.06.002
31. Bao T, Zhang R, Badros A, Lao L (2011) Acupuncture treatment for bortezomib-induced peripheral neuropathy: a case report. Pain Res Treat 2011:920807. https://doi.org/10.1155/2011/920807
32. Garrow AP, Xing M, Vere J, Verrall B, Wang L, Jude EB (2014) Role of acupuncture in the management of diabetic painful neuropathy (DPN): a pilot RCT. Acupunct Med 32(3):242–249. https://doi.org/10.1136/acupmed-2013-010495
33. Bo C, Xue Z, Yi G, Zelin C, Yang B, Zixu W, Yajun W (2012) Assessing the quality of reports about randomized controlled trials of acupuncture treatment on diabetic peripheral neuropathy. PLoS One 7(7):e38461. https://doi.org/10.1371/journal.pone.0038461

34. Lu Z, Luo Z, Jia A, Yu L, Muhammad I, Zeng W, Song Y (2018) Associations of the ABCA1 gene polymorphisms with plasma lipid levels: a meta-analysis. Medicine 97(50):e13521. https://doi.org/10.1097/MD.0000000000013521
35. He GH, Ruan JW, Zeng YS, Zhou X, Ding Y, Zhou GH (2015) Improvement in acupoint selection for acupuncture of nerves surrounding the injury site: electro-acupuncture with Governor vessel with local meridian acupoints. Neural Regen Res 10(1):128. https://doi.org/10.4103/1673-5374.150720
36. Liao HH, Yeh CC, Lin CC, Chen BC, Yeh MH, Chang KM, Yen HR (2015) Prescription patterns of Chinese herbal products for patients with fractures in Taiwan: a nationwide population-based study. J Ethnopharmacol 173:11–19. https://doi.org/10.1016/j.jep.2015.07.014
37. Li S, Zhao J, Liu J, Xiang F, Lu D, Liu B, Yu R (2011) Prospective randomized controlled study of a Chinese herbal medicine compound Tangzhuang ointment for chronic diabetic foot ulcers: a preliminary report. J Ethnopharmacol 133(2):543–550. https://doi.org/10.1016/j.jep.2010.10.040
38. Park JY, Lee J, Jeong M, Min S, Kim SY, Lee H, Park HJ (2014) Effect of Hominis placenta on cutaneous wound healing in normal and diabetic mice. Nutr Res Pract 8(4):404–409. https://doi.org/10.4162/nrp.2014.8.4.404
39. Cho TH, Park KM (2016) Use of acupuncture point injection with placental extract for treatment of complex regional pain syndrome. J Pain Relief 5:246–249. https://doi.org/10.4172/2167-0846.1000246
40. Mayo E (2012) Acupuncture and wound healing. Am J Tradit Chin Vet Med 7(1):45–51
41. Beckmann KH, Meyer-Hamme G, Schröder S (2014) Low level laser therapy for the treatment of diabetic foot ulcers: a critical survey. Evid Based Complement Alternat Med 626127:1. https://doi.org/10.1155/2014/626127
42. Saw A, Kwan MK, Sengupta S (2004) Necrotising fasciitis: a life-threatening complication of acupuncture in a patient with diabetes mellitus. Singap Med J 45(4):180–182. https://www.ncbi.nlm.nih.gov/pubmed/15094988
43. Zhang J, Shang H, Gao X, Ernst E (2010) Acupuncture-related adverse events: a systematic review of the Chinese literature. Bull World Health Organ 88:915–921. https://doi.org/10.2471/BLT.10.076737
44. Dumville JC, Worthy G, Bland JM, Cullum N, Dowson C, Iglesias C et al (2009) Larvaltherapy for leg ulcers (VenUS II): randomised controlled trial. BMJ 338:b773. https://doi.org/10.1136/bmj.b773
45. Nigam Y, Bexfield A, Thomas S, Ratcliffe NA (2006) Maggot therapy: the science and implication for CAM part II—maggots combat infection. Evid Based Complement Alternat Med 3:303–308. https://doi.org/10.1093/ecam/nel022
46. Mumcuoglu KY, Miller J, Mumcuoglu M, Friger M, Tarshis M (2001) Destruction of bacteria in the digestive tract of the maggot of Luciliasericata (Diptera: Calli-phoridae). J Med Entomol 38:161–166. https://doi.org/10.1603/0022-2585-38.2.161
47. Sun X, Jiang K, Chen J, Wu L, Lu H, Wanga A, Wang J (2014) A systematic review of maggot debridement therapy for chronically infected wounds and ulcers. Int J Infect Dis 25:32–37. https://doi.org/10.1016/j.ijid.2014.03.1397
48. Gadelkarim M, Abushouk AI, Ghanem E, Hamaad AM, Saad AM, Abdel-Daim MM (2018) Adipose-derived stem cells: effectiveness and advances in delivery in diabetic wound healing. Biomed Pharmacother 107:625–633. https://doi.org/10.1016/j.biopha.2018.08.013
49. Dong Y, Rodrigues M, Kwon SH, Li X, Sigen A, Brett EA, Elvassore N, Wang W, Gurtner GC (2018) Acceleration of diabetic wound regeneration using an in situ-formed stem-cell-based skin substitute. Adv Healthc Mater 7(17):e1800432. https://doi.org/10.1002/adhm.201800432. Epub 2018 Jul 13
50. Tsang KK, Kwong EW, Woo KY, To TS, Chung JW, Wong TK (2015) The anti-inflammatory and antibacterial action of nanocrystalline silver and Manuka honey on the molecular alternation of diabetic foot ulcer: a comprehensive literature review. Evid Based Complement Alternat Med 2015:218283. https://doi.org/10.1155/2015/218283
51. Almasaudi SB, Al-Nahari AAM, Abd El-Ghany ESM, Barbour E, Al Muhayawi SM, Al-Jaouni S (2017) Antimicrobial effect of different types of honey on Staphylococcus aureus. Saudi J Biol Sci 24(6):1255–1261. https://doi.org/10.1016/j.sjbs.2016.08.007

52. Alam F, Islam MA, Gan SH, Khalil IM (2014) Honey: a potential therapeutic agent for managing diabetic wounds. Evid Based Complement Alternat Med 2014:1–16. https://doi.org/10.1155/2014/169130
53. Adams CJ, Manley-Harris M, Molan PC (2009) The origin of methylglyoxal in New Zealand manuka (Leptospermum scoparium) honey. Carbohydr Res 344(8):1050–1053. https://doi.org/10.1016/j.carres.2009.03.020
54. Tonks AJ, Dudley E, Porter NG et al (2007) A 5.8-kDa component of Manuka honey stimulates immune cells via TLR4. J Leukoc Biol 82(5):1147–1155. https://doi.org/10.1189/jlb.1106683
55. Henriques A, Jackson S, Cooper R, Burton N (2006) Free radical production and quenching in honeys with wound healing potential. J Antimicrob Chemother 58(4):773–777. https://doi.org/10.1093/jac/dkl336
56. Tonks AJ, Cooper RA, Jones KP, Blair S, Parton J, Tonks A (2003) Honey stimulates inflammatory cytokine production from monocytes. Cytokine 21(5):242–247. https://doi.org/10.1016/s1043-4666(03)00092-9
57. Teobaldi I, Stoico V, Perrone F, Bruti M, Bonora E, Mantovani A (2018) Honey dressing on a leg ulcer with tendon exposure in a patient with type 2 diabetes. Endocrinol Diabetes Metab Case Rep 2018:EDM180117. https://doi.org/10.1530/EDM-18-0117
58. Mohamed H, El Lenjawi B, Abu Salma M, Abdi S (2014) Honey based therapy for the management of a recalcitrant diabetic foot ulcer. J Tissue Viability 23(1):29–33. https://doi.org/10.1016/j.jtv.2013.06.001
59. Siavash M, Shokri S, Haghighi S, Mohammadi M, Shahtalebi MA, Farajzadehgan Z (2011) The efficacy of topical Royal Jelly on diabetic foot ulcers healing: a case series. J Res Med Sci 16(7):904–909. https://www.ncbi.nlm.nih.gov/pmc/articles/PMC3263103
60. Abdelatif M, Yakoot M, Etmaan M (2008) Safety and efficacy of a new honey ointment on diabetic foot ulcers: a prospective pilot study. J Wound Care 17(3):108–110. https://doi.org/10.12968/jowc.2008.17.3.28667
61. Surahio AR, Khan AA, Farooq M, Fatima I (2014) Role of honey in wound dressing in diabetic foot ulcer. J Ayub Med Coll Abbottabad 26(3):304–306. http://jamc.ayubmed.edu.pk/index.php/jamc/article/view/1492/519
62. Shukrimi A, Sulaiman AR, Hlim AY, Azril A (2008) A comparative study between honey and Povidone iodine as dressing solution for Wagner type II diabetic foot ulcers. Med J Malaysia 63(1):44–46. https://www.ncbi.nlm.nih.gov/pubmed/18935732
63. Siavash M, Shokri S, Haghighi S, Shahtalebi MA, Farajzadehgan Z (2015) The efficacy of topical royal jelly on healing of diabetic foot ulcers: a double-blind placebo-controlled clinical trial. Int Wound J 12(2):137–142. https://doi.org/10.1111/iwj.12063
64. Imran M, Hussain MB, Baig M (2015) A randomized, controlled clinical trial of honey-impregnated dressing for treating diabetic foot ulcer. J Coll Physicians Surg Pak 25(10):721–725. https://doi.org/10.2015/JCPSP.721725
65. Tsang KK, Kwong EW, To TS, Chung JW, Wong TK (2017) A pilot randomized, controlled study of nanocrystalline silver, Manuka honey, and conventional dressing in healing diabetic foot ulcer. Evid Based Complement Alternat Med 2017:5294890. https://doi.org/10.1155/2017/5294890
66. Eddy JJ, Gideonsen MD, Mack GP (2008) Practical considerations of using topical honey for neuropathic diabetic foot ulcers: a review. WMJ 107(4):187–190. https://www.ncbi.nlm.nih.gov/pubmed/15939005
67. Kateel R, Adhikari P, Augustine AJ, Ullal S (2016) Topical honey for the treatment of diabetic foot ulcer: a systematic review. Complement Ther Clin Pract 24:130–133. https://doi.org/10.1016/j.ctcp.2016.06.003
68. Zhang X, Sun D, Jiang GC (2019) Comparative efficacy of nine different dressings in healing diabetic foot ulcer: a Bayesian network analysis. J Diabetes 11(6):418–426. https://doi.org/10.1111/1753-0407.12871

Modern Phytomedicine in Treating Diabetic Foot Ulcer: Progress and Opportunities

18

Mohamed Ali Seyed and Siddiqua Ayesha

18.1 Introduction

Diabetes mellitus is a severe chronic metabolic disorder observed with hyperglycemic conditions [1], substantially related to morbidity and mortality worldwide and affects health care spending of various countries [2, 3]. There are two commonly categorized types of DM, which are Type 1 (T1DM) (diminished production of insulin) and Type 2 (T2DM) (impaired response to insulin and β-cell dysfunction). Both lead to conditions like hyperglycemia, excessive urine production, compensatory thirst, increased fluid intake, blurred vision, unexplained weight loss, lethargy, and changes in energy metabolism. T2DM very well characterized by increased blood glucose and impaired insulin secretion and its action [3, 4] and constitutes about 90% of the people with diabetes. Physiologically, a drop in the blood glucose level results in decreases in the release of insulin and an increase in glucagon. Previous studies have identified three significant defects associated with the onset of T2DM like increased hepatic glucose production, diminished insulin secretion, and impaired insulin action [5, 6].

18.2 Epidemiology of T2DM

The incidence of diabetes is rapidly increasing worldwide at an alarming rate [7] and its occurrence was increased gradually since the year 1995 from 4% to 5.4% or more by the year 2025 [8] and by 2040 it is predicted to surge over 642 million. The World Health Organization (WHO) continuously cautioned that it would affect

M. A. Seyed (✉)
Department of Clinical Biochemistry, Faculty of Medicine, University of Tabuk, Tabuk, Kingdom of Saudi Arabia

S. Ayesha
School of Public Health SRM University, Chennai, Tamil Nadu, India

M. Zubair et al. (eds.), *Diabetic Foot Ulcer*,
https://doi.org/10.1007/978-981-15-7639-3_18

mostly the developing countries. The organization also estimates that the disorder affects nearly 51–72 million people, which is approximately 42% prevalence increase in the developed nations, however, in the developing countries it goes from 84 to 228 million (170% increase) [8–10]. The International Diabetes Federation (IDF) also estimates the total number of T2DM diabetic subjects to be around 40.9 million in developing countries like China, India, Malaysia, and Saudi Arabia this is further set to rise to 69.9 million by the year 2025 [11, 12]. The vast majority of affected patients in the developing countries are between the age of 45–64 years, while it is >65 years for developed countries [10].

For the past few decades, the diabetes status paradigm from being described as a mild disorder of the aged people to affect now young and middle-aged population of both genders to morbidity and mortality among them. Because of this alarming prevalence of this disorder, it is naturally gaining much in almost all six human-occupied continents of the world [13]. The prevalence of T2DM not only influences the quality of life but also affects vital organs such as the brain, heart, and kidney. Such a problem is seen even more frequently when T2DM is accompanied by hypertension and dyslipidemia and both are known to influence small artery structure and function [14, 15]. In line with this, T2DM patients' small arteries have also shown an enlarged media thickness to lumen diameter ratio compared with normal subjects [16].

18.3 Screening and Diagnosis of T2DM

The obese condition and family history are the two most prominent established risk factors for T2DM, in which the family history predisposes individuals to develop T2DM [17]. Besides the above, unhealthy eating habits, sedentary lifestyle and old age are other risk factors involve in the development of T2DM. Besides the above, high blood pressure elevated cholesterol level, and peripheral insulin resistance are also other factors which caused either by receptor defect or by a post-receptor defect with an insulin-secreting defect [18].

18.3.1 Endothelial Dysfunction Induced by T2DM

Diabetic patients are prone to impair endothelial function, which is an early sign of pro-atherogenic vascular abnormality [19]. Impaired endothelial function is one of the well characterized by a change in endothelium toward reduced vasodilatation and a pro-inflammatory state, which is very much associated with cardiovascular diseases including hypertension, coronary artery, chronic heart failure, peripheral artery disease, diabetes, and chronic renal failure [20]. Various mechanisms involved in the endothelial dysfunction which include reduced vasodilatation, reduced NO generation, oxidative excess, and reduced production of hyperpolarizing factor [21]. Decreased insulin sensitivity leads to the induction of two major pathways emerging from the insulin receptors. The first pathway is phosphoinositide 3-kinase, phosphoinositide-dependent kinase-1, and Akt/protein kinase B leading to marked depression of eNOS. The second pathway is nitrogen activated protein kinase leading to mitogenic effects [22, 23].

Besides the above, hyperglycemic conditions lead to the formation of advanced glycation end-products (AGE), as they play a role to quench nitric oxide (NO) and impair endothelial function [24]. To support this fact, the acute hyperglycemic condition diminishes endothelium-dependent vasodilation in humans in vivo [25]. Hyperlipidemia, specifically hypertriglyceridemia conditions along with low serum high-density lipoprotein (HDL) cholesterol concentration is associated with insulin resistance common in patients with T2DM [26].

18.3.2 Pathophysiology and Complications

The quality of life and characteristic features of T2DM in adult and elderly patients commonly measured by the appearance of symptoms like tiredness, lethargy, and related decreased work performance and fall [27]. Insulin resistance in insulin target cells mainly the liver, skeletal muscle, and adipocytes are considered as an initial characteristic feature among T2DM patients, whereas the following features like increased stimulation and secretion of insulin followed by a gradually diminished function of islet beta-cell reserve demonstrated in chronic condition. Eventually, a complete insulin deficiency state resulted in clinical diabetes [28–30].

It is well demonstrated that T2DM is also associated with numerous microvascular and macrovascular complications [13], where the progressive pathophysiology of T2DM is characterized by declined insulin sensitivity because of decreasing β cell function [31] and decrease of incretin function [32]. Decreased insulin function leads to chronic hyperglycemia and acute glycemic variations that lead to excessive protein glycation and induce oxidative stress [33]. To compensate for the above, Incretin, a group of gastrointestinal hormones that stimulate β-cells and increases the insulin secretion. The long-term complications are macrovascular complications (hypertension, dyslipidemia, myocardial infarction, stroke, etc.), microvascular complications such as diarrhea, diabetic neuropathy, nephropathy, retinopathy, neurogenic disorder, sexual dysfunction, impaired cardiovascular reflexes, and diabetic foot ulcer [27].

18.3.3 Microvascular Complications (MVC)

Diabetic retinopathy (DR) is an MVC, which plays a major in the cause of visual disability and blindness in people with diabetes [34]. Its severity ranges from non-proliferative and pre-proliferative to more severely proliferative DR in which the abnormal growth of new vessels occurs [35]. The prevalence of DR increases with prolonged duration of diabetes [36]. People with DR showed association with younger age onset, tobacco use, insulin treatment, abnormal blood lipid levels, renal disease, elevated homocysteine levels, and a diet high in fat [37–39]. Poor glycemic control is also responsible for DR [40, 41]. The other microvascular alterations associated with DR such as capillary basement membrane thickening, increased permeability of endothelial cells, and formation of microaneurysms, etc. [42, 43].

18.3.4 Diabetic Neuropathy

It is evident that nearly one-half of the diabetic population has a certain form of peripheral neuropathy (PN) [44]. People with diabetes have frequently autonomic neuropathy, including cardiovascular autonomic dysfunction manifested as abnormal heart rate and vascular control [45]. Poor glycemic control, age, duration of diabetes, tobacco use dyslipidemia, and hypertension are responsible for peripheral neuropathy [46]. Hyperglycemia impairs neuronal microvasculature, which is mediated through the abnormal initiation of signaling cascades [47]. However, most of the diagnostic techniques failed to define diabetes-related cardiac autonomic neuropathy. The clinical abnormalities like resting tachycardia, exercise intolerance, resting heart rate variability, slow heart rate, silent myocardial infarction, and increased risk of mortality [48, 49]. Poor maintenance of blood glucose, age, obesity, hypertension, and smoking are the major factors responsible for Cardiac neuropathy among diabetic patients [50].

18.3.5 Diabetic Nephropathy (DN)

Diabetic nephropathy is a serious condition frequently manifested in both T1DM and T2DM patients. Microalbuminuria progresses and terminated in renal failure [51] among diabetic patients. It is presumed that nearly one-fourth T2DM patients express microalbuminuria. Other characteristic features of Diabetic nephropathy are a thickening of glomerular hyperfiltration ultimately leading to glomerular and tubular sclerosis and renal failure [52, 53]. Besides the above, the following such as hyperglycemia, dyslipidemia, and hypertension are also other major causes of diabetic nephropathy.

18.3.6 Macrovascular Complications of Diabetes

Nearly 80% of T2DM patients will develop or die of macrovascular disease [54]. The importance of preventing the macrovascular complications of T2DM has started to receive greater attention. To support this, previous studies have established the encouraging impact of treatments of hypertension on diabetic individuals [34]. The following conditions such as peripheral vascular disease (PVD), coronary artery disease (CAD), and cerebrovascular events (CVA) are termed as macrovascular complications [55]. Although, DM was considered an independent risk factor for the development of atherosclerosis, which in turn responsible for a record number of deaths in patients with T2DM, which accounts for more than 50% of macrovascular complications. Besides the above, the growing population is another major coronary risk factor identified for the CAD epidemic in numerous developing Asian countries including China and India.

Many studies have demonstrated that parallel to the increase in coronary heart disease (CHD) in these countries especially urban and semi-urban areas there has been a tremendous incidence of diabetic-related hypertension, high LDL cholesterol, low HDL cholesterol, and the other metabolic syndrome prevalence [54–56]. Death occurrence among diabetic patients with CAD is greater when compared to their nondiabetic counterparts. Studies have further established the correlation that myocardial infarction in diabetics was more common among diabetic patients with CAD than normal controls [57, 58]. It is interesting to note that diabetics have a fivefold more risk for first MI and a twofold more risk for a recurrent MI than people who previously had an MI but no evidence of hyperglycemia. Diabetic explosions witnessing countries like India and China appear to be more prone to both diabetes and CAD compared to other developing countries [59]. PVD normally defined as a syndrome of the blood vessel, which is not part of the heart or brain. The most common type of PVD, normally detected in lower extremity also called the lower extremity arterial disease (LEAD). Recent evidence suggests that elevated serum triglyceride and dyslipidemia, hypertension, etc. are responsible for 80% of diabetic death worldwide [60].

18.3.7 Cerebrovascular Disease

DM considered one of the well-established risk factors for stroke. The risk is up to two- to fourfold greater in diabetes cases [61]. Diabetic patients, who experienced stroke have more severe neurological lesions and disability [62–65]. Besides the above, other traditional risk factors such as hypertension, dyslipidemia, heart failure, and atrial fibrillation [66] and their increased incidence also contribute to stroke. Hyperglycemia is a potent predictor of fatal and non-fatal stroke [67]. Diabetic retinopathy, proteinuria, microalbuminuria, increased inflammatory markers, and hyperuricemia are other factors contributing to the risk of stroke [67, 68] in people with diabetes.

18.3.8 Peripheral Artery Disease

Peripheral artery disease (PAD), characterized by occlusion of the lower extremity arteries responsible for pain [69] and which result in functional impairments [70] and disability. Diabetics have more chance (15 times) of developing lower extremity amputations when compare to their normal counterparts [71]. In addition, PAD always correlated with the length and severity of the patient's diabetic condition [72, 73]. Hyperglycemia particularly glycation hemoglobin has been shown to be an independent risk factor for PAD [74].

The simplest test available in the clinic to screen PVD is palpitation of peripheral pulses and this is the usual clinical tool to assess the occlusive arteries in peripheries. Although the absence of peripheral, tibial, popliteal, or femoral pulses on peripheral examination are clinically significant [74], one cannot rule out the possibility of using traditional standard techniques such as angiography, color duplex ultrasound, and continuous waveform Doppler [75] for diagnosis of PVD. Hypertension is the primary avertable cause of the two major causes of mortality: coronary artery disease (CAD), and cerebrovascular disease (CVD). Hypertension increases the twofold risk for CAD and sevenfold for CVD and congestive heart attack by fourfold. In addition, studies have also shown that an increase in blood pressure of 5 mmHg is associated with risk for CVD (by 34% increase) and CAD (21%) [76].

18.4 Inflammation Is Associated with Insulin Resistance

Compelling evidence linking inflammation to insulin resistance derives from both epidemiological studies and experimental data in humans and animal models [77, 78]. In a cross-sectional study with the inclusion of 70 healthy individuals aged between 21 and 94 years old showed that with advancing age there was a positive correlation of plasma concentrations of tumor necrosis factor-alpha [79] but shown a negative correlation with whole-body glucose disposal. To support this, in 439 nondiabetic women followed in the Women's Health Study, fasting insulin was strongly correlated with plasma acute-phase reactant C-reactive protein (CRP), with a smaller yet again nonsignificant trend for the pro-inflammatory cytokine, interleukin-6 (IL-6) [77]. In addition, in an analysis of 1008 nondiabetic men and women, a strong association was identified between plasma CRP concentration and insulin sensitivity [80]. Furthermore, a linear rise in CRP levels was noted with T2DM is associated with an augmented risk of cognitive impairment among older T2DM patients with rapid age-related cognitive decline, and a higher incidence of dementia. Although the specific causative factors responsible for cognitive impairment in T2DM are yet to be identified, it is most likely multifactorial one. Inflammatory mediators may, therefore, have a role in the accelerated development of cognitive impairment in people with diabetes either by a direct effect on the brain or through an influence on the development of vascular disease [81].

18.5 Diabetic Foot Ulcer (DFU)

DFU often called a disease of the lower limb or foot ulceration. It often considered as one of the most severe peripheral arterial diseases (PAD), often resulted in amputation because of the combined complications of neuropathy and infection, normally DFU often ignored by patients. However, risks related to this microvascular condition can be taken care of significantly by optimizing glycemic control by early screening/detection and intervention [82].

Diabetic foot infection (DFI) commonly described as the infection caused by various microbial pathogens associated with a tissue injury [83] due to competitive metabolism, toxins, intracellular replication, or antigen–antibody response [84]. Multiple pathogenic microorganisms cause the DFI in DM patients to become very inflamed followed by soreness with delayed wound healing. The causative microorganisms include aerobic bacteria likes *S. aureus*, *S. pyrogens*, *P. aeruginosa*, *P. mirabilis*, *E. coli*, *K. pneumoniae*. Anaerobic bacteria are *C. perfringens*, *B. fragilis*, and yeast such as *C. Albicans* [85].

DFU is one of the most significant and disturbing problems with substantial socioeconomic impact [86]. The occurrence of foot ulceration witnessed worldwide between 4% and 10% of patients; however, the condition is more prevalent among older patients [87, 88] in the developing countries. Infections in DFU patients are difficult to treat because these infected patients have weakness in microvascular circulation, which limits the access of phagocytic engulfing cells to the infected area and results in a poor concentration of antibiotics in the infected tissues [89].

To support the above fact, nearly 85% of all amputations performed in diabetic elderly patients only [90]. Previous studies have estimated that 5% of all patients with diabetes present with DFU history, however, high risks patients who may develop complications of foot ulceration are still existed about 15% [87, 88]. Although neuropathic origins are the most probable causes for foot ulceration, these causes are greatly preventable among T2DM patients especially in the high incident countries in the next 20 years. Would the healing process takes a short time (about 20 weeks) and curable for the neuropathic origin of diabetic patients, whereas neuro-ischemic ulcers take longer and will more often lead to limb amputation [91].

18.5.1 Pathophysiology and Complications of DFU

The important driven factors responsible for the increase in the ailment of DM are vascular problems as well as the delay and failure in the execution of the wound healing phases [92, 93]. Microbial infection often follows diabetic foot ulceration due to vascular complications like insufficiency in oxygen supply, neovascularization, and reduced leukocyte function. It is well characterized that DFU infections are listed as simple cellulitis to more complex chronic osteomyelitis, which is frequently witnessed with hospital admittance and rise in pathogenic microbial infections, which finally lead to the extremity in foot amputation [92–94]. In diabetes patients, mild, moderate, and severe foot infections are all considered serious because of various contributing factors like an open wound, patient's immune deficiency may rapidly extent the infection into the subcutaneous tissue and deeper structures [95]. Impaired microvascular circulation characteristic of diabetes limits transport of phagocytic cells and antibiotics to the infected area, predisposing diabetic patients to more recurrent and potentiate the foot lesions more vulnerable that are more difficult to treat. As a result, it requires careful wound management with surgery [96], topical applications [93] of cream, or suitable medications to correct metabolic defects or intravenous antibiotics [97, 98].

In general, the wound is termed as a disruption in the cellular, anatomical, and functional epithelial continuity of the skin consequent to physical, chemical, thermal microbial, or immunological insult; in other words, it is a disrupted state of the tissue, caused either by physical, chemical, microbial, or immunological insults to normal tissue [99]. According to the current wound forecast, indicate that nearly 6.5 million people suffer from normal chronic wounds worldwide [100, 101].

18.5.2 Processes Involved in Wound Healing

Previous studies have demonstrated that aberrations in the connective tissue, which contribute to the delay or improper wound healing process leading to the formation of DFU specifically the chronic ulcer [102]. Briefly, in all types of wounds, the following four well-coordinated but overlapping phases are involved in the wound healing process, which is hemostasis, inflammation, proliferation, and tissue remodeling or resolution [103–105]. The tissue repair requires the coordination of different cells, growth factors, and cytokines [106]. It begins with the first phase of hemostasis immediately after injury, with vascular constriction and fibrin clot formation, this results in the release of various pro-inflammatory cytokines and growth factors like fibroblast growth factor (FGF), platelet-derived growth factor (PDGF), transforming growth factor (TGF)-β and epidermal growth factor (EGF) [107]. Once the first phase control bleeding and clot formation, then various leukocytes and immune cells like neutrophils, macrophages, lymphocytes sequentially infiltrate and migrate to the affected site by chemotaxis mechanism, followed by the establishment of molecular interactions between them and promote the inflammatory phase [108]. Although these leukocytes and immune cells produce proteases and various reactive oxygen species (ROS), which cause some additional bystander damage [109], however, a significant function of neutrophils in the clearance of invading microbes and cellular debris in the wound or affected site [105, 110]. Besides the above, many studies have established that wound healing processes are influenced or affected by various other factors like infections, nutritional status, medications and hormones, type and sites of wound, and chronic diseases like diabetes [105, 110, 111].

With regard to uncontrolled diabetes, improper wound healing in patients may possibly lead to diabetic foot ulcers or into amputation, especially in poor resource settings. Due to limited awareness and the poor aseptic healthcare condition in wound infection is still a paramount challenging problem faced by developing countries [112]. Besides the above, wound infection is very common in most developing countries because of poor hygienic conditions [113, 114].

Although the precise pathogenesis of poor wound healing in diabetic wounds not adequately understood so far. However, the mechanisms responsible for the delay in wound healing in diabetic patients have been well established [115, 116]. To support the above, many in vivo and clinical investigations have supported the delay in the synthesis of collagen, reduced angiogenesis, and impairment epithelial formation during the proliferative phase [117–120]. Besides the above, other factors implicated in the delayed healing process such as reduced production of necessary growth factors like VEGF, delayed or compromised inflammatory response, reduction in nitric oxide synthase (NOS) activity and excessive protease enzyme activity [121, 122] demonstrated in different phases of the wound healing process [123–127] are yet to be elucidated in detail. Moreover, no approved growth factor and cell therapies are available to treat diabetic foot ulcers or diabetic-related other types of wounds.

18.6 The Role of Medicinal Plants for the Treatment of DM and Wound Healing in DFU

It is well-known that the potential attributes of herbal plants as therapeutics for numerous diseases, which are proven by their mechanism of action practically in all major system of medicine [128]. Impairment in diabetic wound healing is seen as a very severe health problem universally by the health experts despite its association with nonspecific etiology in some cases. Hence, it is essential to consider the value of traditional phytomedicine as one of the right approaches for treatment particularly in poor resource settings [124]. The bioactive principles from various herbal plants contribute their vital role in wound management and care as disinfectants, debridement, and the provision of adequate environment for the natural healing process [129]. The World Health Organization (WHO) has encouraged the use of medicinal plants for the treatment of diabetes and has also recommended for the more verifiable scientific evaluation of the hypoglycemic activities of various plant species [130].

Traditionally most of the Asian and African tropical countries are considered as a reservoir of medicinal plants by employing common knowledge and practice to treat various ailments such as ulcers, boils, sores, and wounds including diabetes [110, 131, 132]. Nearly 10–15% of known 300,000 species of higher plant worldwide have a history of their use for various diseases in the traditional medicine practice [131, 133]. In this regard, many studies have established the beneficial attributes of several species of medicinal plants for therapeutic development considering their availability and low risk nature. In recent years, several plants and their bioactive principles have shown their efficacy in the treatment of T2DM and its complications. Although numerous ethnobotanical reports provide lists of medicinal plants like *Syzygium cumini*, *Momordica charantia*, *Gymnema sylvestre*, *Tinospora cordifolia*, *Ocimum tenuiflorum*, *Allium sativum* L. (Rason)/*Allium cepa* (Onion), *Catharanthus roseus* (Madagascar Periwinkle), and *Pterocarpus marsupium* (Indian Kino) [134, 135] exhibited antidiabetic activities. In addition, a growing number of additional plants like *Aegle marmelos*, *Pterocarpus marsupium*, *Azadirachta indica*, *Asteracantha longifolia*, *Trigonella foenum-graecum* (Fenugreek), *Achyranthes aspera*, *Swertia chirayita* also proven their antidiabetic efficacy. Recently, curcuma longa also gained interest in the metabolic disorder [136], yet the search for additional potential medicinal plants and plant-derived novel drug leads are being explored continuously using advanced techniques for new therapeutic development.

It is evident that applications of herbal derived phytocompounds/bioactive principles have been in use for many decades both by traditional medicine practitioners [137, 138] as well as in the modern system of medicine [137] as therapeutic agents [139]. These compounds have encouraged researchers and pharmaceutical firms to examine the role of medicinal plants to assess their potential wound healing properties and isolate individual chemical entities associated with wound healing. The blood glucose-lowering capacity of some herbal plant extracts has been confirmed in human and animal models of T2DM along with few well-established conventional drugs, which are derivatives of these medicinal plants. An example of that type of therapeutic compound is metformin, a derivative of *Galega officinalis* [140].

Wound healing of DFU is a long awaiting development in health care systems [141]. Even after accomplished wound healing, re-ulcerations occur frequently and commonly lead to minor or major amputation of lower extremities [142]. To treat diabetic foot ulceration, traditional medicine practitioners have employed various practices including medicinal plant applications because of their abilities to promote wound healing and to prevent infection without causing severe side effects [143]. This continued practice and the advent of new efficacious plant-derived traditional medicines have prompted renewed interests in recent years because herbal treatment may be an alternative approach for the treatment of wounds.

The importance of herbal derived bioactive principles and their efficacy against various diseases have drawn global attention as safer alternatives in the management of various infections including diabetic wounds [144]. However, still many anti-diabetic herbal plants not explored in detail, which might provide useful sources for the development of newer drugs or drug leads for T2DM [145]. The available literature on medicinal plants with blood sugar lowering ability is vast with various claims. The purpose of this chapter to highlight and discuss the wound healing efficacy of few prominent medicinal plants and their biologically active substances used to treat diabetes as well as their cellular targets and mechanism of action, this will aid for the better management of diabetic wounds and related microbial infections [144].

Currently, the metformin is the only clinically approved natural antidiabetic drug offered for the treatment of diabetes [140]. This book chapter review aims to outline and discuss the current DM and DFU management approaches with the incorporation of medicinal plants for the prevention as well as for the treatment. Since it is very difficult to comprise all plants and their therapeutic claims with demonstrable evidence in a single book chapter, hence, we have chosen only selected commonly used antidiabetic plants for the benefit of readers.

18.6.1 *Gymnema sylvestre* (Gs)

Gymnema sylvestre **(Gs)** (Fig. 18.1) is a medicinal plant belongs to the family of Asclepiadaceae. Various tropical countries like India, Africa, and Australia uses this herb traditionally for various purposes [146, 147]. Its efficacy indicated that it possesses not only blood sugar-controlling/antidiabetic properties but also shown

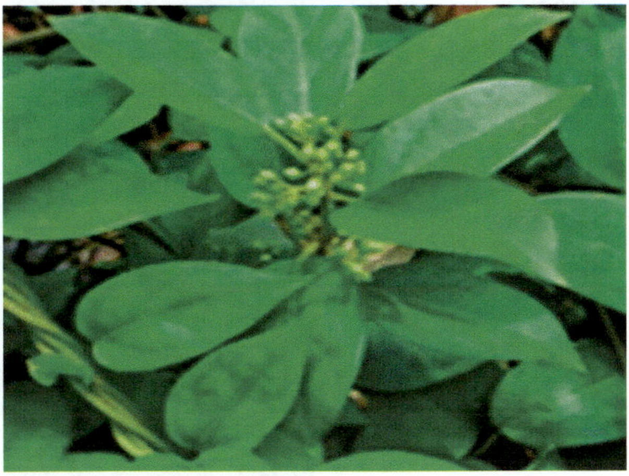

Fig. 18.1 *Gymnema sylvestre* (Gs)

certain benefits like improving urination and stomach ulceration [148–151]. Recent studies have shown that Gymnemic acid molecules, which are a group of triterpenoid saponins [147, 152], alkaloids, acidic glycosides, and anthraquinones [153] responsible for antidiabetic action. Besides the above, the hyperglycemia-induced conditions like rising in urea, uric acid, and creatinine together with decreased glomerular filtration rate were substantially inhibited in the Gs extract treated in diabetic rats [150]. In a clinical study subjected with 22 T2DM patients were given 400 mg Gs extract daily along with their oral hypoglycemic drugs. The study results have shown that almost all patients treated with extract have revealed decreased blood sugar. Nearly 95% of patients (21/22) were able to stop their oral medication and maintain blood sugar control with the Gs extract alone [154]. In addition, another study was postulated that Gs enhance the production of endogenous insulin [155].

18.6.2 *Aegle marmelos*

Aegle marmelos (Fig. 18.2), commonly known as Bael, a plant of Indian continental origin belongs to family Rutaceae [156]. The following bioactive principles such as mucilage, pectin, volatile oil isolated from Bael leaves have demonstrated an excellent antidiabetic property and significantly demonstrated antioxidant activity [157]. In addition, both fruit and root extract showed anti-amoebic and hypoglycemic activities [156]. This plant also exhibited various pharmacological activities by bioactive principles extracted from the root and fruits like alkaloids like aegeline and marmelline, steroids, essential oils, and coumarins such as scoparone, scopoletin, umbelliferone, marmesin, and skimming [158]. Besides the above, xanthotoxol, imperatorin, and alloimperatorin also added in the list. It also contains polysaccharides like galactose, arabinose, uronic acid, and L-rhamnose, which may obtain after hydrolysis. Apart from the above chemical constituents, more than 100 new

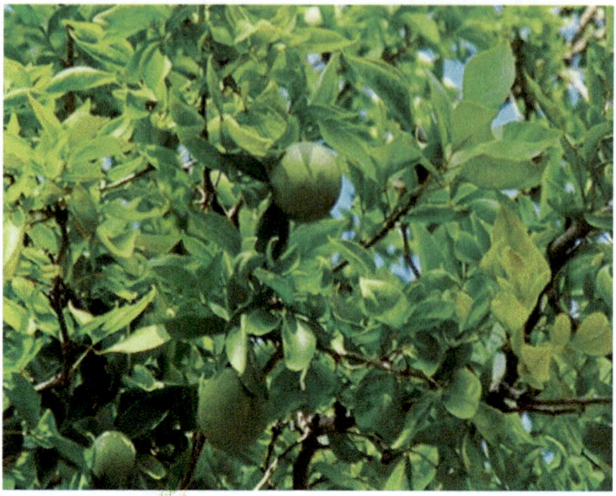

Fig. 18.2 *Aegle marmelos*

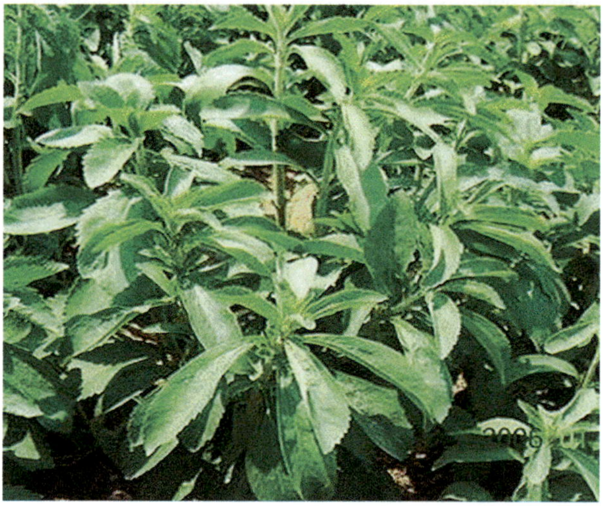

Fig. 18.3 *Pterocarpus marsupium*

compounds have been isolated, the following such as psoralen, marmelide, fagarine, cuminaldehyde, eugenol, marmesinin, marmelosine, luvangetin, auraptene, skimminine, aegelin, lupeol, cineole, citral, citronellal, and tennins have exhibited spectrum of actions against many diseases [159–161].

18.6.3 *Pterocarpus marsupium*

Pterocarpus marsupium (Fig. 18.3) belongs to the family Leguminosae and predominantly grows in most parts of India and Sri Lanka. Previous studies [162, 163] have established that *P. marsupium* as a promising herbal plant because of its antidiabetic efficacy. This plant extract contains various potential phytocompounds. In line with this, the antidiabetic activity of various fractions from the bark was evaluated on lipid profile, blood glucose level, etc. [164, 165]. In addition, an aqueous extract of wood exhibited hypoglycemic activity [166]. The other potentially bioactive compounds are diarylpropane derivative, propterol; stilbene, pterostilbene; hydrochalone, pterosupin; benzofuranone, marsupsin, and polyphenolic compounds exhibit various other pharmacological activities.

18.7 Antidiabetic/Antihyperglycemic/Hypoglycemic Activity

Previous studies [164, 165] have demonstrated that the alcoholic extract of the bark of *P. marsupium* has shown beneficial effects on blood glucose-lowering ability. To support further, an aqueous extract of *P. marsupium* wood and bark was assessed for the antihyperglycemic and hypoglycemic effect in normal and alloxanized diabetic rats [166, 167]. These studies showed that the aqueous extract exhibited a slight but important hypoglycemic effect in normal rats and a significant and clear dose-dependent antihyperglycemic effect evaluated the antihyperglycemic activity of phenolics from *P. marsupium.* The phytocompounds like marsupsin and pterostilbene, which significantly decrease the blood glucose level of hyperglycemic rats [162, 168].

18.7.1 *Momordica charantia* (Karela)

Momordica charantia (*M. charantia*) (Fig. 18.4), also known as bitter melon found throughout India belongs to family Cucurbitaceae [169]. The whole plant, especially the seeds and fruit, has significant pharmacological effects namely, abortifacient, anthelmintic, contraceptive, antimalarial, laxative, dysmenorrhea, eczema, gout, jaundice, leprosy, piles, pneumonia, psoriasis, rheumatism, and scabies [170,

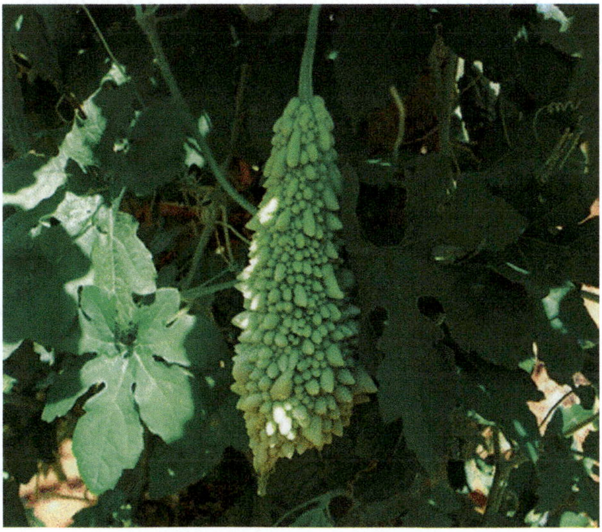

Fig. 18.4 *Momordica charantia*

171]. In many countries and regions, this plant is considered to treat diabetes because it contains many potential phytocompounds with the spectrum of pharmaceutical activities, which include antidiabetic ones [162, 172]. Besides the above, *M. charantia* used broadly as an herbal medication for diabetes [173]. The fresh juice of the unripe fruit of this plant confirmed blood glucose-lowering action in an experimental Streptozotocin (STZ) induced animal models as well as human clinical trials [174]. In this regard, a novel phytochemical inhibits guanylate cyclase enzyme [175]. Other phytochemicals are α- and β-momorcharin, momordin, and cucurbitacin B. Alcohol-derived extract charantin from *M. charantia* consist of mixed steroids, which are more effective than the oral hypoglycemic agents tolbutamide such as tolbutamide, chlorpropamide, and glibenclamide in an animal study [170, 176–179].

Previous studies [180, 181] have confirmed that aqueous extract of *M. charantia* stimulates insulin secretion of cells in pancreatic islets of obese-hyperglycemic mice. Besides the above, it plays a vital role in the regeneration of β-cells in STZ-diabetic rats or recovery of destroyed [182] cells. In addition, polypeptide-P isolated from the bitter gourd in clinical trials showed convincing hypoglycemic activity [172]. The major pure cucurbitane compounds of *M. charantia*, 5,19-epoxy-3,25-dihydroxycucurbita-6,23(E)-diene, and 3,7,25-trihydroxycucurbita-5,23(E)-dien-19-al have been demonstrated to have hypoglycemic effects in the diabetes-induced male ddY mice [183–185] suggested that the antidiabetic mechanism of *M. charantia* extracts may be due to enhancing insulin secretion by the islets of Langerhans, reducing glycogenesis in liver tissue, enhancing peripheral glucose utilization and increasing serum protein levels [181].

18.7.2 *Trigonella foenum-graecum* (Methi)

Trigonella foenum-graecum (Fig. 18.5), belongs to the family of Fabaceae, which is found all over India, its bitter taste seeds are frequently used as a constituent of spices [186–188] and leave as green leafy vegetables in a diet [189]. Traditionally both seeds and leaves have proven their medicinal qualities, as they possess

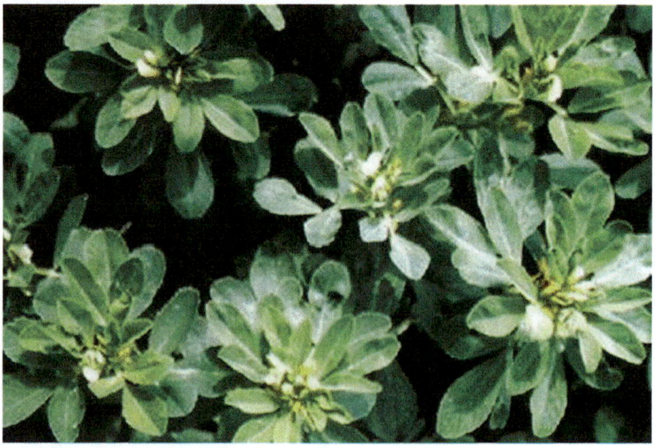

Fig. 18.5 *Trigonella foenum-graecum*

anti-hyperlipidemic and antioxidant properties [186, 190, 191]. In fact, *Trigonella foenum-graecum* seed powder lowered blood sugar levels among diabetic patients [192]. In addition, *Trigonella foenum-graecum* seed powder solution exhibited its potential in improving dyslipidemia in newly diagnosed type II diabetic patients [192]. To support this, study results showed that the *Trigonella foenum-graecum* seed powder solution showed a substantial decrease in TC, TG, and LDL-C levels and an increase in HDL-C level [186, 189].

The components such as saponins, 4-hydroxyleucine/4-hydroxyisoleucine, trigonelline, alkaloid, high fiber [156, 167] and diosgenin [193] are responsible for its various therapeutic potential [194, 195]. Several animal experimental studies have shown that the following active principles such as alkaloid trigonelline, nicotinic acid, and coumarin extracted from a defatted portion of the seed confirmed their antidiabetic potential of *T. foeneum-graecum* [196–198]. Furthermore, fenugreek seed powder exerts have been reported to have neuroprotective effects that probably mediate through a decrease in hyperglycemia and oxidative stress [195, 199]. However, in order to provide adequate confirmation, more research required including comprehensive chemical and pharmacological studies in order to isolate and characterize specific bioactive compounds from *Trigonella foenum-graecum* seed powder [192] and appropriate elucidation of its mechanism of action needs future study.

18.7.3 *Chromolaena odorata*

C. odorata (L.) (Fig. 18.6) King and Robinson is a well-known Devil or Siam weed found in many parts of the world [105]. It is widely, recognized for its traditional wound healing value with another spectrum of pharmacological actions. Although this plant initially identified in Vietnam and named *Eupatorium odoratum* and used exclusively for the treatment of burns, wounds, skin infections, and inflammation [200].

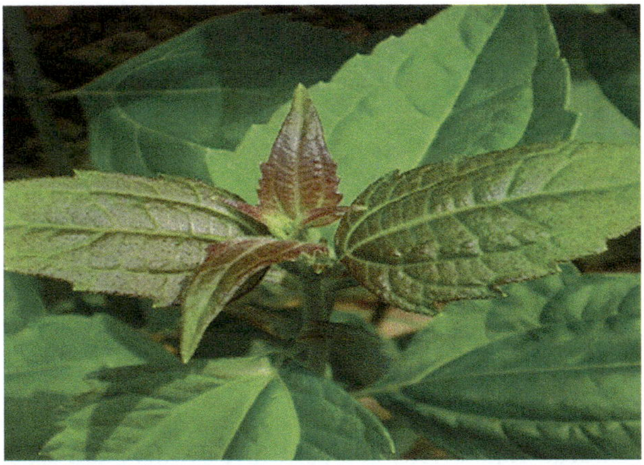

Fig. 18.6 *Chromolaena odorata*

18.7.3.1 Bioactive Principles of *C. odorata*

C. odorata extracts from various parts of the herb exhibit spectrum of pharmacological potentials like antioxidant [201], analgesic, and cytoprotective [202], anti-inflammatory [203], and other medicinally significant properties. Most of the extracts, mostly the leaf derived one facilitates fibroblast and keratinocyte proliferation at wound sites that enhance the healing of wounds [139, 203–205].

Many studies convincing evidence have shown that *C. odorata* exhibited antimicrobial activity against a wide array of pathogens [200, 203, 206–209]. Besides the above, other activities have been demonstrated and verified such as antimalarial, phytopathogenic [210], antiprotozoal [211], anti-biofilm [208], antihepatotoxicity [209], anthelmintic, and wound healing [139, 201, 205]. Adverse drug reactions and the huge expenditure on microbial infections including DFU [211, 212] in many developing and poor resource setting counties had made the management and control of infectious diseases ineffective [213, 214].

Justification: Need for Phytomedicine to Combat Microbial Pathogens For decades until the present, herbal resources, mostly medicinal plants and their extracts derived drug leads are in practice for many medicinal purposes. In the era of reduced therapeutic options to treat multidrug-resistant infections, there is an urgent need to discover new antimicrobial compounds with diverse chemical structures and novel mechanisms of action. Antimicrobials of plant origin have the enormous therapeutic potential [215, 216]. Recently, much attention has directed toward plant extracts and biologically active compounds isolated from popular plant species [105, 139, 205]. The use of medicinal plants plays a vital role in covering the basic health needs in developing countries and these plants may offer a new source of antibacterial, antifungal, and antiviral agents with significant activity against infective microorganisms [217–219]. A recent study by [139] has shown that the ethanolic leaf extract of *C. odorata* showed a relatively larger zone of inhibition in diameter than Streptomycin against all tested organisms.

Phytochemicals such as tannins, flavonoids, alkaloids, and several other aromatic compounds or secondary metabolites such as glycosides, phenols, saponins, and steroids [220–222] have potential curative properties. To support the above claim, the antimicrobial compounds of *C. odorata* (flavonoids) are effective at inhibiting the growth of pathogens by binding to the bacterial cell wall, leading to inhibition of cell wall biosynthesis [213, 223]. In addition, tannins inhibit the growth of many fungi, yeasts, bacteria, and viruses. A recent study [139] also revealed the presence of alkaloids and saponins in the leaf extract further confirming their role in the microbial inhibition.

18.7.4 *Astragalus membranaceus*

Astragalus membranaceus (Fisch.) Bge (Fig. 18.7) belongs to family Leguminosae. Astragali Radix (AR) is a derivative of this plant especially from dried root [224,

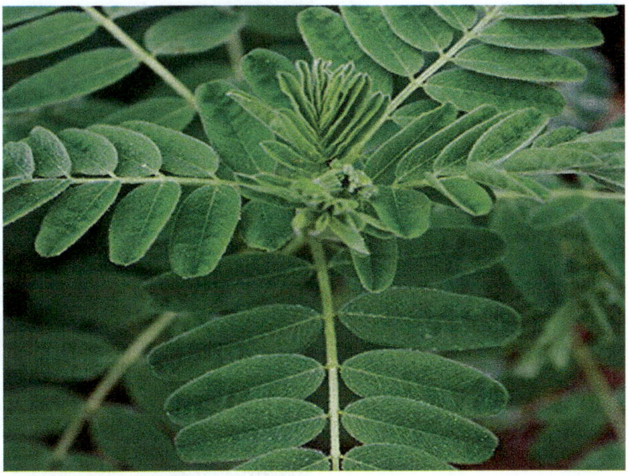

Fig. 18.7 *Astragalus membranaceus*

225] and has been used in Traditional Chinese Medicine (TCM) for hundreds of years to reinforce superficial resistance and promote growth of new tissue [226]. Besides the above, studies have reported its various pharmacological properties such as cardioprotective [227, 228], immunomodulatory [229, 230] as well as insulin-sensitizing [231–233] effects.

With regard to wound healing, a study reported that the aqueous crude extract of AR was demonstrated to promote fibroblast proliferation, both in cell line and in primary culture from diabetic foot ulcer patients, which was considered as the crucial step in wound process [234–237]. The primary constituents of AR include polysaccharides, saponins, flavonoids, amino acids, and trace elements [238, 239]. Saponin and isoflavone-enriched AR extract also promote angiogenesis in human endothelial cells [240] and calycosin was the active angiogenesis-promoting isoflavonoid isolated from AR [241].

18.7.5 *Rehmannia glutinosa libosch*

Rehmannia glutinosa libosch (Fig. 18.8) belongs to family Scrophulariaceae often viewed as safe and chief grade herb practiced in traditional Chinese medicine (TCM). This plant chemical composition contains more than 70 compounds including iridoids, saccharides, amino acid, inorganic ions, as well as other trace elements [242]. The principal compound Rehmanniae Radix (RR), a derivative of the root [243] of this plant played a role in remove pathogenic heat from the blood, nourish “yin” and promote the production of body fluid [244, 245]. Initially, RR recommended by TCM to relieve symptoms of diabetic patients, febrile diseases, skin eruption, and epistaxis [226]. Various scientific studies proved that RR and its active principals possessed a wide spectrum of pharmacological properties on various structures including the nervous system (reviewed by [242]). To support this, a study by [246] has shown that RR extracts inhibiting the progression of diabetic

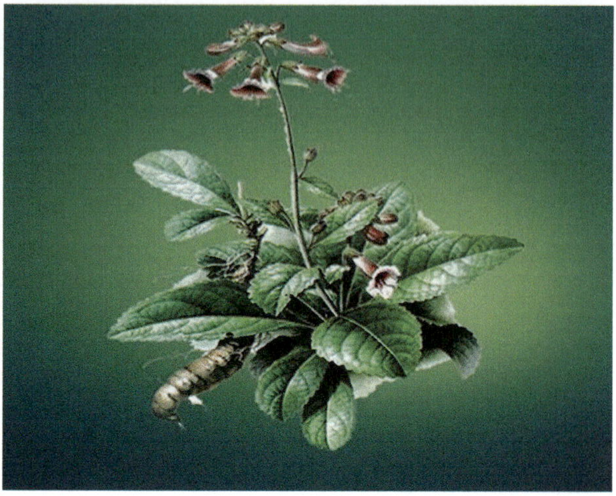

Fig. 18.8 *Rehmannia glutinosa libosch*

nephropathy. More specifically, the aqueous extracts of RR could stimulate fibroblast proliferation [234, 235] and be effective in promoting diabetic foot ulcer healing in rats through the processes of tissue regeneration, angiogenesis, and inflammation control [235, 247, 248]. However, ethanol extract and oligosaccharide fraction demonstrated hypoglycemic activity in streptozotocin (STZ)-induced diabetic rats and glucose-induced hyperglycemic rats, respectively [249, 250]. A study by [118] attempted to evaluate the potencies of individual AR and RR in different mechanistic studies. The study used AR and RR in the ratio of 2:1 and named as NF3. This study carried out to investigate whether herb–herb interaction between AR and RR in NF3 is involved in the diabetic wound healing process or not. In fact, the study results have confirmed that NF3 enhanced diabetic wound healing in rats by various mechanisms such as tissue regeneration, angiogenesis promotion, and inflammation inhibition. To support the above, a report from the clinical study, on the use of two herbal formulae (F1 and F2)/principal component of herbs, RA and RR prevented legs from limb amputation in diabetic patients [251] and were effective in enhancing fibroblast proliferation—the main step in wound healing [234, 252].

18.8 Possible Mechanism of Action of Medical Plants on Wound Healing

In recent years, increasing attention with growing demand and obtainability phytocompounds has encouraged the need to understand the principles responsible for their therapeutic activities and effectiveness. Many studies have reported that bioactive principles contained in herbal plants have growth factor-like activity or has the ability to stimulate an early expression of growth factors [105, 139, 205, 253]. For example, stimulation of fibroblasts has been observed in the wound healing process by plant extracts [254]. In addition, many plant extracts have been known to stop fresh wound bleeding, also inhibit microbial growth, and promote wound healing [247]. Many active compounds enhance the process of wound healing by increasing various activities such as the viability of collagen fibrils, strengthen collagen fibers and increasing the blood circulation, preventing cell damage and/or promoting DNA synthesis [255–257].

To support the above, plant extracts with antioxidant activity play a vital role in promoting the wound healing process as therapeutic agents [139]. The antioxidant activities are mostly associated with the free radical scavenging action of phytocompounds in the extracts acting either singly or synergistically. The following bioactive principles of medicinal plants like alkaloids, flavonoids, triterpenes, tannins, and saponins have exhibited their key roles in wound healing effects [258]. This study report indicates that flavonoids possess both potent antioxidant and free scavenging activities by reducing lipid peroxidation and enhanced vascularity. Tannins plays a vital role in free radical scavenging activity, whereas, triterpenoids and saponins involve in enhancing the wound healing process by wound reduction and enhanced epithelialization [256–258]. Besides the above, trace elements such as zinc and Vitamin C from plant sources contribute to their role in wound healing. For example, zinc acts as a cofactor in many enzymatic reactions including zinc-dependent matrix metalloproteinases, which enhance keratinocyte migration during wound repair, whereas, Vitamin C plays a role in collagen formation [259].

18.9 Concluding Remarks and Future Directions

In summary, DM especially DFU is a debilitating status with a significant loss to quality of life among affected patients mostly in developing countries. Additionally, currently available treatments for this complication are usually not as effective as they brought poor clinical outcomes. This is mainly clarified by the insufficient knowledge of its underlying mechanisms and treatment methods. Although the interest in research and management of DFU has increased in recent years, it is still in the infancy state among diabetes complications in terms of research efforts and resource allocation worldwide despite current treatments inadequate outputs. Additionally, the complexity of its management needs to be addressed on a multidisciplinary approach including the adaptation of phytomedicines with rigorous research approach and appropriate trails that should gather all expertise necessary for the optimal management of each aspect of this complication.

Over the years, globally the use of traditionally herbal plants played a vital role in the treatment of DM specifically T2DM. Numerous types of plant-derived bioactive principles representing various types of chemical compounds such as alkaloids, glycosides, galactomannan, gum, peptidoglycan, glycopeptide, amino acids, and inorganic ions have shown potential therapeutics for diabetes. Therefore, there is plenty of possibility of developing potential antidiabetic drugs from medicinal plants for human use. However, it is still not very clear whether we can use phytomedicine alone as an alternate to combinatorial drug of non-natural origins or as adjuvant drugs along with standard insulin therapy for managing diabetes. In this regard, future investigations are still required to elucidate the comprehensive details of issues such as phytomedicines and properties, an effective dose of each compound, and probable side effects on wound healing processes in diabetic and non-diabetic conditions.

Phytomedicines are important to manage pathological conditions of many diseases including DFU caused by various pathogens and free radicals, as they are nature's gift for not only healing wounds but also contributing to affordable healthcare. Explore the antimicrobial, antioxidant bioactive principles from natural resources; identification and isolation of those natural products are simultaneously presenting enormous scope for their better therapeutic application for treatment of human disease, mainly infection-related complications. Hence, the phytochemical screening and assessment of the antimicrobial, antioxidant activity of medicinal plants play a very important role in identifying new compounds of therapeutic and industrial importance. Therefore it is time for researchers, to identify and explore many currently practicing traditional therapeutic knowledge and medicinal plant sources and interpret them according to the recent advancements to fight against microbial pathogens, reactive oxygen species (ROS), in order to give them a deserving place. This is crucial to its potential future drug design, development, and application for the treatment of wounds in both animal and human medicine and cost-effective health care. In this regard, future studies on the wound healing potential of topical herbal formulations must incorporate careful consideration of the chemical makeup of the final therapeutic product. The future should bring much more high-quality research not only to the area of DFU but also to phytomedicines from basic research to properly conducted clinical trials. Regarding future clinical studies, in addition to the need for thorough consideration of characterization and batch-to-batch reproducibility of topical botanical therapeutics used in the clinic, properly designed randomized controlled trials are suggested.

Besides the above, therapeutic application of cytokines, growth factors and their soluble receptors could be investigated to determine the extent of their involvement and acceptability in wound healing and treatment. Fibrotic processes are continuous and characterized by collagen synthesis, downregulation of degradative enzymes involved in removing scar tissue and fibrosis has been reported to be inhibited by antibodies, peptide receptor antagonists. Research into interactions between fibrotic processes and antibodies could also provide useful information on wound healing. To conclude, a better understanding of the mechanisms of initiation, progression, and resolution of wound healing could lead to the discovery of new therapies that are very much needed. However, despite limitations on the degree and extent of the applications of phytomedicines in the treatment of diabetic wounds, it shows considerable promise and can indeed herald exciting new therapeutic strategies in wound healing. Yet, further research and large clinical trials are recommended to confirm the efficacy and safety of specific medicinal plants and their mechanisms of action, especially on diabetic wound healing.

Competing Interests Authors have declared that no competing interests exist.

References

1. Tierney LM, McPhee SJ, Papadakis MA (2002) Current medical diagnosis & treatment. International edition. Lange Medical Books/McGraw-Hill, New York, NY, pp 1203–1215
2. Bommer C, Heesemann E, Sagalova V, Manne-Goehler J, Atun R, Barnighausen T et al (2007) The global economic burden of diabetes in adults aged 20-79 years: a cost-of-illness study. Lancet Diabet Endocrinol 5(6):423–430
3. American Diabetes Association (2010) Diagnosis and classification of diabetes mellitus. Diabetes Care 33:S62–S69
4. Das SK, Elbein SC (2006) The genetic basis of type 2 diabetes. Cell Sci 2:100–131
5. Stumvoll M, Goldstein BJ, van Haeften TW (2005) Type 2 diabetes: principles of pathogenesis and therapy. Lancet 365(9467):1333–1346
6. Lin Y, Sun S (2010) Current views on type 2 diabetes. J Endocrinol 204(1):1
7. Huizinga MM, Rothman RL (2006) Addressing the diabetes pandemic: a comprehensive approach. Indian J Med Res 124:481–484
8. King H, Auburt RE, Herman WH (1998) Global Burden of Diabetes, 1995–2025: prevalence, numerical estimates, and projections. Diabetes Care 21:1414–1431
9. Ramachandran A, Snehalatha C, Viswanathan V (2002) Burden of type 2 diabetes and its complications – the Indian scenario. Curr Sci 83(12):1472–1476
10. Ramachandran A (2007) Socioeconomic burden of diabetes in India. J Assoc Physicians India 55:9–12
11. Sicree R, Shaw J, Zimmet P (2006) Diabetes and impaired glucose tolerance. In: Gan D (ed) Diabetes atlas. International diabetes federation, 3rd edn. International Diabetes Federation, Belgium, pp 15–103
12. Mohan V, Sandeep S, Deepa R (2007) Indian scenario. Indian J Med Res 125:225–230
13. Wild S, Roglic G, Green A, Sicree R, King H (2004) Global prevalence of diabetes: estimates for the year 2000 and projections for 2030. Diabetes Care 27:1047–1053
14. Timón IM, Collantes CS, Galindo AS, Javier F, Gómez C (2014) Type 2 diabetes and cardiovascular disease: have all risk factors the same strength? World J Diabetes 5(4):444–470
15. Kozakova M, Palombo C (2016) Diabetes mellitus, arterial wall, and cardiovascular risk assessment. Int J Environ Res Public Health 13(2):201. https://doi.org/10.3390/ijerph13020201
16. Rizzoni D, Porteri E, Guelfi D (2001) Structural alterations in subcutaneous small arteries of normotensive and hypertensive patients with non–insulin-dependent diabetes mellitus. Circulation 103:1238–1244
17. Al-Goblan AS, Al-Alfi MA, Khan MZ (2014) Mechanism linking diabetes mellitus and obesity. Diabetes Metab Syndr Obes 7:587–591
18. Gisela W (2005) Insulin and insulin resistance. Clin Biochem Rev 26(2):19–39
19. Alan C, Karin EB (2009) Diabetes and atherosclerosis: is there a role for hyperglycemia? J Lipid Res 50(Suppl):S335–S339
20. Betsy BD (2008) The pathophysiology of cardiovascular disease and diabetes: beyond blood pressure and lipids. Diabet Spectr 21(3):160–165
21. Verma S, Anderson TJ (2002) Fundamentals of endothelial function for the clinical cardiologist. Circulation 105:546–549
22. Cusi K, Maezono K, Osman A, Pendergrass M, Patti ME (2000) Insulin resistance differentially affects the PI 3-kinase- and MAP kinase-mediated signaling in human muscle. J Clin Invest 105:311–320
23. Montagnani M, Ravichandran LC, Chen H, Esposito DL, Quon MJ (2002) Insulin receptor substrate-1 and phosphoinositide-dependent kinase-1 are required for insulin stimulated production of nitric oxide in endothelial cells. Mol Endocrinol 16:1931–1942
24. Zhang L, Zalewski A, Liu Y, Mazurek T, Cowan S (2003) Diabetes-induced oxidative stress and low-grade inflammation in porcine coronary arteries. Circulation 108:472–478

25. Sogawa K, Nagaoka T, Izumi N, Nakabayashi S, Yoshida A (2010) Acute hyperglycemia-induced endothelial dysfunction in retinal arterioles in cats. Invest Ophthalmol Vis Sci 51(5):2648–2655. https://doi.org/10.1167/iovs.09-4070
26. Feng YM, Zhao D, Zhang N, Yu CG, Zhang Q, Thijs L et al (2016) Insulin resistance in relation to lipids and inflammation in type-2 diabetic patients and non-diabetic people. PLoS One 11(4):e0153171
27. Patel P, Macerollo A (2010) Diabetes mellitus: diagnosis and screening. Am Fam Physician 81(7):863–870
28. Seely BL, Olefsky JM (1993) Potential cellular and genetic mechanisms for insulin resistance in common disorders of obesity and diabetes. In: Moller D (ed) Insulin resistance and its clinical disorders. John Wiley & Sons, Ltd, London, pp 187–252
29. Olefsky JM (1999) Insulin resistance and pathogenesis of non-insulin dependent diabetes mellitus: cellular and molecular mechanisms. In: Efendic S, Ostenson CG, Vranic M (eds) New concepts in the pathogenesis of NIDDM. Plenum Publishing Corporation, New York, NY
30. Fritschi C, Quinn L (2010) Fatigue in patients with diabetes: a review. J Psychosom Res 69(1):33–41
31. Kasuga M (2006) Insulin resistance and pancreatic beta cell failure. J Clin Invest 116:1756–1760
32. Knop FK, Vilsbøll T, Højberg PV, Larsen S, Madsbad S, Vølund A et al (2007) Reduced incretin effect in type 2 diabetes: cause or consequence of the diabetic state? Diabetes 56:1951–1959
33. Monnier L, Colette C (2008) Glycemic variability. Should we and can we prevent it? Diabetes Care 31:S150–S154
34. World Health Organization. Diabetes facts. Available from: http://www.who.int/mediacentre/factsheets/fs312/en/index.html. Accessed 13 Dec 2007
35. Harding S (2003) Extracts from "concise clinical evidence": diabetic retinopathy. BMJ 326:1023–1025
36. Escandon JC, Cipolla M (2001) Diabetes and endothelial dysfunction: a clinical perspective. Endocr Rev 22(1):36–52
37. Cusick M, Chew EY, Chan CC (2003) Histopathology and regression of retinal hard exudates in diabetic retinopathy after reduction of elevated serum lipid levels. Ophthalmology 110:2126–2133
38. Romero P, Salvat M, Fernandez J (2007) Renal and retinal microangiopathy after 15 years of follow-up study in a sample of type 1 diabetes mellitus patients. J Diabet Complicat 21:93–100
39. Brazionis L, Rowley K Sr, Itsiopoulos C, Harper CA (2008) Homocysteine and diabetic retinopathy. Diabetes Care 31:50–56
40. Lima VC, Cavalieri GC, Lima MC, Nazario NO, Lima GC (2016) Risk factors for diabetic retinopathy: a case–control study. Int J Retina Vitreous 2:21
41. Simó-Servat O, Hernández C, Simó R (2019) Diabetic retinopathy in the context of patients with diabetes. Ophthalmic Res 62:211–217
42. Carlson EC, Audette JL, Veitenheimer NJ, Risan JA, Laturnus DI, Epstein PN (2003) Ultrastructural morphometry of capillary basement membrane thickness in normal and transgenic diabetic mice. Anat Rec A Discov Mol Cell Evol Biol 271:332–341
43. Hammes HP (2005) Pericytes and the pathogenesis of diabetic retinopathy. Horm Metab Res 37(suppl 1):39–43
44. Juster-Switlyk K, Smith AG (2016) Updates in diabetic peripheral neuropathy. Version 1. F1000 Res 5:F1000 Faculty Rev-738. https://doi.org/10.12688/f1000research.7898.1
45. Vinik AI, Maser RE, Mitchell BD, Freeman R (2003) Diabetic autonomic neuropathy. Diabetes Care 26:1553–1579
46. Dyck PJ, Davies JL, Wilson DM (1999) Risk factors for severity of diabetic polyneuropathy: intensive longitudinal assessment of the Rochester Diabetic Neuropathy Study cohort. Diabetes Care 22:1479–1486

47. Cotter MA, Jack AM, Cameron NE (2002) Effects of the protein kinase C beta inhibitor LY333531 on neural and vascular function in rats with streptozotocin-induced diabetes. Clin Sci (Lond) 103:311–321
48. Cheng YJ, Lauer MS, Earnest CP, Church TS, Kampert JB, Gibbons LW et al (2003) Heart rate recovery following maximal exercise testing as a predictor of cardiovascular disease and all-cause mortality in men with diabetes. Diabetes Care 26:2052–2057
49. Vinik AI, Ziegler D (2007) Diabetic cardiovascular autonomic neuropathy. Circulation 115:387–397
50. Witte DR, Tesfaye S, Chaturvedi N (2005) Risk factors for cardiac autonomic neuropathy in type 1 diabetes mellitus. Diabetologia 48:164–171
51. Brenner BM, Cooper ME, de Zeeuw D, Keane WF, Mitch WE, Parving HH et al (2001) Effects of losartan on renal and cardiovascular outcomes in patients with type 2 diabetes and nephropathy. N Engl J Med 345:861–869
52. Chen S, Hong SW, Iglesias-de la Cruz MC, Isono M, Casaretto A et al (2001) The key role of the transforming growth factor-beta system in the pathogenesis of diabetic nephropathy. Ren Fail 23:471–481
53. van Dijk C, Berl T (2004) Pathogenesis of diabetic nephropathy. Rev Endocr Metab Disord 5:237–248
54. Laakso M (2010) Cardiovascular disease in type 2 diabetes from population to man to mechanisms: the Kelly West Award Lecture 2008. Diabetes Care 33(2):442–449
55. Leung GM, Lam K (2000) Diabetic complications and their implications on health care in Asia. Hong Kong Med J 6:61–68
56. Gupta R, Rastogi P, Sarna M, Sharma SK (2007) Bodymass index, waist-size, waist-hip ratio and cardiovascular risk factors in urban subjects. JAPI 55:621–627
57. Haffner SM, Lehto S, Laakso M (1998) Mortality from coronary heart disease in subjects with type 2 diabetes and in nondiabetic subjects with and without prior myocardial infarction. N Engl J Med 330:229–234
58. Liang H, Vallarino C, Joseph G, Manne S, Perez A, Zhang S (2014) Increased risk of subsequent myocardial infarction in patients with type 2 diabetes: a retrospective cohort study using the U.K. general practice research database. Diabetes Care 37(5):1329–1337
59. Mohan V, Venkatraman VJ, Pradeepa R (2010) Epidemiology of cardiovascular disease in type 2 diabetes: the Indian Scenario. J Diabetes Sci Technol 4(1):158–170
60. Feingold KR, Grunfeld C. Diabetes and dyslipidemia. In: Feingold KR, Anawalt B, Boyce A, et al. 2019 Endotext. South Dartmouth, MA: MDText.com, Inc..; 2000–. Available from: https://www.ncbi.nlm.nih.gov/books/NBK305900/.
61. Centers for Disease Control and Prevention (2020) National diabetes statistics report, 2020. Centers for Disease Control and Prevention, US Department of Health and Human Services, Atlanta, GA
62. Parsons MW, Barber PA, Desmond PM, Baird TA, Darby DG, Byrnes G et al (2002) Acute hyperglycemia adversely affects stroke outcome: a magnetic resonance imaging and spectroscopy study. Ann Neurol 52:20–28
63. Megherbi SE, Milan C, Minier D, Couvreur G, Osseby GV, Tilling K et al (2003) Association between diabetes and stroke subtype on survival and functional outcome 3 months after stroke. Stroke 34:688–694
64. Megherbi R, Molina C, Montaner J (2005) Acute hyperglycemia state is associated with lower tPA-induced recanalization rates in stroke patients. Stroke 36:1705–1709
65. Ribo M, Molina C, Montaner J (2005) Acute hyperglycemia state is associated with lower tPA-induced recanalization rates in stroke patients. Stroke 36:1705–1709
66. Edwin HA, Michael RV, Kathleen HT, John MP (2018) Clinical overview of obesity and diabetes mellitus as risk factors for atrial fibrillation and sudden cardiac death. Front Physiol 9:1847
67. Tun NN, Arunagirinathan G, Munshi SK, Pappachan JM (2017) Diabetes mellitus and stroke: a clinical update. World J Diabetes 8(6):235–248

68. Engstrom G, Stavenow L, Hedblad B (2003) Inflammation-sensitive plasma proteins, diabetes, and mortality and incidence of myocardial infarction and stroke: a population-based study. Diabetes 52:442–447
69. American Heart Association. Peripheral arterial disease risk factors and possible complications. Available from: http://www.americanheart.org/presenter.jhtml?identifier_3020256. Accessed 5 Jan 2008
70. Muller MD, Reed AB, Leuenberger UA, Sinoway LI (2013) Physiology in medicine: peripheral arterial disease. J Appl Physiol 115(9):1219–1226
71. Dickinson PJ, Carrington AL, Frost GS, Boulton AJ (2002) Neurovascular disease, antioxidants and glycation in diabetes. Diabetes Metab Res Rev 18:260–272
72. Jude EB, Oyibo SO, Chalmers N, Boulton AJ (2001) Peripheral arterial disease in diabetic and nondiabetic patients: a comparison of severity and outcome. Diabetes Care 24:1433–1437
73. Al-Delaimy WK, Merchant AT, Rimm EB, Willett WC, Stampfer MJ, Hu FB (2004) Effect of type 2 diabetes and its duration on the risk of peripheral arterial disease among men. Am J Med 116:236–240
74. Fares A, Wang AT, Elraiyah TA, Malgor RD, Rizvi AZ, Lane MA et al (2014) A systematic review for the screening for peripheral arterial disease in asymptomatic patients. J Vasc Surg 61(3):42S–53S
75. Oglat AA, Matjafri MZ, Suardi N, Oqlat MA, Abdelrahman MA, Oqlat AA (2018) A review of medical doppler ultrasonography of blood flow in general and especially in common carotid artery. J Med Ultrasound 26(1):3–13
76. Lastra G, Syed S, Kurukulasuriya LR, Manrique C, Sowers JR (2014) Type 2 diabetes mellitus and hypertension: an update. Endocrinol Metab Clin N Am 43(1):103–122
77. Cowie CC, Rust KF, Byrd-Holt DD, Eberhardt MS, Flegal KM, Engelgau MM (2006) Prevalence of diabetes and impaired fasting glucose in adults in the U.S. population: National Health And Nutrition Examination Survey 1999–2002. Diabetes Care 29:1263–1268
78. Ogden CL, Carroll MD, Curtin LR, McDowell MA, Tabak CJ, Flegal KM (2006) Prevalence of overweight and obesity in the United States, 1999–2004. JAMA 295:1549–1555
79. Milan-Mattos JC, Anibal FF, Perseguini NM, Minatel V, Rehder-Santos P, Castro CA et al (2009) Effects of natural aging and gender on pro-inflammatory markers. Braz J Med Biol Res 52(9):e8392. https://doi.org/10.1590/1414-431x20198392
80. Kim SH, Reaven G, Lindley S (2011) Relationship between insulin resistance and C-reactive protein in a patient population treated with second generation antipsychotic medications. Int Clin Psychopharmacol 26(1):43–47
81. Marioni RE, Strachan MWJ, Reynolds RM, Lowe DGO, Mitchell RJ, Gerry F et al (2010) Association between raised inflammatory markers and cognitive decline in elderly people with type 2 diabetes. Diabetes 59(3):710–713
82. Chowdhary TA, Lasker SS (2002) Complications and cardiovascular risk factors in South Asians and Europeans with early-onset type 2 diabetes. Q J Med 95:241–246
83. White RJ, Cooper R, Kingsley A (2001) Wound colonization and infection: the role of topical antimicrobials. Br J Nurs 10(9):563–578
84. Williams DT, Hilton JR, Harding KG (2004) Diagnosing foot infection in diabetes. Clin Infect Dis 39(2):S83–S86
85. Al-Hegami MA, Alghalibi SMS, Al-Mamari A (2016) Microorganisms responsible of diabetic foot infection in Taiz City, Yemen. Int J Curr Microbiol App Sci 5(7):431–441
86. Citron DM, Goldstein EJC, Merriam CV, Lipsky BA, Abramson MA (2007) Bacteriology of moderate-to-severe diabetic foot infections and in vitro activity of antimicrobial agents. J Clin Microbiol 45(9):2819–2828
87. Lauterbach S, Kostev K, Kohlmann T (2010) Prevalence of diabetic foot syndrome and its risk factors in the UK. J Wound Care 19:333–337
88. Hicks CW, Shalini S, Mathioudakis N, Sherman RL, Hines KF, Black JK et al (2016) Burden of infected diabetic foot ulcers on hospital admissions and costs. Ann Vasc Surg 33:149–158
89. Labro MT (2000) Interference of antibacterial agents with phagocyte functions: immunomodulation or immuno-fairy tales? Clin Microbiol Rev 13(4):615–650

90. Moxey PW, Gogalniceanu P, Hinchliffe RJ, Loftus IM, Jones KJ, Thompson MM et al (2011) Lower extremity amputations—a review of global variability in incidence. Diabet Med 28:1144–1153
91. Katsilambros N, Dounis E, Makrilakis K, Tentolouris N, Tsapogas P (2010) Atlas of the diabetic foot, 2nd edn. Wiley-Blackwell, Oxford
92. Frykberg RG, Wittmayer B, Zgonis T (2007) Surgical management of diabetic foot infections and osteomyelitis. Clin Podiatr Med Surg 24(3):469–482
93. Bader MS (2008) Diabetic foot infection. Am Fam Physician 78(1):71–79
94. Frykberg RG (2002) Diabetic foot ulcers: pathogenesis and management. Am Fam Physician 66(9):1655–1662
95. Lipsky BA, Berendt AR, Deery HG, Embil JM, Joseph WS, Karchmer AW et al (2004) Diagnosis and treatment of diabetic foot infections. Clin Infect Dis 39(7):885–910
96. Nagoba BS, Gandhi RC, Wadher BJ, Rao A, Hartalkar AR, Selkar SP (2010) A simple and effective approach for the treatment of diabetic foot ulcers with different Wagner grades. Int Wound J 7(3):153–158
97. Lipsky BA, Armstrong DG, Citron DM, Tice AD, Morgenstern DE, Abramson MA (2005) Ertapenem versus piperacillin/tazobactam for diabetic foot infections (SIDESTEP): prospective, randomised, controlled, double-blinded, multicentre trial. Lancet 366(9498):1695–1703
98. Lipsky BA, Giordano P, Choudhri S, Song J (2007) Treating diabetic foot infections with sequential intravenous to oral moxifloxacin compared with piperacillin-tazobactam/amoxicillin-clavulanate. J Antimicrob Chemother 60(2):370–376
99. Jones JD, Ramser HE, Woessner AE, Quinn KP (2018) In vivo multiphoton microscopy detects longitudinal metabolic changes associated with delayed skin wound healing. Commun Biol 1:198
100. WHO. Global reports on diabetes. World Health Organization, Geneva. Available from: http://www.who.int.org. Accessed on 12 Dec 2018
101. Wound Management, Forecast to 2021 (March, 2013): Established and emerging products, technologies and markets in the Americas, Europe, Asia/Pacific and Rest of World, http://woundcare-today.com/news/world-at-glance/projected-global-wound-prevalence-by-wound-types
102. Guo S, DiPietro LA (2010) Factors affecting wound healing. J Dent Res 89(3):219–229
103. Gosain A, DiPietro LA (2004) Aging and wound healing. World J Surg 28(3):321–326
104. Mathieu D, Linke J-C, Wattel F (2006) Non-healing wounds. In: Mathieu DE (ed) Handbook on hyperbaric medicine. Springer, Dordrecht, pp 401–427
105. Vijayaraghavan K, Rajkumar J, Seyed MA (2017) Efficacy of Chromolaena odorata leaf extracts for the healing of rat excision wounds. Vet Med 62:565–578
106. Barrientos S, Brem H, Stojadinovic O, Tomic-Canic M (2014) Clinical application of growth factors and cytokines in wound healing. Wound Repair Regen 22(5):569–578
107. Ozgok KMK, Regan JP (2018) Wound healing. StatPearls Publishing, Treasure Island, FL
108. Koh TJ, DiPietro LA (2013) Inflammation and wound healing: the role of the macrophage. Expert Rev Mol Med 13:e23
109. Parkos CA (2016) Neutrophil-epithelial interactions: a double-edged sword. Am J Pathol 186(6):1404–1416
110. Seyed A (2019) A comprehensive review on phyllanthus derived natural products as potential chemotherapeutic and immunomodulators for a wide range of human diseases. Biocatal Agric Biotechnol 17:529. https://doi.org/10.1016/j.bcab.2019.01.008
111. Avishai E, Yeghiazaryan K, Golubnitschaja O (2017) Impaired wound healing: facts and hypotheses for multi-professional considerations in predictive, preventive and personalised medicine. EPMA J 8(1):23–33
112. Hussein J, Mavalankar DV, Sharma S, D'Ambruoso L (2011) A review of health system infection control measures in developing countries. What can be learned to reduce maternal mortality. Glob Health 7:14

113. Datta T, Patra AK, Dastidar SG (2014) Medicinal plants used by tribal population of Coochbehar district, West Bengal, India-an ethnobotanical survey. Asian Pac J Trop Biomed 4(Suppl 1):S478–S482
114. Kramer A, Dissemond J, Kim S, Willy C, Mayer D, Papke R et al (2018) Consensus on wound antisepsis: update 2018. Skin Pharmacol Physiol 31:28–58
115. Lan CCE, Wu CS, Huang SM, Wu IH, Chen GS (2013) High-glucose environment enhanced oxidative stress and increased interleukin-8 secretion from keratinocytes: new insights into impaired diabetic wound healing. Diabetes 62(7):2530–2538
116. Patil MD, Uma G, Fontaine JL, Meneghini L (2018) Does improving glycemic control accelerate healing of diabetic foot ulcers? Diabetes 67(Suppl 1):2218. https://doi.org/10.2337/db18-2218-PUB
117. Xu J, Wu W, Zhang L, Dorsett-Martin W, Morris MW, Mitchell ME et al (2012) The role of microRNA-146a in the pathogenesis of the diabetic wound healing impairment: correction with mesenchymal stem cell treatment. Diabetes 61(11):2906–2912
118. Tam JAC, Lau KM, Liu CL, To MH, Kwok HF, Lai KK (2011) The *in vivo* and *in vitro* diabetic wound healing effects of a 2-herb formula and its mechanisms of action. J Ethnopharmacol 134(3):831–838
119. Caskey RC, Zgheib C, Morris M, Allukiahj M, Dorsett-Martin W, Xu J et al (2014) Dysregulation of collagen production in diabetes following recurrent skin injury: contribution to the development of chronic wound. Wound Repair Regen 22(4):515–520
120. Snyder RJ (2005) Treatment of non-healing ulcers with allografts. Clin Dermatol 23(4):388–398
121. Mangoni ML, McDermott AM, Zasloff M (2015) Antimicrobial peptides and wound healing: biological and therapeutic considerations. Exp Dermatol 15(1):167–173
122. Perez-Gutierrez RM, Vargas RS (2006) Evaluation of the wound properties of *Acalypha langiana* in diabetic rats. Fitoterapia 77(4):286–289
123. Kim LE, Lee JH, Kim SH, Jung Y (2018) Skin regeneration with self-assembled peptide hydrogels conjugated with substance in a diabetic rat model. Tissue Eng 24(1-2):1–15
124. Attah MO, Jacks TW, Jacob A, Eduitem O, John B (2016) The effect of *Aloe vera* on cutaneous wound healing and wound contraction rate in adult rabbits. Nova J Med Biol Sci 5(3):1–8
125. Oso BJ, Abey N, Oyeleke MO, Olowookere B (2019) Comparative study of the *in vitro* antioxidant properties of methanolic extracts of *Chromolaena odorata* and *Ageratum conyzoides* use in wound healings. Int Ann Sci 6(1):8–12
126. Haque MM, Rafiq SS, Ahmed Q, Mostofa M (2003) Treatment of external wounds by using indigenous medicinal plants and patent drugs in guinea pigs. J Biol Sci 11(5):1126–1133
127. Nayak S (2006) Influence of ethanol extract of *Vinca rosea* on wound healing in diabetic rats. J Biol Sci 6(2):51–55
128. Evans WC (2009) Pharmacognosy, 16th edn. Saunders Elsevier, Edinburgh, pp 3–4
129. Firdous SM, Sautya D (2018) Medicinal plants with wound healing potential. Bangladesh J Pharmacol 13(1):41–52
130. Manisha M, Priyanjali D, Jayant L, Saroj G, Thomas PAD (2007) Indian herbs and herbal drugs used for the treatment of diabetes. J Clin Biochem Nutr 40:163–167
131. Ali-Seyed M, Vijayaraghavan K (2019) Nutraceuticals for wound healing: a special focus on Chromolaena odorata as guardian of health with broad spectrum of biological activities. In: Nutraceuticals in veterinary medicine. Springer International Publishing, Cham, pp 541–562. https://doi.org/10.1007/978-3-030-04624-8_36
132. Oguntibeju OO (2019) Medicinal plants and their effects on diabetic wound healing. Vet World 12(5):653–663
133. Barrett M (2007) The hand book of clinically tested herbal remedies, 1st edn. CBS Publishers and Distributers, New Delhi, pp 3–6
134. Bnouham M, Ziyyat A, Mekhfi H, Tahri A, Legssyer A (2006) Medicinal plants with potential anti-diabetic activity - a review of ten years of herbal research (1990-2000). Int J Diabet Metab 14:1–25
135. Gondwe M, Okoro PK, Juta R (2008) Effect of diabetes on kidney. Diabetes 52:283–291

136. Neyrinck AM, Alligier M, Memvanga PB, Névraumont E, Larondelle Y, Préat V, Cani PD, Delzenne NM (2013) Curcuma longa extract associated with white pepper lessens high fat diet-induced inflammation in subcutaneous adipose tissue. PLoS One 8(11):e81252
137. Atanasov AG, Waltenberger B, Pferschy-Wenzig EM, Linder T, Pavel Uhrin CW, Temml V, Wang L, Schwaiger S, Heiss EH, Rollinger JM, Schuster D, Breuss JM, Bochkov V, Mihovilovic MD, Kopp B, Bauer R, Dirsch VM, Stuppner H (2015) Discovery and resupply of pharmacologically active plant-derived natural products: a review. Biotechnol Adv 33(8):1582–1614
138. Yuan H, Ma Q, Ye L, Piao G (2016) The traditional medicine and modern medicine from natural products. Molecules 21(5):559
139. Vijayaraghavan K, Rajkumar J, Seyed MA (2018) Phytochemical screening, free radical scavenging and antimicrobial potential of Chromolaena odorata leaf extracts against pathogenic bacterium in wound infections– a multispectrum perspective. Biocatal Agric Biotechnol 15:103–112
140. Oubre AY, Carlson TJ, King SR, Reaven GM (1997) From plant to patient: an ethnomedical approach to the identification of new drugs for the treatment of NIDDM. Diabetologia 40:614–617
141. Boulton AJ, Vileikyte L, Ragnarson TG, Apelqvist J (2005) The global burden of diabetic foot disease. Lancet 366:1719–1724
142. Mader JK, Haas W, Aberer F, Boulgaropoulos B, Baumann P, Pandis M et al (2019) Patients with healed diabetic foot ulcer represent a cohort at highest risk for future fatal events. Sci Rep 9(1):10325
143. Lankatillake C, Huynh T, Daniel A (2019) Understanding glycaemic control and current approaches for screening antidiabetic natural products from evidence-based medicinal plants. Plant Methods 15:105. https://doi.org/10.1186/s13007-019-0487-8
144. Choudhury H, Pandey M, Hua CK, Mun CS, Jing CK, Kong L et al (2018) An update on natural compounds in the remedy of diabetes mellitus: a systematic review. J Tradit Complement Med 8(3):361–376
145. Salehi B, Ata AV, Anil Kumar N, Sharopov F, Ramírez-Alarcón K, Ruiz-Ortega A et al (2019) Antidiabetic potential of medicinal plants and their active components. Biomolecules 9(10):551. https://doi.org/10.3390/biom9100551. PMID: 31575072; PMCID: PMC6843349
146. Yeh GY, Eisenberg DM, Kaptchuk TJ, Phillips RS (2003) Systematic review of herbs and dietary supplements for glycemic control in diabetes. Diabetes Care 26:1277–1294
147. Kanetkar P, Singhal R, Kamat M (2007) Gymnema sylvestre. A memoir. J Clin Biochem Nutr 41:77–81
148. Tiwari P, Mishra BN, Sangwan NS (2014) Phytochemical and pharmacological properties of Gymnema sylvestre: an important medicinal plant. Biomed Res Int 2014:830285. https://doi.org/10.1155/2014/830285
149. Daisy P, Eliza J, Mohamed Farook KA (2009) A novel dihydroxy gymnemic triacetate isolated from Gymnema sylvestre possessing normoglycemic and hypolipidemic activity on STZ-induced diabetic rats. J Ethnopharmacol 126:339–344
150. Ramkumar KM, Ponmanickam P, Velayuthaprabhu S, Archunan G, Rajaguru P (2009) Protective effect of Gymnema montanum against renal damage in experimental diabetic rats. Food Chem Toxicol 47:2516–2521
151. Grover JK, Yadav S, Vats V (2002) Medicinal plants of India with anti-diabetic potential. J Ethnopharmacol 81:81–100
152. Ye WC, Zhang QW, Liu X, Che CT, Zhao SX (2000) Oleanane saponins from Gymnema sylvestre. Phytochemistry 53:893–899
153. Surveswaran S, Cai YZ, Xing J, Corke H, Sun M (2010) Antioxidant properties and principal phenolic phytochemicals of Indian medicinal plants from Asclepiadoideae and Periplocoideae. Nat Prod Res 24:206–221
154. Ghorbani A (2013) Best herbs for managing diabetes: a review of clinical studies. Braz J Pharmaceut Sci 49(3):413–422. https://doi.org/10.1590/S1984-82502013000300003

155. El Shafey AAM, El-Ezabi MM, Seliem HHM, Ouda HHM, Ibrahim DS (2013) Effect of Gymnema sylvestre R. Br. leaves extract on certain physiological parameters of diabetic rats. J King Saud Univ Sci 25(2):135–141
156. Patel P, Jyoti S, Lokesh S, Narendra P (2012) Aegle marmelos: a review on its medicinal properties. Int J Pharmaceut Phyto Pharmacol Res 01:332–341
157. Sabu MC, Kuttan R (2004) Antidiabetic activity of Aegle marmelos and its relationship with its antioxidant properties. Indian J Physiol Pharmacol 48(1):81–88
158. Abdallah IZA, Salem IS, Abd El-Salam NAS (2017) Evaluation of antidiabetic and antioxidant activity of Aegle marmelos L. Correa fruit extract in diabetic rats. Egypt J Hosp Med 67(2):731–741
159. Dhankhar S, Ruhil S, Balhara M, Dhankhar S, Chhillar A (2011) Aegle marmelos Correa: a potential source of phytomedicine. J Med Plant Res 5(9):1497–1507
160. Laphookhieo S, Phungpanya C, Tantapakul C, Techa S, Tha-in S, Narmdorkmai W (2011) Chemical constituents from Aegle marmelos. J Braz Chem Sac 22(1):176–178
161. Yadav NP, Chanotia CS (2009) Phytochemical and pharmacological profile of leaves of Aegle marmelos Linn. Pharma Rev:144–149
162. Upadhyay OP, Singh RH, Dutta SK (1996) Studies on antidiabetic medicinal plants used in Indian folk-lore. Sac Ayur 48(10):949–955
163. Grover JK, Yadav SP (2004) Pharmacological actions and potential uses of Momordica charantia: a review. J Ethnopharmacol 93:123–132
164. Hariharan RS, Samal KC, Routray KM, Jayakumar RV, Baiju K, Satyavati GV et al (2005) Efficacy of vijayasar (Pterocarpus marsupium) in the treatment of newly diagnosed patients with type 2 diabetes mellitus: a flexible dose double-blind multicenter randomized controlled trial. Diabetol Croat 34(1):13–20
165. Dhanabal SP, Kokate CK, Ramanathan M, Kumar EP, Suresh B (2006) Hypoglycaemic activity of Pterocarpus marsupium Roxb. Phytother Res 20(1):4–8
166. Mukhtar HM, Ansari SH, Ali M, Bhatt ZA, Naved T (2005) Effect of aqueous extract of Pterocarpus marsupium wood on alloxan-induced diabetic rats. Pharmazie 60(6):478–479
167. Rizvi SI, Mishra N (2013) Traditional Indian medicines used for the management of diabetes mellitus. J Diabetes Res 2013:712092. 11 pages. https://doi.org/10.1155/2013/712092
168. Vats V, Grover JK, Rathi SS (2002) Evaluation of anti-hyperglycemic effect of Trigonella foenum-graecum Linn, Ocimum sanctum Linn and Pterocarpus marsupium Linn in normal and alloxanized diabetic rats. J Ethnopharmacol 79:95–100
169. Sathish Kumar D, Vamshi Sharathnath K, Yogeswaran P, Harani A, Sudhakar K, Sudha P et al (2010) A medicinal potency of Momordica charantia. Int J Pharm Sci Rev Res 1(2):018
170. Virdi J, Sivakami S, Shahani S, Suthar AC, Banavalikar MM, Biyani MK (2003) Antihyperglycemic effects of three extracts from Momordica charantia. J Ethnopharmacol 88:107–111. https://doi.org/10.1016/S0378-8741(03)00184-3
171. Dans AML, Villarruz MVC, Jimeno CA, Javelosa MAU, Chua J, Bautista R et al (2007) The effect of Momordica charantia capsule preparation on glycemic control in type 2 diabetes mellitus needs further studies. J Clin Epidemiol 60:554–559. https://doi.org/10.1016/j.jclinepi.2006.07.009
172. Joseph B, Jini D (2013) Antidiabetic effects of Momordica charantia (bitter melon) and its medicinal potency. Asian Pac J Trop Dis 3(2):93–102. https://doi.org/10.1016/S2222-1808(13)60052-3
173. Raman A, Lau C (1996) Anti-diabetic properties and phytochemistry of Momordica charantia L. (Cucurbitaceae). Phytomedicine 2:349–362. https://doi.org/10.1016/S0944-7113(96)80080-8
174. Jayasooriya AP, Sakono M, Yukizaki C, Kawano M, Yamamoto K, Fukuda N (2000) Effects of Momordica charantia powder on serum glucose levels and various lipid parameters in rats fed with cholesterol-free and cholesterol-enriched diets. J Ethnopharmacol 72:331–236
175. Leung L, Birtwhistle R, Kotecha J, Hannah S, Cuthbertson S (2009) Anti-diabetic and hypoglycaemic effects of Momordica charantia (bitter melon): a mini review. Br J Nutr 102:1703–1708

176. Arafat SY, Nayeem M, Jahan S, Karim Z, Reza HM, Hossain MH et al (2016) Ellagic acid rich Momordica charantia fruit pulp supplementation prevented oxidative stress, fibrosis and inflammation in liver of alloxan induced diabetic rats. Orient Pharm Exp Med 16:267–278
177. Ahmed I, Lakhani MS, Gillett M, John A, Raza H (2001) Hypotriglyceridemic and hypocholesterolemic effects of anti-diabetic Momordica charantia (karela) fruit extract in streptozotocin-induced diabetic rats. Diabetes Res Clin Pract 51:155–161
178. Czompa A, Gyongyosi A, Szoke K, Bak I, Csepanyi E, Haines DD et al (2017) Effects of Momordica charantia (Bitter Melon) on ischemic diabetic myocardium. Molecules 22(3):E488. https://doi.org/10.3390/molecules22030488
179. Thent ZC, Das S, Zaidun NH (2018) Emerging trends on drug delivery strategy of Momordica charantia against diabetes and its complications. Curr Drug Deliv 15(4):453–460
180. Huang T, Lu KN, Pai YP, Hsu C, Huang C (2013) Role of GLP-1 in the hypoglycemic effects of wild bitter gourd. Evid Based Complement Alternat Med 2013:625892
181. Jia S, Shen M, Zhang F, Xie J (2017) Recent advances in Momordica charantia: functional components and biological activities. Int J Mol Sci 18(12):E2555. https://doi.org/10.3390/ijms18122555
182. Mahmoud MF, Zahraa F, Ashry Z, El Maraghy NN, Fahmy A (2017) Studies on the antidiabetic activities of Momordica charantia fruit juice in streptozotocin-induced diabetic rats. Pharm Biol 55(1):758–765
183. Harinantenaina L, Tanaka M, Takaoka S, Oda M, Mogami O, Uchida M et al (2006) Momordica charantia constituents and antidiabetic screening of the isolated major compounds. Chem Pharm Bull 54:1017–1021. https://doi.org/10.1248/cpb.54.1017
184. Reyes BAS, Bautista ND, Tanquilut NC, Anunciado RV, Leung AB, Sanchez GC et al (2006) Anti-diabetic potentials of Momordica charantia and Andrographis paniculata and their effects on estrous cyclicity of alloxan-induced diabetic rats. J Ethnopharmacol 105:196–200
185. Fernandes NP, Lagishetty CV, Panda VS, Naik SR (2007) An experimental evaluation of the antidiabetic and antilipidemic properties of a standardized Momordica charantia fruit extract. BMC Complement Altern Med 7:29. https://doi.org/10.1186/1472-6882-7-2
186. Birhane G (2012) Effect of processing on phytochemicals and nutrients composition of fenugreek (Trigonella foenum-graecum L.), and development of value added products. Doctoral dissertation, AAU
187. Meghwal M, Goswami TK (2012) A review on the functional properties, nutritional content, medicinal utilization and potential application of fenugreek. J Food Process Technol 3:181. https://doi.org/10.4172/2157-7110.1000181
188. Khan V, Najmi AK, Akhtar M, Aqil M, Mujeeb M, Pillai KK (2012) A pharmacological appraisal of medicinal plants with antidiabetic potential. J Pharm Bioallied Sci 4:27–42
189. Prasanna M (2000) Hypolipidemic effect of fenugreek: diabetic patients: a clinical study. Indian J Pharm 32:34–36
190. Dangi RS, Lagu MD, Choudhary LB, Ranjekar PK, Gupta VS (2004) Assessment of genetic diversity in Trigonella foenum-graecum and Trigonella caerulea using ISSR and RAPD markers. BMC Plant Biol 4(1):13
191. Gauttam VK, Kalia AN (2013) Development of polyherbal antidiabetic formulation encapsulated in the phospholipids vesicle system. J Adv Pharm Technol Res 4:108–117
192. Geberemeskel GA, Debebe YG, Nguse NA (2019) Antidiabetic effect of fenugreek seed powder solution (Trigonella foenum-graecum L.) on hyperlipidemia in diabetic patients. Clinical study 2019. J Diabetes Res 2019:8507453. 8 pages
193. Saravanan G, Ponmurugan P, Deepa MA, Senthilkumar B (2014) Modulatory effects of diosgenin on attenuating the key enzymes activities of carbohydrate metabolism and glycogen content in streptozotocin induced diabetic rats. Can J Diabetes 38:409–414
194. Joshi DV, Patil RR, Naik SR (2015) Hydroalcohol extract of Trigonella foenum graecum seed attenuates markers of inflammation and oxidative stress while improving exocrine function in diabetic rats. Pharm Biol 53:201–211
195. Mooventhan A, Nivethitha L (2017) A narrative review on evidence-based antidiabetic effect of fenugreek (Trigonella Foenum-Graecum). Int J Nutr Pharmacol Neurol Dis 7:84–87

196. Zia T, Hasnain SN, Hasan SK (2001) Evaluation of the oral hypoglycemic effect of Trigonella foenum-graecum in normal mice. J Ethanopharmacol 75:191–195
197. Mowla A, Alauddin M, Rahman MA, Ahmed K (2009) Antihyperglycemic effect of Trigonella Foenum-Graecum (Fenugreek) seed extract in alloxan-induced diabetic rats and its use in diabetes mellitus: a brief qualitative phytochemical and acute toxicity test on the extract. Afr J Trad Compl Altern Med 6(3):255–261
198. Khlifi S, Jemaa HB, Hmad HB, Abaza H, Karmous I, Abid A et al (2016) Antioxidant, anti-diabetic and antihyperlipidemic effects of Trigonella foenum-graecum seeds. Int J Pharmacol 12(4):394–400
199. Kumar B, Gupta SK, Nag TC, Srivastava S, Saxena R (2012) Green tea prevents hyperglycemia-induced retinal oxidative stress and inflammation in streptozotocin-induced diabetic rats. Ophthalmic Res 47:103–108. https://doi.org/10.1159/000330051
200. Oyetayo VO, Oyetayo FL (2006) Phytochemical screening and antibacterial properties of siam weed, Chromolaena odorata, leaf against aerobic isolates of wound. J Appl Environ Sci 2(1):7–11
201. Vital P, Rivera W (2009) Antimicrobial activity and cytotoxicity of Chromolaena odorata (L. f.) King and Robinson and Uncaria perrottetii (A. Rich) Merr. extracts. J Med Plants Res 3(7):511–518
202. Mahmood AA, Indran M, Salmah I, Sidix K, Suzainur KA (2005) Evaluation of *in vivo* wound healing activity of *Chromolaena odorata* leaf extract on excision wounds model in rats. J Food Technol 3:126–129
203. Chakraborty AK, Sujit R, Umesh KP (2011) Chromolaena odorata. An overview. J Pharm Res 43:573–576
204. Akinmoladun AC, Obuotor EM, Farombi EO (2010) Evaluation of antioxidant and free radical scavenging capacities of some Nigerian indigenous medicinal plants. J Med Food 13:444–451
205. Vijayaraghavan K, Rajkumar J, Seyed MA (2017) Efficacy of *Chromolaena odorata* leaf extracts for the healing of rat excision wounds. Vet Med 62:565–578
206. Kigigha LT, Zige DV (2013) Activity of Chromolaena odorata on enteric and superficial etiologic bacterial agents. Am J Res Commun 1:266–276
207. Stanley MC, Ifeanyi OE, Nwakaego CC, Esther IO (2014) Antimicrobial effects of Chromolaena odorata on some human pathogens. Int J Curr Microbiol App Sci 3:1006–1012
208. Yahya MFZR, Ibrahim MSA, Zawaw WHA, Hamid UMA (2014) Biofilm killing effects of Chromolaena odorata extracts against Pseudomonas aeruginosa. Res J Phytochem 8:64–73
209. Alisi CS, Onyeze GOC, Ojiako OA, Osuagwu CG (2011) Evaluation of the protective potential of Chromolaena odorata Linn. Extract on carbon tetrachloride-induced oxidative liver damage. Int J Biochem Res Rev 1:69–81
210. Sukanya SL, Sudisha J, Prakash HS, Fathima SK (2011) Isolation and characterization of antimicrobial compound from Chromolaena odorata. J Phytol 3:26–32
211. Murthy O, Veerapur VP, Thippeswamy BS, Reddy TN, Rayappa H, Badami S (2013) Anti-diabetic and anti-cataract effects of Chromolaena odorata Linn.; In streptozotocin-induced diabetic rats. J Ethnopharmacol 145(1):363–372
212. Omonije OO, Saidu AN, Muhammad HL (2019) Anti-diabetic activities of Chromolaena Odorata methanol root extract and its attenuation effect on diabetic induced hepatorenal impairment in rats. Clin Phytosci 5:23. https://doi.org/10.1186/s40816-019-0115-1
213. Anyasor GN, Aina DA, Olushola M, Aniyikawe AF (2011) Phytochemical constituents, proximate analysis, antioxidants, anti-bacterial and wound healing properties of leaf extracts of Chromolaena odorata. Ann Biol Res 2:441–451
214. Obey JK, Wright AV, Orjala J, Kauhanen J, Tikkanen-Kaukanen C (2016) Antimicrobial activity of Croton macrostachyus stem bark extracts against several human pathogenic bacteria. J Pathog 2016:1453428. https://doi.org/10.1155/2016/1453428
215. Akinpelu DA, Kolawole DO (2004) Phytochemistry and antimicrobial activity of leaf extract of *Piliostigma thonningii* (Schum). Sci Focus 7:64–70

216. Janarthanam B, Sumathi E (2010) *In vitro* plant regeneration from shoot tip explants of *Exacum travancoricum* Beedi. Plant Tissue Cult Biotech 20:113–118
217. Cespedes CL, El-Hafidi M, Pavon N, Alacorn J (2008) Antioxidant and cardioprotective activities of phenolic extracts from models for fruits of Chilean blackberry Aristotelia chiliensis (Elaeocarpaceae). Maqui Food Chem 107:820–829
218. Reddy BP, Raghavulu SV, Ramakrishna S, Venkateteswarlu Y, Diwan PV (2008) Evaluation of antioxidant and antimicrobial properties of Soymida febrifuga leaf extracts. Phytother Res 22:943–947
219. Sirinthipaporn A, Jiraungkoorskul W (2017) Wound healing property review of siam weed, Chromolaena odorata. Pharmacogn Rev 11(21):35–38
220. Mazid M, Khan TA, Mohammad F (2011) Role of secondary metabolites in defense mechanisms of plants. Biol Med 3:232–249
221. Britto JD, Sebastian SD (2011) Biosynthesis of silver nanoparticles and its antibacterial activity against human. Int J Pharm Sci 5:257–259
222. Ruchi T, Kumaragurubaran K, Rajneesh R, Yashpal SM, Kuldeep D, Sunil KJ (2016) Quorum sensing inhibitors/antagonists Countering food spoilage bacteria-need Molecular and pharmaceutical intervention for protecting current issues of food safety. Int J Pharmacol 12:262–271
223. Lavanya G, Brahmaprakash GP (2011) Phytochemical screening and antimicrobial activity of compounds from selected medicinal and aromatic plants. Int J Sci Nat 2:287–291
224. Li X, Qu L, Dong Y, Han L, Liu E, Fang S et al (2014) A review of recent research progress on the Astragalus Genus. Molecules 19(11):18850–18880
225. Amy GW, Gong RD, Wang HY, Kong XP, Dong TTX, Tsim KWK et al (2018) Evaluation of the pharmaceutical properties and value of Astragali Radix. Medicines (Basel) 5(2):46. https://doi.org/10.3390/medicines5020046
226. State Pharmacopoeia Commission of P.R. China (2010) Pharmacopoeia of the People's Republic of China, vol 1. China Medico-Pharmaceutical Science & Technology Publishing House, Beijing
227. Xu XL, Ji H, Gu SY, Shao Q, Huang QJ, Cheng YP (2008) Cardioprotective effects of Astragali Radix against isoproterenol-induced myocardial injury and its possible mechanism. Phytother Res 22:389–394
228. Zhao P, Su G, Xiao X, Hao E, Zhu X, Ren J (2008) Chinese medicinal herb Radix Astragali suppresses cardiac contractile dysfunction and inflammation in a rat model of autoimmune myocarditis. Toxicol Lett 182:29–35
229. Zhang RP, Zhang XP, Ruan YF, Ye SY, Zhao HC, Cheng QH et al (2009) Protective effect of Radix Astragali injection on immune organs of rats with obstructive jaundice and its mechanism. World J Gastroenterol 15:2862–2869
230. Liu P, Zhao H, Luo Y (2017) Anti-aging implications of Astragalus Membranaceus (Huangqi): a well-known Chinese tonic. Aging Dis 8(6):868–886
231. Xu A, Wang H, Hoo RL, Sweeney G, Vanhoutte PM, Wang Y et al (2009) Selective elevation of adiponectin production by the natural compounds derived from a medicinal herb alleviates insulin resistance and glucose intolerance in obese mice. Endocrinology 150:625–633
232. Hoo RL, Wong JY, Qiao C, Xu A, Xu H, Lam KS (2010) The effective fraction isolated from Radix Astragali alleviates glucose intolerance insulin resistance and hypertriglyceridemia in db/db diabetic mice through its anti-inflammatory activity. Nutr Metabol 7:67–78
233. Juan YC, Kuo YH, Chang CC, Zhang LJ, Lin YY, Hsu CY et al (2011) Administration of a decoction of sucrose- and polysaccharide-rich Radix Astragali (huang qi) ameliorated insulin resistance and fatty liver but affected beta-cell function in type 2 diabetic rats. Evid Based Compl Altern Med 2011:349807. https://doi.org/10.1155/2011/349807
234. Lau T, Chan YW, Lau CP, Chan CM, Lau C, Fung KP et al (2007) Investigation of the effects of Chinese medicine on fibroblast viability: implications in wound healing. Phytother Res 21:938–947. https://doi.org/10.1002/ptr.2191
235. Lau TW, Chan YW, Lau CP, Lau KM, Lau CBS, Fung KP et al (2009) Radix Astragali and Radix Rehmanniae the principal components of two anti-diabetic foot ulcer herbal formulae,

elicit viability-promoting effects on primary fibroblasts cultured from diabetic foot ulcer tissues. Phytother Res 23:809–815
236. Kim J, Moon E, Kwon S (2014) Effect of Astragalus membranaceus extract on diabetic nephropathy. Endoc Diabet Metab Case Rep 2014:140063. https://doi.org/10.1530/EDM-14-0063
237. Cui K, Zhang S, Jiang X, Xie W (2016) Novel synergic antidiabetic effects of Astragalus polysaccharides combined with Crataegus flavonoids via improvement of islet function and liver metabolism. Mol Med Rep 13:4737–4744
238. Ma X, Shi Q, Duan J, Dong T (2002) Chemical analysis of Radix Astragali (Huangqi) in China: a comparison with its adulterants and seasonal variations. J Agric Food Chem 50:4861–4866. https://doi.org/10.1021/jf0202279
239. Yu QT, Qi LW, Li P, Yi L, Zhao J, Bi Z (2007) Determination of seventeen main flavonoids and saponins in the medicinal plant Huang-qi (Radix astragali) by HPLC-DAD-ELSD. J Sep Sci 30:1292–1299
240. Zhang Y, Hu G, Lin HC, Hong SJ, Deng YH, Tang JY et al (2009) Radix Astragali extract promotes angiogenesis involving vascular endothelial growth factor receptor-related phosphatidylinositol 3-kinase/Akt-dependent pathway in human endothelial cells. Phytother Res 23:1205–1213
241. Tang JY, Li S, Li ZH, Zhang ZJ, Hu G, Cheang LC et al (2010) Calycosin promotes angiogenesis involving estrogen receptor and mitogen-activated protein kinase (MAPK) signaling pathway in zebrafish and HUVEC. PLoS One 5:e11822. (Electronic Resource)
242. Zhang RX, Li MX, Jia ZP (2008) Rehmannia glutinosa: review of botany chemistry and pharmacology. J Ethnopharmacol 117:199–214
243. Li ZF, Yang YQ, Xie DF, Zhu LF, Zhang DG, Lin WX (2012) Identification of autotoxic compounds in fibrous roots of Rehmannia (Rehmannia glutinosa Libosch.). PLoS One 7(1):e28806. https://doi.org/10.1371/journal.pone.0028806
244. Shi CJ, Wen XS, Gao HF, Liu ZH, Xu XK, Li LF et al (2016) Steamed root of Rehmannia glutinosa Libosch (Plantaginaceae) alleviates methotrexate-induced intestinal mucositis in rats. J Ethnopharmacol 183:143–150
245. Gong W, Zhang N, Cheng G, Zhang Q, He Y, Shen Y et al (2019) Rehmannia glutinosa Libosch extracts prevent bone loss and architectural deterioration and enhance osteoblastic bone formation by regulating the IGF-1/PI3K/mTOR pathway in streptozotocin-induced diabetic rats. Int J Mol Sci 20:3964
246. Yokozawa T, Kim HY, Yamabe N (2004) Amelioration of diabetic nephropathy by dried Rehmanniae Radix (Di Huang) extract. Am J Chin Med 32:829–839
247. Lau TW, Sahota DS, Lau CH, Chan CM, Lam FC, Ho YY et al (2008) An in vivo investigation on the wound-healing effect of two medicinal herbs using an animal model with foot ulcer. Eur Surg Res 41:15–23
248. Lau TW, Lam FF, Lau KM, Chan YW, Lee KM, Sahota DS et al (2009) Pharmacological investigation on the wound healing effects of Radix Rehmanniae in an animal model of diabetic foot ulcer. J Ethnopharmacol 123:155–162
249. Zhang R, Zhou J, Jia Z, Zhang Y, Gu G (2004) Hypoglycemic effect of Rehmannia glutinosa oligosaccharide in hyperglycemic and alloxan-induced diabetic rats and its mechanism. J Ethnopharmacol 90:39–43
250. Waisundara VY, Huang M, Hsu A, Huang D, Tan BK (2008) Characterization of the antidiabetic and antioxidant effects of Rehmannia glutinosa in streptozotocin-induced diabetic Wistar rats. Am J Chin Med 36:1083–1104
251. Wong MWN, Leung PC, Wong WC (2001) Limb salvage in extensive diabetic foot ulceration-a preliminary clinical study using simple debridement and herbal drinks. Hong Kong Med J 7(4):403–407
252. Nunan R, Harding KG, Martin P (2014) Clinical challenges of chronic wounds: searching for an optimal animal model to recapitulate their complexity. Dis Model Mech 7(11):1205–1213

253. Phan TT, Hughes MA, Cherry GW (2001) Effects of an aqueous extract from the leaves of Chromolaena odorata on the proliferation of human keratinocytes and on their migration in an in vitro model of epithelialization. Wound Repair Regen 9(4):305–313
254. Suguna L, Singh S, Sivakumar P, Sampath P, Chandrasekaran G (2002) Influence of Terminalia chebula on dermal wound healing in rats. Phytother Res 16(3):227–231
255. Esimone CO, Nworu CS, Jackson CL (2009) Cutaneous wound healing activity of a herbal ointment containing the leaf extract of Jatropha curcas. Int J Appl Res Nat Prod 1(4):1–4
256. Okoli CO, Akah PA, Okoli AS (2007) Potentials of leaves of Aspilia africana in wound care: an experimental evaluation. BMC Complement Altern Med 27(3):24
257. Majumder M, Nayeen N, Kamati JV, Asad M (2005) Evaluation of Tectona grandis leaves for wound healing activity. Pak J Pharm Sci 20(2):120–124
258. Thakur R, Jain N, Pathak R, Sandhu SS (2011) Practices in wound healing studies of plants. Evid Based Complement Alternat Med 2011:1–17
259. Suntar P, Koca U, Akkol EK, Yilmazer D, Alper M (2011) Assessment of wound healing activity of the aqueous extracts of Calutea cilicica. Evid Based Complement Alternat Med 2011:1–7. Accessed 16 May 2018

Management of Diabetic Foot Ulcer by *Hirudo medicinalis*, the "Healing Leech"

19

Sumbul Rehman

19.1 Introduction and Prevalence

Diabetic Foot Ulcer (DFU) is a chronic open wound on the bottom of the foot, a most common lower extremity complication of prolonged and poorly controlled blood sugar level in 15–25% of diabetes patients [1]. It occurs due to two main severe complications viz. Diabetic neuropathy and peripheral vascular disease. Among this, 14–25% of patients got complications to an extent that it needs to be amputated due to complications [2], and thus it has become the leading cause of nontraumatic lower extremity amputations in the USA. And it is observed that at every 30 s, a lower limb amputation is carried out due to diabetes throughout the world. The mortality rate due to diabetic foot gangrene is just next to that of cancer.

Diabetic foot ulcer is more prevalent in men as compared to women with a fasting blood sugar level of 220 mg (%) [2]. Mostly found in Native Americans, African Americans, Hispanics [3], and older men, patients using insulin or with diabetic-related multiple organopathy like kidney, eye, or heart. The use of alcohol or tobacco or being overweight may also play an important role in its progression.

With the continuous uncontrolled rise in blood sugar level, numerous problems arise which lead to vessel diseases that limit or prevent blood from reaching the toes, fingers, hands, and feet. When blood flow becomes severely restricted, the affected tissue can die. This is the leading cause of amputation among people with diabetes. Losing a digit or limb due to complications from diabetes is a major concern for millions of people worldwide. The most effective way to stop this process is to increase circulation to the affected tissues without the risk of blood clots. Various clinical studies have reported that leech therapy can play a vital role in healing the ulcer.

S. Rehman (✉)
Department of Ilmul Advia (Unani Pharmacology), Faculty of Unani Medicine, Aligarh Muslim University, Aligarh, Uttar Pradesh, India

M. Zubair et al. (eds.), *Diabetic Foot Ulcer*,
https://doi.org/10.1007/978-981-15-7639-3_19

19.1.1 DFU in Type 1 and Type 2 Diabetes Mellitus

Diabetic foot ulcer is a chronic ulcer, chronicity in terms of its nonhealing after appropriate treatment for 3 months, and is unable to heal even after continuous treatment for 12 months and its grading varies with complication [4]. It is usually found to be of grade 4 or 5.

For many years diabetic wound ulcer was classified as per Meggitt-Wagner ulcer classification system (Table 19.1) [5].

Wagner's classification was later revised by Brodsky [6], to assess the depth of the lesion and ischemic changes in DFUs, to ease the treatment modalities in diabetic neuropathy (Table 19.2).

- *Depth of lesion*—Graded from 0 (when there is no break in the skin) to 3 (presence of abscess, or exposed bone, osteomyelitis), and 4 (necrotic foot area) to 5 (entire foot get necrotic).
- *Ischemic changes*—Graded from A (No Ischemia) to D (Complete Gangrene).

And recently diabetic foot classification is remodified, as it gets beyond ulceration too and infection may or may not be present in DFU. So, as diabetes has been classified as type 1 and type 2 diabetes mellitus; its complication has been classified into three (Table 19.3) [7].

Among these Type 1 diabetic foot complications accounts for 86.6–91.06% admission to the hospitals that may occur individually or in combination and thus become the major cause of amputation.

Table 19.1 Meggitt-Wagner classification of foot ulcers

Grade	Description of the ulcer
0	Pre- or post-ulcerative lesion completely epithelialized
1	Superficial, full-thickness ulcer limited to the dermis, not extending to the subcutis
2	Ulcer of the skin extending through the subcutis with exposed tendon or bone and without osteomyelitis or abscess formation
3	Deep ulcers with osteomyelitis or abscess formation
4	Localized gangrene of the toes or the forefoot
5	Foot with extensive gangrene

Table 19.2 Bodsky's modification in Wagner classification of wound ulcers

	0	1	2	3	4	5
A	Callus or scar	Superficial wound	Wound penetrating to tendon/capsule	Wound penetrating to bone/joint	Necrotic foot areas	Necrotic foot, entire
B	Infection	Infection	Infection	Infection	Infection	Infection
C	Ischemia	Ischemia	Ischemia	Ischemia	Ischemia	Ischemia
D	Infection + ischemia	Infection + ischemia	Infection + ischemia	Infection + ischemia	Infection + ischemia	Infection + ischemia

Table 19.3 Classification of diabetic foot ulcer based on lesions

S. No.	Type of lesions observed	Type of diabetes	Nature of ulcer
1.	Cellulitis, wet gangrene, abscess, necrotizing fasciitis, osteomyelitis, etc.	Type 1 diabetes foot complication	Infective DFU
2.	Nonhealing ulcers, peripheral arterial disease, hammer toes, entrapment neuropathies, diabetic neuro-osteoarthropathy, etc.	Type 2 diabetes foot complication	Non-infective DFU
3.	Like-charcot foot with infected ulcer, nonhealing ulcer with osteomyelitis, etc.	Type 2 diabetes foot complication	Mixed DFU

19.1.2 Pathophysiology and Clinical Presentation of DFU

Along with the severity of glucose level in the blood with time, its formation is due to the combinatorial factors such as foot deformity, traumatic conditions, lesser blood flow toward the extremities, neuropathy which lead to reduced or complete lack of sensations. Presence of vascular diseases worsens the condition, as the ability of the body to fight infection already got reduced due to diabetes and it further got complicated by reducing its ability to heal at the site and thus there always remains a chance for an infection.

Prolonged Sugar level with associated complications proceeds to develop cracks in the feet which turn into chronic wound ulcers, as a result of a combination of growth factor fabrication, accumulation of collagen, fibrosis, and abnormal pressure. It is soon encroached by the inflammatory response which lasts longer, inflammatory cells like neutrophils; macrophages, T-lymphocytes, fibroblasts, and prostaglandin E2 (PGE2) secrete enzymes that result in pain, redness, warmth, and swelling indispensable for the healing cascade [8]. And DFU is characterized by a series of exasperated and extended inflammatory response.

It is clinically manifested by loss of sensation in lower extremities; redness and swelling at the bottom of the foot along with some exudate of purulent odor. To confirm, superficial pain perception along with temperature, light, and pressure sensation is examined. Sometime when peripheral neuropathy predominates it is represented as muscle cramps in both the limbs along with burning sensation; pins and needles; shooting, sharp, or stabbing pains; which aggravate at night often worse, which are usually present in peripheral neuropathy [5]. In such cases, Neuropathy Symptom Score (NSS) is adopted which is considered a high predictive value to screen for peripheral neuropathy in diabetes [9].

As tissue death cannot be reversed, surgical removal of the affected tissue (debridement) or amputation of the limb is the only treatment option left when gangrene has advanced. Thus foot ulceration precedes 85% of diabetes-related amputations in the USA [10]. But researches have shown that its development can be prevented and amputation rate can be minimized by some preventions or following some alternate therapies like leech therapy/Hirudinotherapy.

19.1.3 Prophylaxis and Treatment of DFU in Molecular Science

DFUs are associated with complexities of vascular disease and ischemia which delays healing. Atherosclerosis along with ischemia contributes to amputation in 90% diabetic patients [8]. Capillary thickening produces inelasticity, vasoconstriction and condition worsened with the over-loaded microbial growth; so, its treatment becomes more perplex as lack of sterility delays healing.

It seems to be a great challenge to manage the wound if some basic principles are not routinely followed. So, paramount care is needed while thoroughly examining the patient's condition. A comprehensive systemic approach to assess and treat by elucidating underlying areas of concern need to be specifically addressed which leads to favorable outcomes. Due to variation in the complexity of the diabetic patient and wound condition, it is mostly represented by variation in clinical condition. In such cases, a multidisciplinary approach, molecular as well as holistic approach is recommended to attain higher success rate in improving patient condition. Medical/holistic management of the patient must commence concurrently with wound management [11].

Diabetic patients recurrently need improved control of their hyperglycemia, renal insufficiency, sustenance, and other associated medical comorbidities that may adversely distress the healing of wound. DFU can be prevented by following regular podiatric care immediately and its treatment always aims to reduce the risk of infection and amputation and thus, improving the quality of life and reduce health care costs. It can be attained if the emphasis is given on healing, faster the healing, lesser will be the chances for an infection.

The key to successful wound healing is regular podiatric medical care to ensure the following "gold standard" of care taken sequentially:

- Off-loading—reducing the pressure from the area.
- Removal of the dead skin debris.
- Proper cleaning and use of medications in dressings or therapies of the ulcer.
- Use of antibiotics, if infected.
- Improving blood circulation.
- Prevention of infection.
- Management of blood glucose level and other health ailments associated.
- Surgery: though a number of noninfected foot ulcer can be treated without any surgeries, but in some cases, certain excision of bone(s) is needed to be done to reduce the pressure on the affected site or to correct the deformity like bony unions, hammertoes.

Earlier it was a practice "to let the wound open." But in the present era with polluted air, this will worsen the condition. It is quite evident that open wounds give a nice diet for microorganism present in the air and give rise to infection. So, they must be kept covered and moist by dressings with proper topical medications. Healing time varies with the available condition of ulcer, but appropriate wound management enhances the speed of the healing process [8, 12].

Although allopathic medicine offers an enormous amount of treatment modalities to heal the ulcer in every respect including lumbar sympathectomy or spinal cord stimulation as a part of neurovascular interventions; negative pressure wound therapy (NPWT), electromagnetic stimulation or enhanced local oxygen therapy for local mechanical therapy; vasoactive growth factors or tissue-engineered skin product for topical therapy; systemic therapy with hyperbaric oxygen or intravenous therapy with agents such as prostaglandins [12–16].

Besides the higher cost and time taken to heal DFU before it reaches the dreadful condition of being amputated, these nonhealing diabetic wounds remain to mystify. And unfortunately, in spite of having all such great scientific technologies, newer strides observed in technological innovations with a wide range of treatment for wounds in the present century, these ulcers remain to perplex and encounter the healers [16, 17].

It demands non-surgical approaches to be introduced to aid the wound management [18]. So, an attempt should be made to combine it with the traditional practices that were followed in ancient times to overcome such dreadful conditions along with the present-day treatment. It is evident that wound healing can be enhanced by improving blood circulation to the ulcerated site which can be attained with non-invasive methods like Medical leech therapy (MLT).

19.2 Therapeutic Bleeding by Medicinal Leech Therapy (MLT)/Hirudinotherapy: A Medical Basis

19.2.1 Historical Background

Since ancient times, physicians formed the elite, the upper crust of the medical system from where the bloodletting through leech therapy arrived. Being a humankind's belief about "blood" which flows through the veins of history, it was observed that nature expulsion of blood in the form of menstruation lead to an idea of therapeutic bleeding—phlebotomy; and thus bloodletting was performed by venesection, wet cupping or leeching. It sounds to be a traditional practice of Medieval era, but studies of the nineteenth century confirm its scientific use in certain health ailments.

Leech like hematophagous animals have been used since ancient times for a series of biologically active compounds present in their saliva especially the anticoagulant factor, which prevent blood clotting. Historically, their use date backs to ancient Egypt and the beginning of civilization by ancient Egyptians, Indians, Arabs, and Greeks [19]. Promising property of its substantial use in medicine lies in its own meaning, as the word "Leech" is derived from an AngloSaxon word "Laece" which means "to heal" and thus they are used since then as a means of local depletion (bloodletting) [20, 21]. Historically they are first reported by a pupil of Aesculapius, Themison (80–40 BC) in Greece and the oldest therapeutic book about leech is Leech-dom [22]. Avicenna (980–1037 AD)-an eminent Unani Physician also delineated in his famous encyclopedia "Canon of Medicine," that leech can suck blood from deep veins which cannot be reached by the conventional wet cupping and he acclaimed leeching for skin diseases. Later, it is reported to be found in a painting in an Egyptian Tomb of around 1500 BC, and in twelfth century, Abdul Latif Baghdadi also cites its therapeutic use after surgery. Ibn Maseehi (1233–1286 AD) has also detailed about the two forms of leeches in his treatise "*Umda Fi Jarahat*"—detailed basic treasure of surgery and differentiated the medical leeches from the nonmedical (poisonous) ones according to their shape and color [23]. It was also well mentioned in the literature of Ayurvedic System of Medicine as evident in Sushruta Samhita [19, 51, 52]. Renaissance of its medical journey reached its zenith in seventeenth and eighteenth century AD in Europe, while it was in use by Arabs for bloodletting.

It predates the medieval era by a substantial chunk of time, although their popularity does not remain to be constant, it varied with time. Their revival from the benighted era reached its zenith in early nineteenth century and reached to its peak in Europe between 1825 and 1850 to an extent that supplies become exhausted, 50,000 leeches were used during the course of 1831 by the Manchester Royal Infirmary, in the UK, in France "Leech Farms" were unable to meet the demand and in 1833, over 41,500,000 leeches were imported into France, and only nine or ten million exported. In one of the instances Richard Arnold, a Savannah physician, in 1838 complain regarding the cost of leech to be "only in the reach of the rich," when they were sold at 50 cents each [20, 24]. Later they were used by the physicians of the emperor and influential academic surgeons, but then it saw a downfall toward the end of the century, as it become associated with lay therapist and quackery.

With the advent of "germ theory," the western medicine reached to its peak, and the leech therapy was considered as "the myth of the past" and gradually lost the favor. Bloodletting using leeches and other methods enjoyed resumption in the early nineteenth century, particularly in France, when in 1922 Surgeon Termier recommended direct application of leech, and he described it as "hirudinization of the blood," renowned scientist Bottenberg also established the general indication of leech therapy in 1935 [25]. Later, MLT enjoyed an International come back in 1960 when many scientific researches took interest in their use for microsurgeries because of their promising effect shown in postoperative venous congestion and graft rejections. And, it was on such a big scale that a specific medicinal leech farm first of its kind was established in Swansea in 1981 by Dr. Roy Sawyer which now supplies leeches to the hospitals all over the world [23]. Leech therapy further got the new impulse of treatment modality after initial publications by Upton's group in 1980s [25, 26].

Researches remain to be continued for its beneficial use in many clinical conditions. And, it was found to be effective in sustaining retrieval of compromised microvascular free tissue transfer, and it was observed that the salvage of compromised, venous congested tissues can be improved by early application of leech. They help to improve blood flow to regions where it has slowed or stopped, thus prevent tissue death. This caused a renaissance of leech therapy and now they are used for their therapeutic value globally. Although many complaints were made regarding the continuous oozing of blood from the site of leech bite even after its withdrawal, but later this phenomenon was explained by John Berry Haycroft, a

Birmingham chemist in 1884. He discovered the presence of an anticoagulant "hirudin" which is injected by the leeches in the blood that keeps it flowing through the capillaries [27].

And the twenty-first century has revealed a number of studies, which confirms its efficacy in many health ailments like circulatory disorders, skin diseases, arthritis, etc. Now, leech sale and its use have been permitted, only for its use in microsurgeries and plastic surgeries by the Food and Drug Authority of USA (FDA) [26].

19.2.2 Medicinal Leeches

There are more than 600 leech species which belong to the Class Hirudinea which in habitat aquatic (ponds, streams, lake, and the sea) as well as moist terrestrial regions. They are widespread in many parts of the world with great abundance in North America, Europe, and Southeast Asia. Among various species present globally, European medical leech *Hirudo medicinalis*—specifically known as "Healing Leech," is preferred over American species *Hirudo decora*, as it sucks less blood through its superficial incision. There are other species too, which vary in length and their ability to suck the blood used for therapeutic bloodletting such as *Hirudinaria manillensis*, *Hirudo nipponia*, *Hirudo verbena*, and *Hirudo orientalis* [28] (Fig. 19.1).

Hirudo medicinalis belong to the Phylum Annelida; a family of "fresh-water parasitic invertebrates." They are hermaphrodite, multi-segmented, carnivorous worms having sucker-blade like three jaws with tiny rows of around 100 teeth in each jaw, which pierce host skin to slit the skin of the host. Contaminants present around cause the stress to the leech, as a result, a slimy mucous secretion lies over their body.

19.2.3 Medicinal Leech Storage, Its Application and Removal

Medicinal leech should always be collected from an authentic supplier. Throughout Europe, it is supplied by an International Swansea-based company Biopharm which was established in Hendy, South Wales (U.K) in 1812, from where it is moved in 1984. They are supplied in a specialized container having gel for short transference or distilled, non-chlorinated water for long transport. From Leech farm to be used

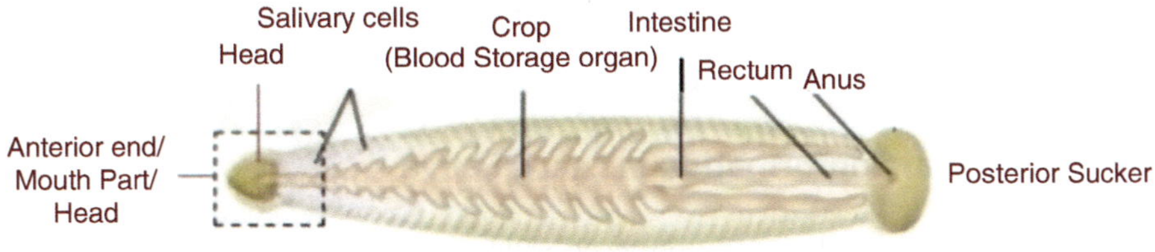

Fig. 19.1 Anatomical description of *Hirudo medicinalis*

for therapeutic purpose FDA recommends to maintain 10–15 leech per plastic/glass container having fresh distilled water; water volume/leech should not be less than 0.7 L. A very small percentage of salt is added as directed and kept at 4 °C in a cool dark place with a minimal perforation in the jar. The water of the jar should be replaced after alternate days depending upon the turbidity. Before, their therapeutic use they should be taken out at normal RT to regain their active motility [29].

Before application inclusion criterion along with specific bio-markers hematologic evaluation must be checked. Then only, it should be applied in a proper hygienic and sterile condition.

As a part of protocol of wound management skin is washed thoroughly with sterile water. Leech is taken out with a pair of long non-toothed forceps from the container (it is preferred that leech should be docile, which can be attained if it is applied immediately when it is taken out from refrigerator). Sometime, it needs a plastic syringe with plunger removed; in which leech is placed and inverted over the wound site, and sometime it directly attaches itself to the wound site. In some cases, blood droplets from a small prick helps in their attachment over the site. Proper supervision is always needed to restrict it to the site only, unnecessary movement can be avoided by restricting their movement by dampened gauze [30].

On a single application, live leeches attach themselves, by the suckers present at both the ends to the target area on the patient undergoing treatment. The narrow anterior end is the mouth with around 300 teeth in three sets of jaws, which leave a Y-shaped scar later [31]. Instantly it releases hirudin, a potent anticoagulant along with anesthetic and other chemical agent present in its saliva; after which it grow thrice of its size after sucking up to 15–20 mL of blood in rhythmic contractions during 10–30 min in a single feed, after which it usually drop itself [32]. If it fails to do so, a flat slim blunt blade is intervened in between the skin and the anterior sucker; once it is achieved the leech body is slightly holded by the posterior end too, and is put back in the separate container. Sometime 5% topical cocaine can be used to paralyze it and get it to detach from the skin. It should never be forcibly detached to avoid skin excoriation. They are discarded as per the protocol of bio-hazardous waste, immersed in 70% ethanol for 5–10 min.

Hirudin along with other co-factors causes blood thinning and vasodilatation which cause bleeding to be continued for 8–10 h, after its removal. During this time, it should be washed thoroughly and some protocols suggest the use of heparin to prolong bleeding [30] while some suggest hydrogen peroxide to control the effect of anticoagulant [33]. It varies with patient condition, so regular observation of color and appearance of tissue site along with vital signs and blood count should be monitored throughout the process. Prolonged treatment in large area of skin may demand blood transfusion.

19.2.4 Natural Conformation in Leech Saliva

Extensive research studies done on leech saliva have confirmed that it is rich in active biomolecules that act in multiple ways. There are more than 20 molecules whose mechanism of action is well defined as anticoagulant, anti-inflammatory,

Hirudin
Hyaluronidase
Calin
Destabilase
Aapyrase
Eglin
Bdellins
Decorsin
Hirustasin

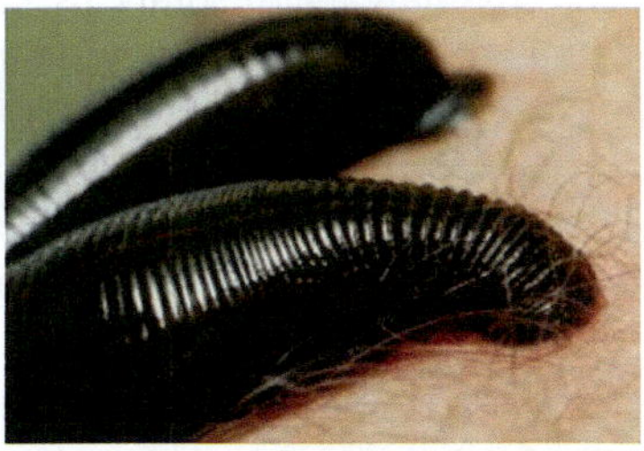

Guamerin
Piguamerin
Gallin: Potent thrombin inhibitor
Gamma-Glutamyl Transpeptidase
Platelet Active factor Antagonist.
Ornithin rich peptide active
Acetylcholine
Histamine
Enzymes like fibrinase and collagenase

Fig. 19.2 Potential bioactive ingredients of leech saliva

analgesic, platelet inhibitory, thrombin regulatory, antimicrobial, etc. but still much is to be explored before making any strong assumption. Just after their attachment to the host skin, they release all these biologically active compounds in balanced set and along with 100 different types of peptides and proteins [34]; it includes the following which gets released into the bloodstream for health benefit (Fig. 19.2):

Hirudin (an antithrombotic factor), Hyaluronidase (a diffusing substance which increases the permeability of connective tissues to absorption by reducing the viscosity), Calin (suppresses the adhesion of platelets to collagen and act as antithrombotic), Destabilase (lysozyme with glycosidase potential, act as antibacterial as well as thrombolytic), Apyrase (Nonspecific Platelet Aggregate Inhibitor), Eglin (Inhibitor of alpha-chymotrypsin, subtilisin, chymosin, granulocyte proteinases, elastase, and cathepsin G), Bdellins (Plasmin Inhibitor), Decorsin (acts as an antagonist of platelet glycoprotein II b-III a and is a potent inhibitor of platelet aggregation), Hirustasin (a specific inhibitor of the blood coagulation Factor Xa), Guamerin (Human leukocyte elastase inhibitor), Piguamerin (inhibits plasma and tissue kallikrein and trypsin), Gallin (thrombin inhibitor), Gamma-Glutamyl Transpeptidase, Platelet Active factor Antagonist (important compound for the treatment of thromboembolic disorders and inflammation), Ornithine rich peptide active. Besides these, it also contains acetylcholine, histamine like vasodilators that prolong bleeding time. Certain enzymes like fibrinase and collagenase that reduce scar tissue and adhesions and help reduce fibroblast formation in hypertrophic scars and keloids [28, 34–36, 38, 39].

They collectively act as

- Local anesthetic
- Local vasodilator
- Anticoagulant agents (hirudin)
- Analgesic and anti-inflammatory
- Platelet aggregation inhibitors (calin, saratin, for instance)
- Collagen inhibitors that prevent its adhesion on surface

They trigger the immune system also to do the work and thus all these collectively prevent clotting and improve circulation, and prevent tissue death. The leeches leave behind small, Y-shaped wounds that usually heal without leaving a scar. Medicinal leeches most often come from Hungary or Sweden (Fig. 19.3).

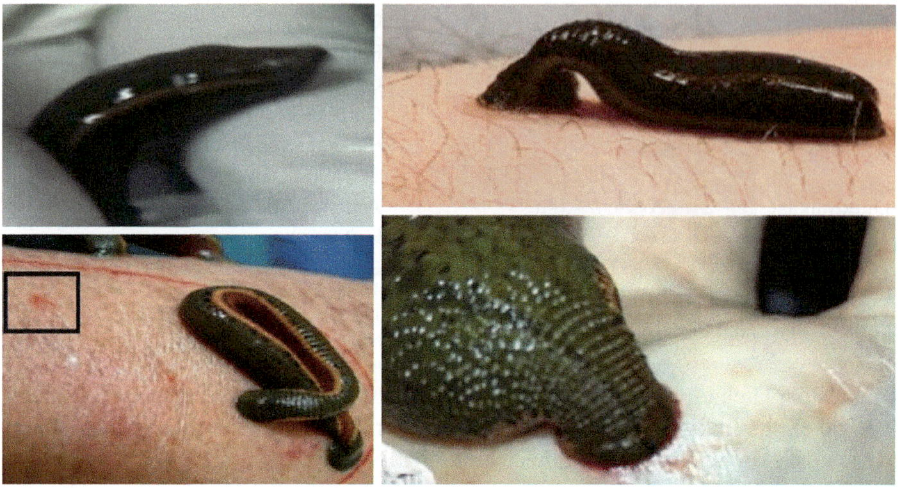

Fig. 19.3 Leech attachment to the skin through its anterior sucker leaving Y-shaped scar

19.2.5 Therapeutic Property of Medicinal Leech Therapy (MLT)

MLT, which was once considered to be an eternal part of the traditional system of medicine viz. Ayurveda and Unani System of Medicine substantially benefitted many practitioners following allopathic medicine too. And a revival in its use is observed due to its simple and inexpensive means of preventing complications and for the common aim of providing benefit to the mankind to treat nervous system abnormalities, dental problems, skin diseases, plastic or reconstructive surgeries, and infections.

And now, past many years leech therapy preferably referred as hirudino therapy is used to treat a wide range of conditions by medical professionals. Like the post-operative treatment of a scalp avulsion as reported by Henderson et al., in 1983 [37]; Russia in the 1900s found newer uses of leeches for the treatment of hypertension, migraines, phlebitis, varicose veins, arthritis, hemorrhoids, and ovarian cysts and in the USA, plastic surgeons used them to drain blood from wounds after limb amputation. In 1970s their demand revived again to its heights of popularity after the success got in finger reattachment procedures and soft tissue surgeries of the face, and later in various other plastic or reconstructive surgeries, specifically due to their ability of preventing scab formation. It is due to the presence of an anticoagulant that they secrete into wound which allows them to heal from inside outward. Small leeches were preferred to be used after microsurgeries on the face or neck.

Alleged benefits of medicinal leeches have been substantially extended after the exploration of various chemicals present in the leech saliva, that are now been used by the pharmaceutical companies for their use in various medical conditions that can be improved by their proper use like in high-risk cases of limb amputations as a complication of diabetes, circulatory disorders to treat blood clots and varicose

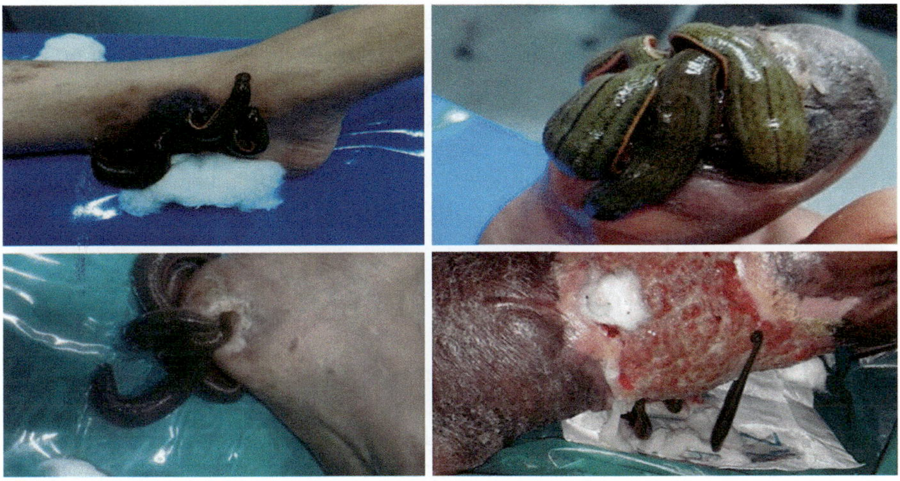

Fig. 19.4 Leeches applied on diabetic foot ulcer

vein; for preserving soft tissues and promoting healing after facial reconstructive surgeries like forehead, nose, lip, cheeks. Its effect on blood clotting further helps to heal naturally and completely leaving behind minimal or no scar (Fig. 19.4).

19.2.6 Therapeutic Uses

MLT has been used efficiently for the treatment of circulatory diseases, as various clinical forms of coronary heart disease, stable angina, and postinfarction cardiosclerosis has also been reported [28, 38–43] which to an extent confirm the inhibition of platelet aggregation by the chemicals present in leech saliva.

Baskova et al. [41] also confirm their on the endothelial vasomotor function of medium and small resistance arteries. Further, he studied that its effect is not just the local, but it is a systemic effect which normalizes stiffness of the arterial wall. This process is supposed to involve the salivary cell secretion of the medicinal leech, which is able to raise the NO level both in cells and in extracellular fluid and to activate *e-NOS* and *n-NOS*, as it has been shown recently in the culture of human vascular endothelial cells (HUVEC).

There is also evidence by Gasic et al. [44] where salivary gland extract showed anti-metastatic effect which can be attributed to the anti-platelet-aggregating, anticoagulant, and anti-proteolytic enzyme activities present in leech saliva. Ammar and his co-workers [45] also proved its efficacy in prostate cancer through in vitro and in vivo antitumor activity with no apparent side effects. It can be attributed to its ability to inhibit cellular proliferation, prevention of cellular adhesion, and anti-inflammatory properties. Although its activity may vary with different types of cancer. Further, due to its proven anti-inflammatory and anesthetic properties, it can be used to reduce tenderness and pain in joint diseases like osteoarthritis [46].

Other claims made for MLT includes its use in the treatment of migraine, infertility, baldness sinusitis, glaucoma, chronic renal failure, hepatitis, cystitis, Alzheimer's disease, and many more [47–50]. Although due to its therapeutic properties specifically due to the bioactive molecules in its saliva, it is mentioned to be used in various health ailments as mentioned by many [47–50], but the story may not be true always, unless and until it is scientifically verified. So, before using it clinically it should be scientifically re-validated for its claim made.

19.2.7 Contraindications

Hirudinotherapy is an easy remedy which involves a lower end risk of side effects, compared to other. So, people with anemia, blood clotting conditions, or compromised arteries are not considered as candidates for leech therapy. And so, are the children under the age of 18 years old, pregnant women and immune-compromised people are also usually advised to avoid it. Further, it can be harmful in other conditions too, if used wrongly. So, it is always advised to use a healthy, fresh leech and patient should be told well, before the procedure to be done, to restore the mental condition while the blood oozes out from the wound.

Sometime it is observed that blood continues to ooze out from the leech bite site in spite of leech removal; so it should be treated accordingly. In some cases, leeches move out to other area of the body, which may cause unnecessary blood loss; so a continuous supervision is necessary (Fig. 19.5).

19.3 Healing Ulcer in Diabetes

Medicinal Leech therapy can help in the healing of the ulcer by improving blood circulation along with other chemicals present in leech saliva that work as co-factors in diabetic wound ulcer healing. Several case studies have reported its use successfully. MLT has been a traditional practice in various evidence-based medicine; and in Ayurveda also it is followed successfully; like in an observational single case

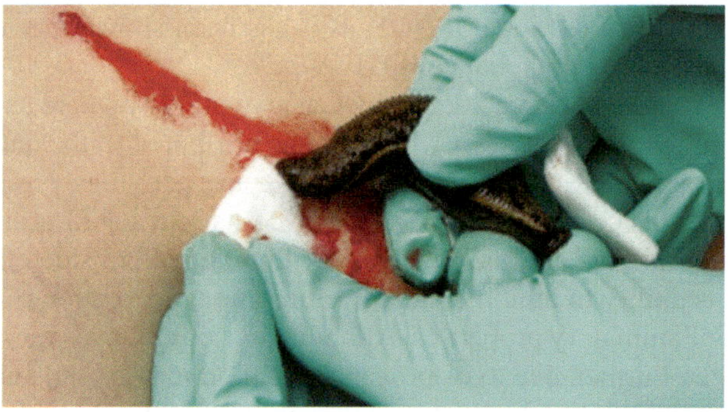

Fig. 19.5 Blood oozing out from the attached leech site

done without control at an Ayurvedic Hospital in Mumbai (India) [51]. In the study done by Dwivedi, he discussed the case of a 45-year-old male diabetic patient having inflamed infected DFU on both the foot at Planter surface; with pus, bleeding purulent smell was treated with MLT. Along with the general care for wound with Ayurvedic therapy and control of diabetes with western medicine, leech therapy was employed. It was used weekly in four sittings for 30 days; using three leeches at the wound site. Follow-up was taken regularly and the changes in clinical features were noted, it is well documented photographically weekly and the DFU get completely cured. Rampure [52] have also discussed a case study of 52-year-old male patient, being cured with leech therapy as a part of Ayurvedic Panchkarma. Four leeches were applied once a week on the nonhealing irregular inflamed ulcer with mild pus discharge at the left ankle joint after proper antidiabetic treatment which was properly healed after 30 days.

Similarly as per the Unani system of medicine, Zaidi [53] has also illustrated wound healing by leech therapy in a 60-year-old diabetic lady along with Unani medicine used as blood purifier and deobstruent. Foot ulcer was of fifth grade that was almost turned into gangrene with severe foul smell in the necrosed area and causing much pain in the left foot; thus was in all facing the prospects of amputation. Hirudinotherapy was followed for a period of 20 days that minimize the painful condition and helped in almost complete healing during the course of 3–5 months, with complete removal of necrosed area [53].

Follower of Alternative and Complementary Medicine in Iran, Hajtalebi [54] also details about a case study done on 58-year-old diabetic patient having two chronic wound of Stage II/Grade III on the right foot and was left for amputation. After proper anti-hyperglycemic control over sugar level along with medicinal herbs, he was able to successfully cure the foot ulcer within 60 days. It was done by application of 10–12 leeches being placed inside and around the wound during 16 sessions after every 2–4 day. Another study mentioned by the same author in 2017, also re-confirms the use of leech therapy in DFU [55]. As mentioned by the author a 74-year-old lady with a prolonged history of 20 years with diabetes was treated in such a severe condition when all allopathic medicines were exhausted before uncontrolled blood sugar level and sepsis and as it was not responding to any such treatment, it was left for amputation only. The patient had a severely infected cyanosed sore on the big toe of her right foot, for at least 2 months, and the unadorned inflammation was spread over the other fingers and continued to the ankle. In the meantime, she was provided with the present-day treatment, which did not benefit her and the suffering of the patient was increased along with the wound condition that worsened day after day. Physician started the treatment by giving dietotherapy, along with medicinal herbs, and modern blood sugar control drugs. Leech therapy was used to treat the ulcer using six medium-sized leeches in ten sessions, once after 3 days inside and around the wound and after ten sessions the wound was found to be completely healed and the blood sugar also came to the controlled conditions in 40 days of treatment.

19.4 Conclusion

Several successful clinical stories elaborating on the logistic pathway behind the therapeutic efficacy; that leech therapy can be used widely in healing the diabetic wound ulcer and the rate of amputation can be minimized to an extent. Established mechanism of action for its medicinal value lies in the pharmacological synergy which occurs among the chemicals present in leech saliva where hyaluronidase and collagenase got released after leech bite, histamine like molecule further cause vasodilatation, concurrently blood coagulation is inhibited by the combined inhibition of platelet aggregation, coagulation cascade, and kinin activity along with inhibition of inflammatory reactions under analgesia. So, a combination of traditional therapies like Medicinal leech therapy which act in many ways to treat not only the wound, but also reducing the associated complications, along with the synthetic antidiabetic drug can provide with 'patient's healing. Still, Molecule based community at a large is skeptical about most of the claims made by holistic based healers, but scientific researches going on leech therapy are showing a promising role in the treatment. And so, they are relied upon, since centuries as an essential part of medical care. The present-day scientists have limited their role and leeching nowadays is being used only in microsurgeries to relieve the venous congestion. An enormous amount of therapeutic property lies in their saliva, which needs to be explored further. So that they could be relied upon and used for medical care needed.

References

1. Antonopoulos AS, Siasos G, Konsola T, Oikonomou E, Tentolouris N, Kollia C, Gouliopoulos N, Zografos T, Papavassiliou AG, Tousoulis D (2015) Arterial wall elastic properties and endothelial dysfunction in the diabetic foot syndrome in patients with type 2 diabetes. Diabetes Care 38(11):e180–e181. https://doi.org/10.2337/dc15-1042
2. Almaramhy H, Mahabbat NA, Fallatah KY, Al-Ahmadi BA, Al-Alawi HH, Guraya SY (2018) The correlation of fasting blood glucose levels with the severity of diabetic foot ulcers and the outcome of treatment strategies. Biomed Res 29(9):1961–1967. https://doi.org/10.4066/biomedicalresearch.29-18-502
3. Bessie A, Young BA, Maynard C, Reiber G, Boyko EJ (2003) Effects of ethnicity and neuropathy on lower-extremity amputation risk among diabetic veterans. Diabetes Care 26(2):495–501. https://doi.org/10.2337/diacare.26.2.495
4. Kahle B, Hermanns HJ, Gallenkemper G (2011) Evidence-based treatment of chronic leg ulcers. Dtsch Arztebl Int 108(14):231–237. https://doi.org/10.3238/arztebl.2011.0231
5. Alexiadou K, Doupis J (2012) Management of diabetic foot ulcers. Diabet Ther 3:4. https://doi.org/10.1007/s13300-012-0004-9
6. Robinson AH, Pasapula C, Brodsky JW (2009) Surgical aspects of the diabetic foot. J Bone Joint Surg (Br) 91(1):1–7
7. Jain AKC (2016) Type 1 diabetic foot complications. J Diabet Foot Complic 8(1, 3):17–22
8. Gianino E, Miller C, Gilmore J (2018) Smart wound dressings for diabetic chronic wounds. Bioengineering (Basel) 5(3):51. https://doi.org/10.3390/bioengineering5030051
9. Meijer JW, Smit AJ, Sonderen EV, Groothoff JW, Eisma WH, Links TP (2002) Symptom scoring systems to diagnose distal polyneuropathy in diabetes: the Diabetic Neuropathy Symptom score. Diabet Med 19:962–965. https://doi.org/10.1046/j.1464-5491.2002.00819.x

10. Dillingham TR, Pezzin LE, MacKenzie EJ (2002) Limb amputation and limb deficiency: epidemiology and recent trends in the United States. South Med J 95:875–883
11. Frykberg RG, Banks J (2015) Challenges in the treatment of chronic wounds. Adv Wound Care (New Rochelle) 4(9):560–582. https://doi.org/10.1089/wound.2015.0635
12. Anonymous. https://www.apma.org/diabeticwoundcare. Accessed 30 Mar 2020
13. Agale SV (2013) Chronic leg ulcers: epidemiology, aetiopathogenesis, and management. Chron Ulc Updat Epidemiol Physiopathol Ther 2013:413604. https://doi.org/10.1155/2013/413604
14. Collins L, Seraj S (2010) Diagnosis and treatment of venous ulcer. Am Fam Physician 81(8):989–996
15. Everett E, Mathioudakis N (2018) Update on management of diabetic foot ulcers. Ann N Y Acad Sci 1411(1):153–165. https://doi.org/10.1111/nyas.13569
16. Medical Advisory Secretariat (2006) Negative pressure wound therapy: an evidence-based analysis. Ont Health Technol Assess Ser 6(14):1–38
17. Armstrong DJ, Boulton AJM, Bus SA (2017) Diabetic foot ulcers and their recurrence. N Engl J Med 376(24):2367–2375. https://doi.org/10.1056/NEJMra1615439
18. Enoch S, Grey JE, Harding KG (2006) ABC of wound healing. Non-surgical and drug treatments. BMJ 332(7546):900–903. https://doi.org/10.1136/bmj.332.7546.900
19. Lone AH, Ahmad T, Anwar M, Habib S, Sofi G, Imam H (2011) Leech therapy - a holistic approach of treatment in Unani (Greeko-Arab) medicine. Anc Sci Life 31(1):31–35. PMID: 22736888 PMCID: PMC3377041
20. Hyson JM (2005) Leech therapy: a history. J Hist Dent 53(1):25–27
21. Stapelberg M-M (2015) Through the darkness: glimpses into the history of western medicine. Chapter 3: Phlebotomy, purges and other medical marvels. Crux Publisher, London
22. Panda AK, Debnath SK (2012) Effectiveness of leech therapy in Gambhira Vata-Rakta (Acute Gout): a pilot study. J Homeopat Ayur Med 1:108. https://doi.org/10.4172/2167-1206.1000108
23. Neelofer, Khan KZ, Sheerani FS (2018) Leech therapy in non-healing ulcer. A case study. Int J Med Sci Innov Res 3(6):69–74
24. Whitaker IS, Rao J, Izadi D, Butler PE (2004) Historical article: Hirudo medicinalis: ancient origins of, and trends in the use of medicinal leeches throughout history. Br J Oral Maxillofac Surg 42(2):133–137
25. Abdullah S, Dar LM, Rashid A, Tewari A (2012) Hirudinotherapy/Leech therapy: applications and indications in Surgery. Arch Clin Exp Surg 1:172–180
26. Munshi Y, Ara I, Rafique H, Ahmad Z (2008) Leeching in the history--a review. Pak J Biol Sci 11(13):1650–1653. https://doi.org/10.3923/pjbs.2008.1650.1653
27. Sunil KS, Aradhyamath S, Hiremath S (2015) Concept of Leech therapy. Int J Ayur Med 3(8):2559–2563
28. Abdualkader AM, Ghawi AM, Alaama M, Awang M, Merzouk A (2013) Leech therapeutic applications. Indian J Pharm Sci 75(2):127–137. https://doi.org/10.4103/0250-474X.115456
29. Singh SK, Rajoria K (2019) Medical leech therapy in Ayurveda and biomedicine – a review. J Ayur Integr Med. https://doi.org/10.1016/j.jaim.2018.09.003
30. Marsden MB, Ng A (2014) Hirudotherapy: a guide to using leeches to drain blood from tissue. Clin Pharm 6:69
31. Mumcuoglu KY (2014) Recommendations for the use of leeches in reconstructive plastic surgery. Evid Based Complement Alternat Med 2014:205929. https://doi.org/10.1155/2014/205929
32. Ghosh S (2019) Relevance of leech therapy in contemporary medicine: a mini-review. Quest Int J Med Health Sci 2(1):8–12. Available from: http://www.qiup.edu.my/wpcontent/uploads/2019-3.pdf
33. John S (2018) How to remove a Leech (and how to avoid them in the first place). The Manual
34. Baskova IP, Zavalova LL, Basanova AV (2004) Protein profiling of the medicinal leech salivary gland secretion by proteomic analytical methods. Biochemistry (Mosc) 69:770–775. https://doi.org/10.1023/B:BIRY.0000040202.21965.2a
35. Zaidi SMA, Jameel SS, Zaman F, Jilani S, Sultana A, Khan SA (2011) A systematic overview of the medicinal importance of sanguivorous leeches. Altern Med Rev 16(1):59–65

36. Hildebrandt JP, Lemke S (2011) Small bite, large impact–saliva and salivary molecules in the medicinal leech, *Hirudo medicinalis*. Naturwissenschaften 98:995–1008
37. Henderson HP, Matti B, Laing AG, Morelli S, Sully L (1983) Avulsion of the scalp treated by microvascular repair: the use of leeches for post-operative decongestion. Br J Plast Surg 36:235–239
38. Sig AK, Guney M, Uskudar Guclu A, Ozmen E (2017) Medicinal leech therapy-an overall perspective. Integr Med Res 6(4):337–343. https://doi.org/10.1016/j.imr.2017.08.001
39. Porshinsky BS, Saha S, Grossman MD, Beery Ii PR, Stawicki SPA (2011) Clinical uses of the medicinal leech: a practical review. J Postgrad Med 57:65–71
40. Baskova IP, Isakhanyan GS (2004) Hirudotherapy: science and practice. Monolit, Moscow
41. Baskova P, Pavlova IB, Parfenov AS (2014) Analysis of the effects of medicinal leech on arterial function in elderly volunteers by means of photoplethysmography with angioscan. Hum Physiol 40(2):214–219. https://doi.org/10.1134/S0362119714020029. ISSN 0362-1197
42. Isakhanyan GS (1991) Girudoterapiya v klinike vnutrennikh boleznei (Hirudotherapy in the clinical picture of internal diseases). Aiastan, Yerevan
43. Isakhanyan GS, Tumasyan KS, Mkrtchyan LS (1991) Influence of hirudotherapy on platelet aggregation in acute myocardial infarction patients. Krovoobrashchenie 24:32
44. Gasic GJ, Iwakawa A, Gasic TB, Viner ED, Milas L (1984) Leech salivary gland extract from Haementeria officinalis, a potent inhibitor of cyclophosphamide- and radiation-induced artificial metastasis enhancement. Cancer Res 44(12):5670–5676
45. Ammar AE, Hassona MH, Meckling GR, Chan LG, Chin MY, Abdualkader A, Alaama M, Merzouk A, Helaluddin A, Ghawi A, Kucuk O, Guns ES (2015) Assessment of the antitumor activity of leech (*Huridinaria manillensis*) saliva extract in prostate cancer. Cancer Res 75(15 Suppl):Abstract nr 5130. https://doi.org/10.1158/1538-7445.AM2015-5130. Abstract. In: Proceedings of the 106th Annual Meeting of the American Association for Cancer Research. 2015. Philadelphia, PA. Philadelphia (PA). AACR
46. Rai PK, Singh AK, Singh OP, Rai NP, Dwivedi AK (2011) Efficacy of leech therapy in the management of osteoarthritis (Sandhivata). Ayu 32(2):213–217. https://doi.org/10.4103/0974-8520.92589
47. Ansari S, Nil F, Jabeen A, Sultana A, Khan QA (2019) Post-auricular leech therapy reduced headache & migraine days in chronic migraine. J Drug Deliv Therapeut 9(1-s):75–80. https://doi.org/10.22270/jddt.v9i1-s.2345
48. Whitaker IS, Cheung CK, Chahal CAA, Karoo ROS, Gulati A, Foo ITH (2005) By what mechanism do leeches help to salvage ischaemic tissues. A review. Br J Oral Maxillofac Surg 43:155–160
49. Das BK (2014) An overview on hirudotherapy/leech therapy. Ind Res J Pharm Sci 1:33–45
50. Singh AP (2010) Medicinal leech therapy (hirudotherapy): a brief overview. Complement Ther Clin Pract 16:213–215
51. Dwivedi AP (2012) Case study of leech application in diabetic foot ulcer. Int J Res Ayur Pharm 3(5):748–751. https://doi.org/10.7897/2277-4343
52. Rampure N, Channabasavanna BM, Mallikarjun (2017) Jaloukavacharana in diabetic foot ulcer - a case study. J Ayur Integr Med Sci 2(3):274–278
53. Zaidi SMA (2016) Unani treatment and leech therapy saved the diabetic foot of a patient from amputation. Int Wound J 13:263–264. https://doi.org/10.1111/iwj.12285
54. Hajtalebi H, Iurigh HK, Hajtalebi HR (2016) Treatment of diabetic foot ulcer in a 58-year old Turkman patient. Trad Integr Med 1(4):151–159
55. Hajtalebi H, Khani Iurigh H, Hajtalebi H (2017) Treatment of diabetic foot ulcer in a 74-year-old female patient based on Iranian traditional medicine in Bojnurd. Asian J Clin Case Rep Trad Altern Med 1(1–2):1–10. https://doi.org/10.22040/ajcrtam.2017.24881

Nanotechnology and Diabetic Foot Ulcer: Future Prospects

20

Mohammad Azam Ansari, Khursheed Ali, Zeba Farooqui, Hanan A. Al-Dossary, Mohammad Zubair, and Javed Musarrat

20.1 Introduction

Diabetes was discovered independently in several parts of the world prior to the time there were no physicians or chemists. Interestingly, the discovery of diabetes was made by observing that insects tend to attract toward the sweet urine of certain diseased persons [1]. In 2010, the International Diabetes Federation (IDF), claimed four million deaths under the age groups of 20–79 years, globally [2]. In 2013, rapid growth in the prevalence of diabetes was observed affecting 382 million people worldwide [3] with a figure of 30.3 million affected individuals in the USA alone in 2015 [4]. According to the World Health Organization (WHO), diabetes

The original version of this chapter was revised. The correction to this chapter can be found at https://doi.org/10.1007/978-981-15-7639-3_21

M. A. Ansari (✉) · H. A. Al-Dossary
Department of Epidemic Disease Research, Institute for Research and Medical Consultations (IRMC), Imam Abdulrahman Bin Faisal University, Dammam, Kingdom of Saudi Arabia

K. Ali
Faculty of Agricultural Sciences, Department of Agricultural Microbiology, Aligarh Muslim University, Uttar Pradesh, Aligarh, India

Z. Farooqui
College of Pharmacy, University of Houston, Houston, TX, USA

M. Zubair
Department of Medical Microbiology, Faculty of Medicine, University of Tabuk, Tabuk, Kingdom of Saudi Arabia

J. Musarrat
Faculty of Agricultural Sciences, Department of Agricultural Microbiology, Aligarh Muslim University, Uttar Pradesh, Aligarh, India

School of Biosciences and Biotechnology, Baba Ghulam Shah Badshah University, Rajouri, Jammu & Kashmir, India

M. Zubair et al. (eds.), *Diabetic Foot Ulcer*,
https://doi.org/10.1007/978-981-15-7639-3_20

holds the status of a chronic disease associated with lengthening of hyperglycaemic conditions due to inability or complete irreversible damage of insulin exuding pancreatic cells [5]. During the 1980s, the WHO classified diabetes as insulin-dependent diabetes mellitus (IDDM) or type 1 diabetes, and non-insulin-dependent diabetes mellitus (NIDDM) or type 2 [6]. In 1997, the classification of diabetes was updated as mere type 1 and type 2 diabetes while discarding IDDM and NIDDM by the WHO [7]. According to medical acquaintances, diabetes crops up due to prolonged hyperglycaemic conditions arising due to some abnormalities surfacing in the normal functioning of the pancreatic cells. In fact, pancreatic α- and β-cells are dedicated to sustain blood glucose (BG) levels in the bloodstream of healthy individuals. Strictly, an increased BG concentration signals the β-cells of the pancreas for the secretion of the hormone insulin which in-turn stimulates the processes of hepatic glucose uptake and extra-hepatic glucose uptake from the blood. On the contrary, when BG level falls below a minimum threshold, α-cells of the pancreas are signaled for the secretion of hormone glucagon which stimulates hepatocytes for the breakdown of stored glycogen into glucose and releasing it into the bloodstream, thereby attaining normal glycemic levels [8]. The defects in insulin-secreting pancreatic β-cells are characterized by metabolic disorder, resulting in elevated BG concentrations. One such anomaly is called type 1 diabetes mellitus (T1DM), which arises due to an autoimmune disorder, characterized by complete destruction of the insulin-secreting β-cells and its survivors are completely dependent on exogenous insulin [9]. In general, the documented medico-literature reports normal BG levels to be in a constricted range of 70–110 mg/dL after 2–3 h of a meal or undergoing an overnight fast [10]. Besides, type 2 diabetes mellitus (T2DM) is characterized either by the inability of the pancreas to secrete sufficient insulin or insensitivity of insulin or a combination of both. The prolonged hyperglycaemic (BG > 120 mg/dL) patients are prone to develop multiple health complications such as neuropathy, retinopathy, nephropathy, peripheral vascular disease, and coronary heart disease. Conversely, in case of hypoglycemia (BG < 60 mg/dL), the low BG level reflects anxiety, perspiring, an extreme appetite which may lead to lethargy, coma, and sometimes even death. Strictly speaking, the level of BG within the salutary window of 60–120 mg/dL is the hallmark of sustaining a healthy life.

Besides, DFUs are generally identified as a chronic microbial infection site due to the manifestation of a wide range of pathogens. *Staphylococcus aureus* and *Pseudomonas aeruginosa* are of the frequently identified bacteria which readily form chronic biofilm matrices in order to evade bactericidal effects and accumulate antibiotic resistant against a broad range of conventional antibiotic agents. Thus, the clinical management of multiple drug-resistant (MDR) bacteria-infected DFUs become very challenging. Interestingly, among the modern therapeutics modalities, metal or metal oxide-based nano-formulations and antibiotic-nanoparticles (NPs) assemblies are being debated hotly as an alternative and promising remedy against MDR, globally. Nevertheless, this chapter precisely highlights a landscape of the current trends of NPs based therapies against biofilm-forming MDR bacteria and infected DFUs healing.

20.2 Diabetic Foot Ulcer (DFU)

Diabetic foot ulcer (DFU) is a "corollary of snags" of diabetes mellitus (DM) which eventually leads to constrained mobility, amputations, and even death. One of the most vital features of DFS is diminished sensitivity to pain after primary damage. The affected person does not show normal pain-averting manners or respond for "timely urgent help." Besides these, dysregulation in any of the progression's escorts to deferred or non-curable phenotypes as commonly evident in DFUs. Thus, the dysregulated metabolism in diabetics leads the development of adverse secondary pathophysiological outcomes affecting multi-organ system imposing multifaceted complications [11]. DFU is one of the most distressing unremitting complications of diabetes which is developed in 26.1 million people, globally [12]. A DFU is often a low-affair inching, unproblematic surprise that blankets a sudden rising flood of complications in its dark portals. In medical terminology, DFU is defined as a deep tissue inflicted infection, ulceration, and/or destruction allied with neurological aberrations and varying degrees of peripheral vascular disease in the lower limb of the patients with DM. The durational incidence of DFUs arrays from 19% to 34% of total diabetic patients [12]. Estimated 15–25% of the diabetics are at major risk to develop DFUs [13], which may later result in the most dreaded consequence in the 108,000 lower limb amputations performed per year in the USA [4], due to lack effective therapies. The 1-year progression past amputation is poor, resulting in the mortality rate of about 44% [14]. According to Jeffcoate et al. [15], highlighted the practice of effective and advanced wound management therapies can play a crucial role in healing the chronic DFUs up to 59% without amputation.

20.3 DFUs Classification

The salient characteristics of ulcers such as location, appearance, size, and depth provide scope to map the progress during healing. Beyond this physical assessment, the chronic wounds, i.e., DFUs are subjected to their etiological verification, for neuropathic, ischemic, or neuro-ischemic symptoms [16], and, hence provide bases to classify the ulcers accordingly [17]. In general, delayed healing effects are assigned to the peripheral vascular complications due to increased wound depth which likely augment infections. Nevertheless, it is a proper classification which addresses the challenges generally faced by clinicians. Albeit, the intriguing field of DFUs prompted the clinicians and scientists to categorized DFUs through proper classification parameters such as (1) location of ulcer, (2) depth of wounds, (3) neuropathy, and (4) ischemia [18] to facilitate interdisciplinary understanding.

Following are the most importantly used classification systems

1. University of Texas classification
2. Wagner-Armstrong grades classification
3. Brodsky depth-ischemic classification
4. International working group classification

20.3.1 University of Texas Classification

The classification of the University of Texas (UT) establishes an informative bridge between infection peripheral arterial diseases (PAD) [19, 20]. The UT classification uses numerical 0, 1, 2, and 3 to depict the pre- or post-ulcerative lesions, the involvement of tendon, capsule, and bone, reaching tendon or capsule and reaching bone or joint, respectively. Similarly, alphabets A, B, C, and D are used to indicate the presence or absence of infection and ischemia (A = absence of both, B = infection only, C = ischemia only, D = both).

20.3.2 Wagner-Armstrong Grades Classification

Wagner-Armstrong grading classification is an integrated system that explains the deepness of the lesions according to Wagner with precise information on infection and PAD well in accordance with the UT classification. Hence, the collective cataloging is consigned as Wagner-Armstrong classification but readily avoided in case of severe deformities such as ischemia and associated infections [19, 20].

20.3.3 Brodsky Depth-Ischemic Classification

Brodsky, a foot and ankle specialist modified Wagner-Armstrong grading classification system highlighting the subtle but accurate differences between the lesions of grade 2 and 3 and the vascularity of foot with respect to the grade of prescribed treatment grade [21].

20.3.4 International Working Group Classification

In 2001, the International Working Group (IWG) on diabetic foot devised a risk assessment scheme in order to assure the plausible complications [22]. Later, the IWG devised scheme was widely accepted, predicting, and classifying the diabetics prone to develop foot problems [23].

20.3.5 PEDIS Classification System

The PEDIS classification system developed by IWG on Diabetic Foot, to only targets DFUs via three medico-pathological conditions namely wound, infection, and ischemia in well-coordinated evaluation approach [24], however, it lacks a general description of wound, loss of tissue and the limb salvageability. Later, this system was described in reference to specific concerns of infection with an exceptional follow-up scheme in 2012 IDSA (Clinical Practice Guideline for the Diagnosis and Treatment of Diabetic Foot Infections) and 2014 WIfI classification method [25].

20.3.6 Kobe Classification

In 2011, the Department of Plastic Surgery, Kobe University, Japan, published a four-level classification system popularly known as Kobe classification. This system is primarily based on the etiology and treatment of [26].

20.4 DFU Global Epidemiology

The global prevalence of DM has been estimated around twofold in respect to the threshold line of 2.8% in 2000 to 4.4% by 2030, devastating nearly 350 million individuals [27]. In reference to the diabetes epidemic [28], it can be argued that the increase in DFUs patients is due to the rapid pace growing number of people with DM. Within western countries, approximately 10% of the total population suffers from diabetes [29], at the rate of around 3% and 0.1% per year new episodes of DFUs and active Charcot foot, respectively [30, 31].

Importantly, the prevalence of DFUs is 1.6–6.3% while having lifetime risk about 15–25% [13], indicates that one million of 50 million inhabitants of a country may become DFUs patient lifetime. Surprisingly, alone in USA, the cost of diabetes in 2012 was $245 billion however 43% of total cost spent in the medical care of diabetics. The total medical care expenditures of people living without diabetes are surprisingly 2.3-fold lesser as compared to diabetics [32]. Comparatively, the huge expenditures in diabetes clinical management can be assigned to nearly 6.7 million diabetics who are surviving with DFUs or infections out of 785 million of diabetes-associated outpatient calls between 2007 and 2013 [33].

20.5 Etiology and Pathophysiology of DFU

In 1818, Mott provided the first recognizable description of a neuropathic ulcer. According to the description, sole of diabetic's foot experiences (1) hardening of surrounding cuticle, (2) loss of insensitivity to a great level diminishing all modalities of sensation and, (3) palpable ankle pulses with, (4) warm, pink, and the dry foot itself [34]. Due to loss of sensations, a person with diabetes often remains unaware about the formation of lesions until notices the discharge of pus or blood. Nevertheless, the determination of a DFU etiology is carried out by taking primary characteristics of ulcers such as depth, size, appearance, location, etc. Secondly, a lesion is supposed to be categorized neuropathic, ischemic, or neuro-ischemic [35]. The etiology of DFUs is therefore closely integrated with the incidence of peripheral neuropathy and repetitive trauma due to painful walking activities with DFU foot [36], which therefore later leads the structural deformations, compromised joint movements and even partial foot amputations as liabilities of peripheral neuropathy to diabetics. Strictly speaking, in case of the diabetic foot, concentrated pressure area due to abnormal weight-bearing and shear forces enhance the risk of ulcer development [37–39]. In 1983, Brand highlighted that the discrete shear forces for a long period of time can augment local inflammation, focal tissue ischemia, and destruction, which eventually prompt the ulceration [40].

20.5.1 Pathophysiology of DFU

Like multifaceted etiology of DFUs, a normal foot lesion involves simultaneous action of a multicomponent milieu while converting into a chronic DFU [18]. Also, diabetic neuropathy is one of the general complications of diabetes and has emerged as one of the major causes of substantial morbidity and increased mortality [41].

20.5.1.1 Neuropathy

Diabetic peripheral neuropathy (DPN), popularly known as loss of sensation, frequently occurs in diabetics' is one of the most common complications amongst several neuropathic syndromes which is activated as main DFU initiating factor [42]. DPN is a multifaceted entity that encompasses (1) focal and multifocal neuropathies, e.g., mononeuropathy, amyotrophy, radiculopathy, multiple lesions mononeuritis multiplex and entrapment and, (2) symmetrical neuropathies, such as autonomic and acute sensory [43, 44]. According to Tesfaye et al. [45], DPN is a proportional, length-dependent sensorimotor polyneuropathy that induces metabolic and micro-vessel variations in response to exposure chronic hyperglycemia and cardiovascular risk descriptions. Furthermore, the presence of diabetic retinopathy and nephropathy in diabetics suggests that polyneuropathy is an attributable trait for diabetes.

20.5.1.2 Microangiopathy

The functional changes in microvascular function such as endothelial dysfunction and abnormal neurovascular control decrease the blood flow into DFU significantly causing a delay in wound healing [46, 47]. Specifically, the involvement of endothelial proliferation in diabetics can cause arteriolar occlusion [48]. Besides, a wide range of structural and functional abnormalities such as the gaseous and nutrient exchange between blood and tissue cells observed affecting the cutaneous microcirculation across different capillary beds over the disease time [49]. Overall, it can be articulated that the impaired microvascular function affects the direct or indirect healing of DFUs.

20.5.1.3 Delayed Wound Healing

The process of wound healing does meet its end where a wound is closed, but continues till complete healing. In fact, the wound curative mechanism is a highly dynamic process involving the overlapping of hemostasis, proliferation, inflammation, and re-modeling that engrosses multiple cell types (like keratinocytes, endothelial cells, fibroblasts, macrophages, and neutrophils). In DFUs, the deregulation in any of these factors contributes macro- and microvascular, neuropathic, immune functions, and biochemical malfunctions which result significantly in the delay of healing process [41, 50]. Besides these intrinsic factors, the evolution of DFU also involves some parallel extrinsic aspects such as callous formation, repeated trauma, excessive pressure, and wound infection [51, 52]. Beyond, MicroRNA profiling of epidermis and dermal fibroblasts of diabetic foot skin (DFS) and healthy nondiabetic foot skin (NFS) highlighted the presence of subtle genomic changes such as deregulation of five miRNAs and upregulation of MiR-31-5p and miR-31-3p in DFS [52].

20.5.1.4 Infections

Infection is the most important factor complexing foot ulcer clinical management. However, besides ischemia, many factors such as peripheral neuropathy [53], and vascular insufficiency [54], contribute ulceration in the diabetic foot. For instance, medical occult ulcers form insidiously subterranean to the callus [55, 56]. Besides, an array of soft associated abnormalities including edema, abscess, ulcer, arthritis, and cellulitis were found commonly in the diabetic foot [57, 58]. Furthermore, infected ulcers or soft tissue infections lead to osteomyelitis which extends to the bones [59]. On an average, about 15% of diabetic foots suffer from osteomyelitis [57, 58]. Soft tissue infection is important because >90% osteomyelitis in DFUs results from the spread of soft tissue infection [60]. Besides these, more than 60% of all infections are caused by microbial biofilms [61] as per recent report of the National Institute of Health (NIH). Overall, the severity of infections in DFUs is subjected to their sign and extent of inflammation and depth of infected tissue, as per PEDIS validated classifications of diabetic foot infection and Infectious Diseases Society of America (IDSA). In DFUs, the bacterial infection causes multilayer microbial matrix formation, popularly known as biofilms, provides the resistant to antimicrobials agents and contributes to delaying wound healing [62, 63].

Nevertheless, DFUs generally in diabetics are at greatest risk maintaining microbial infection and hence clinicians evaluate such types of lesions for the possibility of infection [64, 65]. Purulent drainage of pus along with other inflammatory signs including erythema, induration, inflammation, pain, softness is a potential indicator of infection. However clinical signs on juncture contradict the implication and severity of infection. For example, fever at 102 °F indicates the wound is deeper with a serious infection and maintains extensive necrosis, pus, and cellulitis in diabetic foot, whereas, 12–35% patients hospitalized for limb-threatening infection have significant fever [64, 65].

20.6 Microbiome and DFU

20.6.1 Microbiology of DFU

The DFU microbiome can be defined as the totality of microflora, their genomes, and interactions within multilayered microenvironment commonly known as biofilm. In general, chronic lesions or wounds are prone to develop polymicrobial biofilms which are composed of Corynebacterium, Pseudomonas, and Staphylococcus [66–68]. The DFU microbiome is often regarded as playing pivotal role in delayed lesion healing [66] by attenuating the antimicrobial effects therapeutic agents potentially by modifying or shielding their respective targets. Recently, Wolcott et al. [69] have studied 2963 microbiomes from chronic wounds including DFUs, and found a large number of anaerobic bacteria while Staphylococcus followed by Pseudomonas as the most prevalent microbes. Besides, Gardner et al. [70] specifically explored the biodiversity and bioburden of the DFU microbiome of 52 patients using 16S rRNA gene PCR method and identified Staphylococcus in about 94% of DFUs and both anaerobes and Proteobacteria to the tune of 100% of these wounds [69]. This study has also highlighted the fact that the diversity DFU microbiome significantly varies as a reduction of anaerobes and Proteobacteria as lesion depth decreases.

Therefore, it would be appropriate to say that the DFU microbiomes possess intrinsic potential to be translated certainly while being influenced by external factors because an open DFU cavity often contains numerous bacteria of either commensal or colonizing nature, some of which holds the capacity of becoming invasive pathogens [71]. Slater et al. [72] have observed that wound depth beyond the bone can yield the recovery of same microorganisms in swab as well as deep tissue samples, whereas, only 65% organisms can be recovered from swab specimens compared to deep tissues cultures with the exemption of Corynebacterium species likely as colonizers or contaminants [73]. Thus, clinicians require standard interpretation criteria for whether a microorganism is potentially invasive or colonizer. At the same time, the limb-threatening infections (LTI) and non-limb-threatening-infections (NLTI) in diabetics also reflected significant microbial diversity. For instance, NLTI with no earlier antimicrobial therapy maintains Staphylococcus aureus and group B streptococci specifically [74–76]. Precisely, S. aureus isolated from NLTI patients also found to accumulate methicillin-resistant (MRSA) in the soft tissue of ulcers as compared to the skin [74]. In 2010, Lipsky et al. [77] have also observed an increase from 11.6% to 21.9% in MRSA prevalence in diabetes patients between 2003 and 2007 [77]. While, LTIs were observed generally polymicrobial in type yielding on an average of 2.3–5.8 bacterial species per deep tissue culture from a single lesion sample including both Gram-positive cocci and Gram-negative rods cells [71, 74, 78–80]. Strictly, MRSA, streptococci, Enterobacter species, Proteus species, Klebsiella species, *Escherichia coli*, and *Pseudomonas aeruginosa* were prominent among these clinical infections. Among the anaerobes, Prevotella species, Pepto streptococcus species and Bacteroides species, including those of the *B. fragilis* group, are more often recovered [81, 82].

20.6.2 Biofilm and Antimicrobial Resistance in DFU

The growing concern of antibiotic-resistant strains [83, 84], embedded in highly complex and multicomponent biofilm matrices, has led IDSA (Infectious Diseases Society of America), assigning *Enterococcus faecium*, *Staphylococcus aureus*, *Klebsiella pneumoniae*, *Acinetobacter baumannii*, *Pseudomonas aeruginosa*, and Enterobacter species as "ESKAPE pathogens" due to ever-changing dynamics of the host and decreasing treatment regimen against them [85]. In general,

Staphylococcus aureus (Gram-positive) and *Pseudomonas aeruginosa* (Gram-negative) are assigned as potential biofilm producers in many chronic infections, due to their resistance to antibiotics [86, 87]. Albeit, there is no doubt that the antibiotics can work well provided the bacteria are in their planktonic state. Contrarily, chronic wounds such as DFU often acquire organized aggregates or coexisting clusters of bacteria in biofilm matrices which are comprised of liquid polysaccharides, proteins, and extracellular DNA (eDNA), which constitute the extracellular polymeric substances [88]. Therefore, the formation of biofilms in chronic wounds can be argued as a core reason for the failure of about 65–80% antibiotic treatment modalities and causes delays in wound healing [89–91].

According to Wang et al. [92], despite target specific acceleration of tissue engineering to halt the normal orchestrated and schemed course of wound healing cascades (including hemostasis, inflammation, proliferation, and remodeling), >25% diabetics of survived limb amputation due to chronic DFUs [93, 94]. Recently, Ch'ng et al. have suggested the role of polymicrobial bacterial biofilms as the likeliest reason for delayed healing in prolonged chronic infection [95], by sustaining the influx of pro-inflammatory cells and impede host response parallel [96–98]. The community of bacterial biofilms most commonly composed of *Staphylococcus*, *Pseudomonas*, and *Corynebacterium* [66, 68], and irreversibly adhered to the tissue surface in wounds by getting embedded self-produced extracellular polymeric substances (EPS) matrix [99]. This EPS often shields the bacteria in biofilms to rescue from antibiotics and host innate immune cells in order to create an immediate microenvironment for bacteria to accumulate resistant by either mutation or gene transfer [62]. Precisely, there is >50% higher risk of biofilm formation in chronic wounds in diabetics compared to nondiabetics [89, 100–102], because on an average a >90% of such wounds can provoke excessive inflammation by the activation of immune complexes causing long-standing release of inflammatory cytokines, thus slowing the cutaneous wound healing [103, 104]. Nevertheless, as a usual chronic wound type, DFU does not encompass the normal course of healing cascades due to polymicrobial biofilms infections.

20.7 Risk Factor and Prevention of DFUs

20.7.1 Risk Factors

Foot ulceration is around 25% high [13] and 40–80% frequent [105] in diabetic patients causing a huge risk of morbidity and mortality. The study of Lavery et al. [106] highlighted the peril of hospitalization with the lower-extremity amputation reported to be approximately 56-fold and 155-fold higher in diabetics with DFUs compared to diabetics without DFU, respectively. Furthermore, according to the Centre for Disease Control and Prevention, alone in the USA, diabetes has become a devastating complication causing blindness in adults at an average rate of 24,000 individuals per year [107], whereas, around 43% diabetics enter for dialysis and transplantation [108]. Besides, twofold to sixfold diabetic population is more likely to develop risk of heart disease, whereas and twofold to fourfold more likely to have a stroke as compared to nondiabetics. Drastically, diabetes can result in 15-fold to 40-fold greater risk of amputations in diabetics compared to nondiabetics which were estimated the loss of 82,000 limbs per year due to diabetes [109]. Typically, in diabetics, the epidemiology of individual risk factors such as diabetic peripheral neuropathy (DPN) an impairment of nerves that alters autonomic, motor, and sensory functions [42], the compromised vascular system believed to contribute both macro- and microvascular peripheral vascular disease, resulting in ischemic limb because of the abridged healing capacity of wounds itself [110], and musculoskeletal deformities such as a presence or absence of hammertoe or bunion play a major role in ulceration pathway in respect to negative and positive pressure and friction [111].

20.7.2 Treatment Modalities

Treatment of DFU infections is a complicated and economically cumbersome job that requires long-term medications and hospitalization. Indeed, treatment of DFU infections is teamwork including experienced physicians, surgeons, podiatrists, and competent and trained dressing nurses. Therefore, an average treatment cost of a DFU with Wagner grade I in five industrialized countries was estimated at $3096 in 2010; however, if complications come to amputation, the cost will rise to almost $107,900 [112]. Beyond, evaluation of DFUs begins with a detailed clinical history and physical examination. The standard wound care however is a multifaceted procedure which includes debridement, unloading of DFU, use of appropriate antibiotics schedules, and advanced dressings, etc. However, the superficial topical dressings, lotions, ointments, and acellular matrices may proffer some advantages depending on the wound environment, but many wounds deserve refined and sophisticated therapies in addition to the standard curative modalities to accomplish complete wound closure [113]. Nevertheless, the latest treatment modalities are based on necrotic debris removal, infection control, and relieve in chronic pressure on DFUs. In addition to antibiotic therapy, the treatment of DFUs has been developed through bioengineered tissue engraftment in order to accelerate the wound healing process by releasing required growth factors, cytokines, and other proteins adequately [114]. Also, the less toxic, hazardous, and expensive biomaterials accelerate wound healing and control infection, which can be envisioned as novel treatment modality [115]. Both synthetic and natural polymers are underlined to investigate their intrinsic therapeutic potential to trigger the regeneration of damaged dermal and epidermal tissues [116].

Besides, in view of antibiotic based treatment modalities, advanced technologies such as DNA microarray and multiplex real-time PCR are in use nowadays to analyze both virulence and resistance of microbial strains [117, 118]. Thus, systemic antibiotic therapy is required to control DFU infection clinically but not appraised as the lone cure [120–122]. To date, different systemically active antibiotic agents such as ertapenem, linezolid, doripenem, dalbavancin, ceftobiprole, tigecycline, or daptomycin [123–126] have shown significant antimicrobial activities against the bacterial isolates of DFU.

20.7.3 Preventive Management

Diabetes patients unfortunately develop multiple complications such as peripheral vascular disease, chronic renal disease, ulcerations, gastrointestinal diseases, or cardiac diseases. Therefore, an organized multi-disciplinary DFU care team is needed to manage the prevention and cure of diabetes patients via predictive, preventive, and mechanistic strategies. In view of historical background, Dr. Elliot P. Joslin (Joslin Diabetes Centre, USA established in 1952) reviewed that DFU complications deserve a team of specialists in order to manage DFU infections [127]. This is very obvious since the ultimate target is the complete healing of wound and limb salvage while curing DFUs. However, there are several inexpensive and feasible strategies which can play a crucial part in the clinical management of DFUs such as, (1) assembling of a competent diabetic foot care team, (2) strong commitment to delivering the highest quality health care, (3) psychosocial and educational trainings for to DFUs and, (4) underscoring the role of footwear and the state of the art techniques in the prevention of DFUs.

Generally, the term "quality health care" is the indicator of quality assurance essentials which reflect the commitment of "undertaking the right thing at the right time in the right way for the right person" intending to have the best achievable results [119]. According to this quality paradigm, the quality care of DFU patient, in fact, encompasses via four matrices and the three of them are process-based channels, namely the evaluations which provide adequate facilities at the correct time and the apt accomplishment of the services. The fourth evaluation requires the "best results" outcome assessment [128].

Beyond, individuals with diabetes and DFUs face traumatic events such as elevated levels of mental stress, anxiety, feeling of helplessness, and temporary conditions of cognitive perplexity while going through the course of diabetes [129, 130]. Specially, the four periods merit unique mention like the onset of diabetes, maintenance, and prevention of health, early commencement of complications, and the phase of illness where complications dominate [130, 131]. Therefore, motivation and patients' trainings to create adequate skills to take care of itself play a vital job in the prevention of DFUs. In fact, diabetes patients with DFUs must understand all the instructions of DFUs preventive and caring guidelines.

Furthermore, diabetes and diabetes complications provoke progressive developments in foot structures and their functions. The morphological changes majorly observed in the tissues of foot–ankle complex [132–134]. Precisely, these changes in tissues affect the tendons and ligaments, cartilage, muscles, peripheral sensory system, skin, foot morphology, and patient's weight due to a complex cascade of intrinsic events. Besides these, for instance, if a diabetic is seriously compromised, the most important challenge is the prevention of ulcerative infections. For this, the primary preventive measure to be taken is dialog with the patient for proper, containment, and shielding footwear rather than remedial. According to peripheral neuropathy based investigations, the proper footwear is intended to (1) redistribute the plantar pressure in order to shun highly localized and contained pressure peak, (2) reduce the friction and abrasion, (3) deterrence of mechanical and thermal trauma and (4) the restoration or maintenance of foot function during walk. Thus, the function of footwear in the avoidance of diabetic foot complications is taken as a serious preventive action.

20.8 Nanotechnology as an Innovative Approach for Accelerating Wound Healing in DFU

20.8.1 Nanotechnology and DFU

As defined by the World Health Organization (WHO), Diabetic foot is an "ulceration of foot associated with neuropathy and different grades of ischemia and infection" that leads to tissue breakdown. Treatment for diabetic foot ulcer includes dressings, infection management with antibiotics, wound debridement, off-loading, and surgical revascularization [135, 136]. Recently, modern approaches to wound dressing received great attention. These dressing can release peptides, therapeutic agents, growth factors (GFs), stem cells, and other bioactive substances that afford the favorable microenvironment for successful healing and curing by controlling wound humidity and soaking up excess exudates.

Such dressings could reduce inflammatory cytokines and excessive protease levels while amplifying the GFs in the wound biochemical environment, thus, decreasing tissue degradation and enhance tissue formation [137]. However, in developing countries, people still use natural substances (herbs, plant extracts, honey) in the treatment of infections including diabetic wounds. In cases of persistent DFU conditions that do not respond to standard treatment procedures, skin grafting including autograft, allograft, xenograft, and bioengineered skin substitutes (artificial skin), are considered as alternative options [138]. Despite these interventions, approximately 40–70% of chronic ulcer patients remain unhealed. For the patients with impaired or delayed wound healing ability, new strategies/methods need to be developed for the acceleration of wound healing process, decreasing the infection and reduction in the scar formation.

During the past few decades, nanotherapeutics have emerged as one of the promising strategies to overcome the chronic and persistent nature combined with the associated complications of non-repairing wounds. Nanoparticles (NPs) facilitate the targeted delivery of active drugs that are usually not bioavailable in vivo due to short half-life, poor solubility, and/or leakage from the spot of the wound. The major advantage of nanoparticles-based treatment is the high surface area to volume ratio which increases the degrees of probability of interaction with biological target and offers improved penetrating ability to the wounds. Nanoparticle-based drug delivery allows a controlled release of the drug that let the continuous interaction between drug and target. There are two key criteria of nanomaterials employment in wound healing: (1) nanomaterials with inherent therapeutic properties advantageous for wound healing (2) nanomaterials as delivery medium for therapeutics. Silver, gold, copper, zinc oxide, cerium oxide, yttrium oxide, titanium dioxide, carbon-based nanoparticles and nanoparticles bearing nitric oxide are most studied

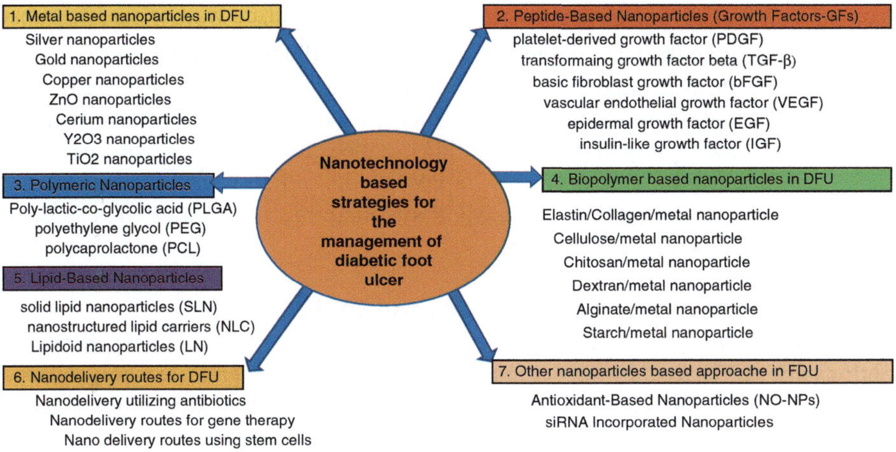

Fig. 20.1 Various nanotechnology-based strategies and approaches for the treatment and management of diabetic foot ulcer

metallic and non-metallic nanoparticles for wound healing due to their inherent antibacterial properties. Different nanotechnology-based strategies for the treatment, cure, and management of diabetic foot ulcers have been shown in Fig. 20.1.

20.8.2 Nanoparticles for Treatment of DFU

20.8.2.1 Metal Nanoparticles and DFU

Silver nanoparticles (AgNPs) are the most studied nanoparticles in wound care management because of their known antibacterial effects [139]. The antibacterial effects of Ag are mediated by the interaction of Ag^+ with three main constituents of the bacterial cell viz. (1). peptidoglycan composed cell wall, (2) bacterial DNA and, (3) proteins and enzymes involved in essential cellular processes such as electron transport chain (ETC). In addition, AgNPs have shown to be anti-inflammatory in property and promotes wound healing by reducing the release of cytokine, thereby, decreasing the infiltration of lymphocyte and mast cell [140, 141]. Dressing impregnated with AgNPs have shown to be efficient in wound healing in diabetic mice [142]. Likewise, gold nanoparticles (AuNPs) have been widely studied for medical applications. Leu et al. [143] combined AuNPs with the antioxidant epigallocatechin gallate (EGCG) and α-lipoic acid (ALA) hastening the diabetic wound healing by the regulation of inflammation and angiogenesis. In another attempt, researchers synthesized antimicrobial Au nanodots that inhibited the growth of MDR bacteria and promoted healing in the rodent wound model [144]. The antimicrobial peptide surfactin was found to be self-assembled on Au nanodots by hydrophobic interactions with the molecules of 1-dodecanethiol that served as the capping agent on the Au nanodots. The NPs demonstrated much higher antibacterial wound healing effect against MDR bacteria (like methicillin-resistant *S. aureus*) infected wound than the free surfactin. This enhanced effect is due to the capability of the fabricated NPs to disintegrate the bacterial membrane. Copper NPs (CuNPs) have also gained special attention in managing diabetic foot ulcer infection. Recently, Xiao et al., synthesized copper-based metal-organic framework NPs (Cu-MOFNPs), which are known to degrade rapidly in protein solutions, can be customized for slow release of Cu^{2+}, minimizing its toxicity and improving its efficacy of healing DFUs. Incorporation of folic acid with Cu-MOFNPs enabling the controlled release of Cu^{2+} enhanced biocompatibility [94].

20.8.2.2 Metal Oxide Nanoparticles and DFU

Metal oxide NPs (ZnO, TiO_2, CeO_2, and Y_2O_3) are among the most attractive options for DFU as they are comprised of essential mineral elements for the human body. ZnO NPs are effectively used for wound healing as their own strong antibacterial properties and can stay at the wound site for a longer time period, thus, escalating the healing process. In a recent study, Steffy et al. [145] biosynthesized ZnO nanoparticles that displayed strong bactericidal properties against multidrug resistant strains isolated from DFU. CeO_2NPs have strong free radical scavenging properties [146]. Further, Ce atom has dual oxidation state +4 and +3, meaning that its reduction from the oxidation state of Ce^{4+} to Ce^{3+} resulting in oxygen vacancy. This improves the potential of the CeO_2NPs of healing DFUs followed by free radical scavenging activity. Y_2O_3NPs are nontoxic to neutrophils and macrophages. Also, Y_2O_3NPs require maximum free energy for the formation of oxide from yttrium than other metal oxides, hence it is considered for the treatment of DFU [147].

20.8.2.3 Biopolymer Based Nanoparticles in DFU

20.8.2.3.1 Cellulose and Its Derivatives/Metal Nanoparticle for DFU

The wound healing ability of cellulose is reported in several studies as it can accelerate the healing process via the release of numerous growth factors (GFs). Cellulose-based materials integrated with antibacterial and antimicrobial agents are designed which can be used for healing diabetic wounds. Cellulose acetate nanofibers embodied with AgNPs were used as wound dressing showed high production of collagen ensuring its use as wound healing material [148]. Bamboo cellulose nanocrystal based nano-bio-composite hydrogels soaked with AgNPs effectively heal diabetic wound in mice by decreasing inflammation with concomitantly generating collagen [149]. A bacterial cellulose incorporated with AuNPs was also studied as a healing material prepared as nanocomposites [150]. These nanocomposites material showed magnificent antibacterial properties with outstanding moisture retention ability.

20.8.2.3.2 Chitosan/Metal Nanoparticle for DFU

Chitosan is a cationic polymer that can interact with anionic components of microbial cell membranes resulting in the disruption of the membrane and other intracellular constituents. A fusion composite of PLGA NPs entrenched in chitosan nanofibers was studied to deliver dual growth factors (VEGF and PDGF) exhibiting improved wound healing via VEGF mediated angiogenesis and PDGF interceded tissue regeneration [151]. AgNPs collagen/chitosan scaffold [152], scaffold containing colloid Au/chitosan [153], chitosan-based Cu nanocomposite [154] are also studied for their wound healing application.

20.8.2.3.3 Dextran/Metal Nanoparticle for DFU

Dextran based hydrogels are very soft and pliable and were able to encourage complete skin regeneration without any addition of GFs and cytokines [155]. AgNPs incorporated dextran hydrogel was tested against Bacillus cereus for its antibacterial effect and concluded to be an effective antibacterial material with adequate biocompatibility and biodegradability [156]. Păunica-Panea et al. [157] prepared dextran and collaged based composite incorporated with ZnO as antimicrobial agent having potential for skin regeneration and wound healing.

20.8.2.3.4 Alginate/Metal Nanoparticle for DFU

Alginate is a biopolymer that is readily used in the treatment of diabetic wound incorporation of NPs on alginate-based hydrogel that has been reported to improve wound healing process. Mohandas et al. [158] developed alginate hydrogel/ZnO NPs composite bandage. The prepared nanocomposite exhibited improved antibacterial activity and enhanced.

20.8.2.3.5 Elastin/Collagen/Metal Nanoparticle for DFU

Akturk et al. [159] designed composites of collagen/gold nanoparticles for rapid wound healing and in vivo study showing that the gold nanoparticles were biocompatible with the cells of skin tissue. The scaffolds of elastin and silk fibroin have been developed for the treatment of burns and it was found that porous scaffolds were mechanically stable, biocompatible, and most importantly mimicked the properties of extracellular matrix (ECM). Further, it has been tested and found that these porous structures accelerate and improve the healing and finally confirmed that it suits excellent wound healing material [160]. Kawabata et al. [161] developed a novel wound healing material in form of silk elastin sponge. In vivo study shows that silk elastin fastens the healing process and thus it can be applied to various wounds that are difficult to treat with the aqueous solution [161].

20.8.2.3.6 Starch/Metal Nanoparticle for DFU

Starch is a carbohydrate biopolymer macromolecule and found in abundance in potato, rice, wheat, cassava, and maize. Due to its biocompatible nature, easy availability, low cost, renewability, nontoxic and thermoplastic nature, it is used in various biomedical applications such as drug delivery systems, stents, scaffolds of tissue engineering, orthopedic surgery, and bone cement [162–166]. Antimicrobial hydrogel containing starch coated with copper nanoparticles has been developed by Villanueva et al. [167] exhibit a great potential of using it as wound healing material.

20.8.3 Lipid Based Nanoparticles

There are various lipids based NPs which show promising effect against chronic wounds. Nanostructured lipid carriers (NLC) and Solid lipid nanoparticles (SLN) are potent drug delivery systems attracting much interest as efficient and nontoxic carriers for various active compounds [168–172]. These nanoparticles have been tested in vivo for topical administration of growth factors by administering recombinant human epidermal growth factor (rhEGF) encapsulated SLN and NLC. These NLC-rhEGF and SLN-rhEGF showed enhanced efficiency of encapsulation and a faster rate of wound closure [173]. Wound dressings embedded with Ag sulfadiazine loaded SLNs were developed in the treatment of skin lesions [174]. Furthermore, SLNs have been tested for delivering other bioactive molecules such as opioids like morphine [175], resveratrol [176] for wound healing [177, 178]. PLGA NPs were used to transport rhEGF for the enhancement of the closure of full-thickness diabetic wounds [179]. Proteoliposome was also tested to deliver growth factor co-receptors along with growth factors that showed increased re-epithelization and angiogenesis [180]. Phenytoin-loaded lipid nanostructured carrier was found to be enhancing the healing of neuropathic DFUs [181].

20.8.4 Antioxidant Based Nanoparticles (NO-NPs)

The biomedical application of nitric oxide (NO) in the treatment of chronic ulcers has emerged because of their antibacterial and antibiofilm activity against a number of bacterial sp. It has been reported that NO induces angiogenesis, re-epithelialization, fibroblast, and collagen synthesis and increases the level of growth factors and inflammatory cells [182]. Blecher et al. [183] reported that post-topical application of NO-NPs in diabetic mice, NO-NPs accelerated the closure of the wound with high level of blood vessels, increased content of collagen fibroblasts and reduced inflammatory cells. In a similar in vivo study, it has also been reported that NO-NPs hasten the wound healing, mediate propagation, and resettlement of fibroblasts with increased collagen expression and elevate the level of anti-inflammatory cytokines along with TGF-β (transforming growth factor-beta) in diabetic mice [184].

20.8.5 siRNA-Based Nanoparticles

Kasiewicz and Whitehead [185] investigated that the topical application of siTNFα-loaded LNPs compacted the expression of TNFα in nondiabetic wounds by 54% at 500 nM dose, whereas 250 nM affected about 43% gene silencing in diabetic mice and they observed that the siTNFα-loaded LNPs closed the wound in diabetic mice faster than control wounds by reducing the duration and severity of chronic diabetic wounds [185]. In another study, Kasiewicz and Whitehead [186] reported that lipidoid loaded-siTNF-α NPs downregulates the TNF-α and MCP-1 expression and accelerate the closure of DFUs. Kim and Yoo [187] developed MMP-2 siRNA-incorporated linear polyethylenimine (LPEI) complex onto a nano-fibrous mesh which efficiently suppressed the level of MMP-2, promoting and accelerating the wound healing in diabetic murine wounds [187]. Randeria et al. [188] constructed GM3S (ganglioside-monosialic acid 3-synthase) thiolated-siRNA conjugated with AuNPs. The constructed GM3S SNA, efficiently accelerated the relocation and propagation by diminishing the level of ganglioside GM3S and, consequently accelerating the wound healing in type 2 diabetic wound model.

20.9 Nanodelivery Routes for DFU

20.9.1 Nanodelivery Utilizing Antibiotics for DFU Treatment

Treatment of DFUs through antibiotics faces several challenges due to the increase in antibiotic-resistant strains. Reformulations of antibiotics using nanoparticles provide a promising solution against antibiotic resistance, toxicity stability, and solubility. Chakraborty et al. [189] tested the efficacy of folic acid coupled nano-sized-chitosan vehicle loaded with drug vancomycin against drug-resistant *S. aureus*. As folic acid is a vital nutrient required for nucleotide synthesis by bacteria, it mediates the transport of vancomycin loaded chitosan nanoparticles into the cytoplasm via endocytosis. Chitosan, gelatine, and EGCG NPs have been incorporated in polyglutamic acid and gelatin hydrogels enclosing activated carbon fibers with gentamicin, to create a wound dressing for enhancing rejuvenation and inhibition of microbial growth [190].

20.9.2 Nanodelivery Routes for Gene Therapy in DFU

Sustained gene delivery therapy has attracted many researchers as a promising option for the treatment of DFU. The gene therapy can deliver growth modulating genes to the cells at the wound site, thus assist in the improvement of the reparative process. Several nonviral vectors such as PLGA and others have been developed to improve the efficiency of gene therapy [191].

20.9.3 Nano Delivery Routes Using Stem Cells in DFU

It has been suggested that the amalgamation of stem cells props up angiogenesis and re-epithelialization in chronic wounds [182]. The nanotechnology-modified stem cells showed enhanced and improved production of hVEGF, cell viability, and engraftment into the target tissues. After implantation of scaffolds seeded with VEGF-expressing stem cells (hMSCs and hESdCs), about twofold to fourfold higher vessel concentration was observed in comparison to the control cells. It has been suggested that direct delivery of MSCs (mesenchymal stem cells)/nano scaffold to the wound can induce the fast death of the cell [192]. Hamdan et al. [193] proposed that the nano scaffold/BM-MSC (Bone marrow-derived mesenchymal stem cells) nanocomposite exhibits useful novel advance for wound cure and skin generation in acute full-thickness skin wounds [193]. Thus, nanotechnology-based delivery of stem cells may play an imperative role in the therapeutic management of DFU [191].

20.10 Conclusion and Future Prospects

In conclusion, it is observed that the microbial infections, accumulation of bacterial biofilm, and development of chronic ulceration in diabetics are coherent events which all together lead complicates the treatment of DFUs. Furthermore, the accumulation of MDR in causative bacterial strains has accentuated the challenges of DFUs treatments. Systematic reviews on DFUs treatment highlights that clinical management is a huge economic burden, globally. Recently, nanotechnological-based nano-formulation and nanodelivery techniques using nanoparticles have revolutionized the medical field for the diagnosis and treatment of various microbial infections and other diseases. The various nanodelivery systems such as nanoparticles drug delivery systems, peptides-based delivery systems, biopolymer-based systems, polymeric gene delivery systems, stem cell delivery systems, and free radical scavenging systems by exploring nanotechnology are found to be very effective and gained worldwide popularity as an alternative for the treatment of bacterial infections and DFUs. Therefore, the summary of nano-formulations development and their remedial impacts against MDR and wound healing presented herein encourages the clinicians and researchers to device novel yet inexpensive, less risky, and more promising antibacterial formulations.

References

1. Free HM, Free AH (1984) Analytical chemistry in the conquest of diabetes. Anal Chem 56(6):664A–684A
2. International Diabetes Federation (IDF). Morbidity and mortality. http://atlas.idf-bxl.org/content/diabetes-mortality. Accessed March 2010
3. Guariguata L, Whiting DR, Hambleton I, Beagley J, Linnenkamp U, Shaw JE (2014) Global estimates of diabetes prevalence for 2013 and projections for 2035. Diabetes Res Clin Pract 103(2):137–149
4. National Diabetes Statistics Report (2017) Estimates of diabetes and its burden in the United States. Centers for Disease Control and Prevention, U.S. Department of Health and Human Services, Atlanta, GA, p 2017
5. World Health Organisation (W.H.O). Health topics: diabetes. http://www.who.int/topics/diabetes_mellitus/en/. Accessed March 2010
6. Quon MJ, Cochran C, Taylor SI, Eastman RC (1994) Noninsulin-mediated glucose disappearance in subjects with IDDM. Discordance between experimental results and minimal model analysis. Diabetes 43(7):890–896
7. Tesfaye S, Stevens LK, Stephenson JM, Fuller JH, Plater M, Ionescu-Tirgoviste C et al (1996) Prevalence of diabetic peripheral neuropathy and its relation to glycaemic control and potential risk factors: the EURODIAB IDDM complications study. Diabetologia 39(11):1377–1384

8. Balakrishnan NP, Rangaiah GP, Samavedham L (2011) Review and analysis of blood glucose (BG) models for type 1 diabetic patients. Ind Eng Chem Res 50(21):12041–12066
9. Matthews D, Meston N, Dyson P, Shaw J, King L, Pal A (2008) Medication. In: Diabetes: the facts, 1st edn. Oxford University Press, Oxford, p 5376
10. Makroglou A, Li J, Kuang Y (2006) Mathematical models and software tools for the glucose-insulin regulatory system and diabetes: an overview. Appl Numer Math 56(34):559–573
11. Lázaro-Martínez JL, Aragón-Sánchez J, Alvaro-Afonso FJ, García-Morales E, García-Álvarez Y, Molines-Barroso RJ (2014) The best way to reduce reulcerations: if you understand biomechanics of the diabetic foot, you can do it. Int J Low Extrem Wounds 13(4):294–319
12. Armstrong DG, Boulton AJ, Bus SA (2017) Diabetic foot ulcers and their recurrence. N Engl J Med 376:2367–2375
13. Singh N, Armstrong DG, Lipsky BA (2005) Preventing foot ulcers in patients with diabetes. JAMA 293(2):217–228
14. Fortington LV, Geertzen JH, van Netten JJ, Postema K, Rommers GM, Dijkstra PU (2013) Short and long term mortality rates after a lower limb amputation. Eur J Vasc Endovasc Surg 46:124–131
15. Jeffcoate WJ, Chipchase SY, Ince P et al (2006) Assessing the outcome of the management of diabetic foot ulcers using ulcer-related and person-related measures. Diabetes Care 29(8):1784–1787
16. Margolis DJ, Kantor J, Berlin JA (1999) Healing of diabetic neuropathic foot ulcers receiving standard trcaimeiit. A meta-analysis. Diabetes Cure 22:692–695
17. Kaufman J, Breeding L, Rosenberg N (1987) Anatomical location of acute diabetic foot infection: its influence on the outcome of treatment. Am J Surg 53:109–112
18. Armstrong DG, Lavery LA (1998) Diabetic foot ulcers: prevention, diagnosis and classification. Am Fam Physician 57:1325–1332
19. Wagner FW Jr (1981) The dysvascular foot: a system for diagnosis and treatment. Foot Ankle 2:64–122
20. Armstrong DG, Lavery LA, Harkless LB (1998) Validation of a diabetic wound classification system. The contribution of depth, infection, and ischemia to risk of amputation. Diabetes Care 21:855–859
21. Brodsky JW (1999) The diabetic foot. In: Mann RA, Coughlin MJ (eds) Surgery of the foot and ankle, 7th edn. Mosby-Year Book, St Louis, MO
22. Peters EJ, Lavery LA (2001) Effectiveness of the diabetic foot risk classification system of the international working group on the diabetic foot. Diabetes Care 24:1442–1447
23. Schaper NC (2003) International Consensus on the diabetic foot and practical guidelines on the management and the prevention of the diabetic foot. International Working Group on the diabetic foot. Curr Diab Rep 3:475
24. Karthikesalingam A, Holt PJ, Moxey P, Jones KG, Thompson MM, Hinchliffe RJ (2010) A systematic review of scoring systems for diabetic foot ulcers. Diabet Med 27:544–549
25. Mills JL Sr, Conte MS, Armstrong DG, Pomposelli FB, Schanzer A, Sidawy AN et al (2014) The society for vascular surgery lower extremity threatened limb classification system: risk stratification based on Wound, Ischemia, and foot Infection (WIfI). J Vasc Surg 59:220–34.e1-2
26. Terashi H, Kitano I, Tsuji Y (2011) Total management of diabetic foot ulcerations—Kobe classification as a new classification of diabetic foot wounds. Keio J Med 60:17–21
27. Wild S, Roglic G, Green A, Sicree R, King H (2004) Global prevalence of diabetes: estimates for the year 2000 and projections for 2030. Diabetes Care 27(5):1047–1053
28. Edmonds M, Foster A (2000) The high-risk foot. In: Managing the diabetic foot. Blackwell Science, London, pp 35–44
29. Daousi C, MacFarlane IA, Woodward A, Nurmikko TJ, Bundred PE, Benbow SJ (2004) Chronic painful peripheral neuropathy in an urban community: a controlled comparison of people with and without diabetes. Diabet Med 21(9):976–982
30. Hall GC, Carroll D, Parry D, McQuay HJ (2006) Epidemiology and treatment of neuropathic pain: the UK primary care perspective. Pain 122(1–2):156–162

31. The Diabetes Control and Complications Trial Research Group (1993) The effect of intensive treatment of diabetes on the development and progression of long-term complications in insulin-dependent diabetes mellitus. N Engl J Med 329(14):977–986
32. American Diabetes Association (2013) Economic costs of diabetes in the U.S. in 2012. Diabetes Care 36(4):1033–1046
33. Skrepnek GH, Mills JL, Lavery LA, Armstrong DG (2017) Health care service and outcomes among an estimated 6.7 million ambulatory care diabetic foot cases in the U.S. Diabetes Care 40(7):936–942
34. Mott VA (1818) A case of circular callous ulcer in the bottom of the foot. Med Surg Reg NY 1:129
35. Bowling FL, Abbot CA, Harris WE et al (2012) A pocket sized disposable device for testing the integrity of sensation in the outpatient setting. Diabet Med 29:1550–1552
36. Armstrong DG, Peters EJ, Athanasiou KA, Lavery LA (1998) Is there a critical level of plantar foot pressure to identify patients at risk for neuropathic foot ulceration? J Foot Ankle Surg 37(4):303–307
37. Cavanagh PR, Ulbrecht JS, Caputo GM (1996) Biomechanical aspects of diabetic foot disease: aetiology, treatment, and prevention. Diabet Med 13(Suppl 1):S17–S22
38. Lavery LA, Vela SA, Lavery DC, Quebedeaux TL (1996) Reducing dynamic foot pressures in high-risk diabetic subjects with foot ulcerations. A comparison of treatments. Diabetes Care 19(8):818–821
39. Lavery LA, Lavery DC, Quebedeax-Farnham TL (1995) Increased foot pressures after great toe amputation in diabetes. Diabetes Care 18(11):1460–1462
40. Brand PW (1983) The diabetic foot. In: Ellenberg M, Rifkin H (eds) Diabetes mellitus, theory and practice, 3rd edn. Medical Examination Publishing, New York, NY, pp 803–828
41. Eming SA, Martin P, Tomic-Canic M (2014) Wound repair and regeneration: mechanisms, signaling, and translation. Sci Transl Med 6(265):265sr6
42. LeQuesne P, Parkshouse N, Faris I (1991) Neuropathy. In: Faris I (ed) The management of the diabetic foot, 2nd edn. Churchill Livingstone, Edinburgh, p 41
43. Thomas PK (1973) Metabolic neuropathy. J Roy Coll Phys (Lond) 7:154–174
44. Pop-Busui R, Boulton AJ, Feldman EL, Bril V, Freeman R, Malik RA, Sosenko JM, Ziegler D (2017) Diabetic neuropathy: a position statement by the American Diabetes Association. Diabetes Care 40(1):136–154
45. Tesfaye S, Vileikyte L, Rayman G, Sindrup S, Perkins B, Baconja M et al (2011) on behalf of the Toronto Expert Panel on Diabetic Neuropathy. Painful diabetic peripheral neuropathy: consensus recommendations on diagnosis, assessment and management. Diabetes Metab Res Rev 27:629–638
46. Defronzo RA, Ferrannini E, Keen H, Zimmet P (2004) International textbook of diabetes mellitus. In: Dinh TL, Veves A (eds) The diabetic foot, 3rd edn. John Wiley & Sons, Ltd., New York, NY, pp 1315–1332
47. Calvet MH, Yoshikawa TT (2001) Infections in diabetes. Infect Dis Clin N Am 15:407e18
48. Flynn MD, Tooke JE (1992) Aetiology of diabetic foot ulceration: a role for the microcirculation? Diabet Med 9(4):320–329
49. Moura LI, Dias AM, Carvalho E, de Sousa HC (2013) Recent advances on the development of wound dressings for diabetic foot ulcer treatment--a review. Acta Biomater 9(7):7093–7114
50. Sargen MR, Hoffstad O, Margolis DJ (2013) Geographic variation in Medicare spending and mortality for diabetic patients with foot ulcers and amputations. J Diabetes Complicat 27(2):128–133
51. Tsourdi E, Barthel A, Rietzsch H, Reichel A, Bornstein SR (2013) Current aspects in the pathophysiology and treatment of chronic wounds in diabetes mellitus. Biomed Res Int 2013:385641
52. Ramirez HA, Liang L, Pastar I, Rosa AM, Stojadinovic O, Zwick TG et al (2015) Comparative genomic, MicroRNA, and tissue analyses reveal subtle differences between non-diabetic and diabetic foot skin. PLoS One 10(8):e0137133

53. Horowitz JD, Durham JR, Nease DB, Lukens ML, Wright JG, Smead WL (1993) Prospective evaluation of magnetic resonance imaging in the management of acute diabetic foot infections. Ann Vasc Surg 7(1):44–50
54. Edmonds ME, Roberts VC, Watkins PJ (1982) Blood flow in the diabetic neuropathic foot. Diabetologia 22(1):9–15
55. Murray HJ, Young MJ, Hollis S, Boulton AJ (1996) The association between callus formation, high pressures and neuropathy in diabetic foot ulceration. Diabet Med 13(11):979–982
56. Gooding GA, Stess RM, Graf PM, Moss KM, Louie KS, Grunfeld C (1986) Sonography of the sole of the foot. Evidence for loss of foot pad thickness in diabetes and its relationship to ulceration of the foot. Investig Radiol 21(1):45–48
57. Marcus CD, Ladam-Marcus VJ, Leone J, Malgrange D, Bonnet-Gausserand FM, Menanteau BP (1996) MR imaging of osteomyelitis and neuropathic osteoarthropathy in the feet of diabetics. Radiographics 16(6):1337–1348
58. Moore TE, Yuh WT, Kathol MH, el-Khoury GY, Corson JD (1991) Abnormalities of the foot in patients with diabetes mellitus: findings on MR imaging. AJR Am J Roentgenol 157(4):813–816
59. Bamberger DM, Daus GP, Gerding DN (1987) Osteomyelitis in the feet of diabetic patients. Long-term results, prognostic factors, and the role of antimicrobial and surgical therapy. Am J Med 83(4):653–660
60. Gold RH, Tong DJ, Crim JR, Seeger LL (1995) Imaging the diabetic foot. Skelet Radiol 24(8):563–571
61. Kim L (2001) Riddle of biofilm resistance. Antimicrob Agents Chemother 45(4):999–1007
62. Mah TFC, O'Toole GA (2001) Mechanisms of biofilm resistance to antimicrobial agents. Trends Microbiol 9(1):34–39
63. Shahi SK, Kumar A (2015) Isolation and genetic analysis of multidrug resistant Bacteria from diabetic foot ulcers. Front Microbiol 6:1464
64. Lipsky BA et al (2012) Infectious Diseases Society of America clinical practice guideline for the diagnosis and treatment of diabetic foot infections. Clin Infect Dis 54(12):e132–e173
65. Lipsky BA et al (2004) A report from the international consensus on diagnosing and treating the infected diabetic foot. Diabetes Metab Res Rev 20(Suppl 1):S68–S77
66. Misic AM, Gardner SE, Grice EA (2014) The wound microbiome: modern approaches to examining the role of microorganisms in impaired chronic wound healing. Adv Wound Care (New Rochelle) 3(7):502–510
67. Zeeuwen PL, Boekhorst J, van den Bogaard EH, de Koning HD, van de Kerkhof PM, Saulnier DM et al (2012) Microbiome dynamics of human epidermis following skin barrier disruption. Genome Biol 13(11):R101
68. Redel H, Gao Z, Li H, Alekseyenko AV, Zhou Y, Perez-Perez GI et al (2013) Quantitation and composition of cutaneous microbiota in diabetic and nondiabetic men. J Infect Dis 207(7):1105–1114
69. Wolcott RD, Hanson JD, Rees EJ, Koenig LD, Phillips CD, Wolcott RA et al (2016) Analysis of the chronic wound microbiota of 2,963 patients by 16S rDNA pyrosequencing. Wound Repair Regen 24(1):163–174
70. Gardner SE, Hillis SL, Heilmann K, Segre JA, Grice EA (2013) The neuropathic diabetic foot ulcer microbiome is associated with clinical factors. Diabetes 62(3):923–930
71. Sapico FL, Canawati HN, Witte JL, Montgomerie JZ, Wagner FW, Bessman AN (1980) Quantitative aerobic and anaerobic bacteriology of infected diabetic feet. J Clin Microbiol 12(3):413–420
72. Slater RA, Lazarovitch T, Boldur I, Ramot Y, Buchs A, Weiss M et al (2004) Swab cultures accurately identify bacterial pathogens in diabetic foot wounds not involving bone. Diabet Med 21(7):705–709
73. Pellizzer G, Strazzabosco M, Presi S, Furlan F, Lora L, Benedetti P et al (2001) Deep tissue biopsy vs. superficial swab culture monitoring in the microbiological assessment of limb-threatening diabetic foot infection. Diabet Med 18(10):822–827

74. Lipsky BA, Pecoraro RE, Larson SA, Hanley ME, Ahroni JH (1990) Outpatient management of uncomplicated lower-extremity infections in diabetic patients. Arch Intern Med 150(4):790–797
75. Lipsky BA, Pecoraro RE, Wheat LJ (1990) The diabetic foot. Soft tissue and bone infection. Infect Dis Clin N Am 4(3):409–432
76. Caputo GM, Ulbrecht JS, Cavanagh PR, Juliano PJ (2000) The role of cultures in mild diabetic foot cellulitis. Infect Dis Clin Pract 9:241–243
77. Lipsky BA, Tabak YP, Johannes RS, Vo L, Hyde L, Weigelt JA (2010) Skin and soft tissue infections in hospitalised patients with diabetes: culture isolates and risk factors associated with mortality, length of stay and cost. Diabetologia 53(5):914–923
78. Scher KS, Steele FJ (1988) The septic foot in patients with diabetes. Surgery 104(4):661–666
79. Citron DM, Goldstein EJ, Merriam CV, Lipsky BA, Abramson MA (2007) Bacteriology of moderate-to-severe diabetic foot infections and in vitro activity of antimicrobial agents. J Clin Microbiol 45(9):2819–2828
80. Grayson ML, Gibbons GW, Habershaw M, Freeman DV, Pomposelli FB, Rosenblum BI et al (1994) Use of ampicillin/sulbactam versus imipenem/cilastatin in the treatment of limb-threatening foot infections in diabetic patients. Clin Infect Dis 18(5):683–693
81. Gerding DN (1995) Foot infections in diabetic patients: the role of anaerobes. Clin Infect Dis 20(Suppl 2):S283–S288
82. Johnson S, Lebahn F, Peterson LR, Gerding DN (1995) Use of an anaerobic collection and transport swab device to recover anaerobic bacteria from infected foot ulcers in diabetics. Clin Infect Dis 20(Suppl 2):S289–S290
83. Bassetti M, Merelli M, Temperoni C, Astilean A (2013) New antibiotics for bad bugs: where are we? Ann Clin Microbiol Antimicrob 12:22
84. Boucher HW, Corey GR (2008) Epidemiology of methicillin-resistant Staphylococcus aureus. Clin Infect Dis 46:S344–S349
85. Boucher HW, Talbot GH, Bradley JS, Edwards JE, Gilbert D, Rice LB et al (2009) Bad bugs, no drugs: no ESKAPE! An update from the Infectious Diseases Society of America. Clin Infect Dis 48:1–12
86. Marrie TJ, Nelligan J, Costerton JW (1982) A scanning and transmission electron microscopic study of an endocardial pacemaker lead. Circulation 66:1339–1341
87. Singh PK, Schaefer AL, Parsek MR, Moninger TO, Welsh MJ, Greenberg EP (2000) Quorum-sensing signals indicate that cystic fibrosis lungs are infected with bacterial biofilms. Nature 407:762–764
88. Davies D (2003) Understanding biofilm resistance to antibacterial agents. Nat Rev Drug Discov 2:114–122
89. Costerton J, Lewandowski W, Caldwell Z, Korber DE, Lappin-Scott HM (1995) Microbial biofilms. Annu Rev Microbiol 49:711–745
90. Hall-Stoodley L, Costerton JW, Stoodley P (2004) Bacterial biofilms: from the natural environment to infectious diseases. Nat Rev Microbiol 2:95–108
91. Passerini LO, Lam K, Costerton JW, King EG (1992) Biofilms on indwelling vascular catheters. Crit Care Med 20:665–673
92. Wang J, Chen XY, Zhao Y, Yang Y, Wang W, Wu C et al (2019) pH-Switchable antimicrobial nanofiber networks of hydrogel eradicate biofilm and rescue stalled healing in chronic wounds. ACS Nano 13:11686–11697
93. Boulton AJ, Kirsner RS, Vileikyte L (2004) Neuropathic diabetic foot ulcers. N Engl J Med 351:48–55
94. Xiao J, Zhu Y, Huddleston S, Li P, Xiao B, Farha OK, Ameer GA (2018) Copper metal-organic framework nanoparticles stabilized with folic acid improve wound healing in diabetes. ACS Nano 12:1023–1032
95. Ch'ng JH, Chong KK, Lam LN, Wong JJ, Kline KA (2019) Biofilm-associated infection by enterococci. Nat Rev Microbiol 17:82–94
96. van Asten SA, La Fontaine J, Peters EJ, Bhavan K, Kim PJ, Lavery LA (2016) The microbiome of diabetic foot osteomyelitis. Eur J Clin Microbiol Infect Dis 2:293–298

97. Pastar I, Nusbaum AG, Gil J, Patel SB, Chen J, Valdes J et al (2013) Interactions of methicillin resistant Staphylococcus aureus USA300 and Pseudomonas aeruginosa in polymicrobial wound infection. PLoS One 8(2):e56846
98. Messad N, Prajsnar TK, Lina G, O'Callaghan D, Foster SJ, Renshaw SA et al (2015) Existence of a colonizing Staphylococcus aureus strain isolated in diabetic foot ulcers. Diabetes 64(8):2991–2995
99. Hu D, Li H, Wang B, Ye Z, Lei W, Jia F et al (2017) Surface-adaptive gold nanoparticles with effective adherence and enhanced photothermal ablation of methicillin-resistant Staphylococcus aureus biofilm. ACS Nano 11:9330–9339
100. Fitzgerald RH, Mills JL, Joseph W, Armstrong DG (2009) The diabetic rapid response acute foot team: 7 essential skills for targeted limb salvage. Eplasty 9:e15
101. Boulton AJ, Armstrong DG, Albert SF, Frykberg RG, Hellman R, Kirkman MS et al (2008) Comprehensive foot examination and risk assessment. A report of the Task Force of the Foot Care Interest Group of the American Diabetes Association, with endorsement by the American Association of Clinical Endocrinologists. Phys Ther 88(11):1436–1443
102. Bjarnsholt T, Kirketerp-Moller K, Jensen PO, Madsen KG, Phipps R, Krogfelt K et al (2008) Why chronic wounds will not heal: a novel hypothesis. Wound Repair Regen 1:2–10
103. Wolcott RD, Rhoads DD, Dowd SE (2008) Biofilms and chronic wound inflammation. J Wound Care 17:333–341
104. Leaper D, Assadian O, Edmiston CE (2015) Approach to chronic wound infections. Br J Dermatol 173:351–358
105. Prompers L, Huijberts M, Schaper N, Apelqvist J, Bakker K, Edmonds M et al (2008) Resource utilisation and costs associated with the treatment of diabetic foot ulcers. Prospective data from the Eurodial Study. Diabetologia 51:1826–1834
106. Lavery LA, Armstrong DG, Wunderlich RP, Mohler MJ, Wendel CS, Lipsky BA (2006) Risk factors for foot infections in individuals with diabetes. Diabetes Care 29:1288–1293
107. Centers for Disease Control and Prevention. National diabetes fact sheet. http://www.cdc.gov/diabetes/pubs/estimates.htm
108. American Diabetes Association. Facts and figures. https://www.diabetes.org/info/facts/facts_nephropathy.jsp
109. American Diabetes Association. Facts and figures. https://www.diabetes.org/info/facts/facts_CVD.jsp
110. Faris I (1991) Vascular disease. In: Faris I (ed) The management of the diabetic foot, 2nd edn. Churchill Livingstone, Edinburgh, p 9
111. Grant WP, Sullivan R, Sonenshine DE et al (1997) Electron microscopic investigation of the effects of diabetes mellitus on the Achilles tendon. J Foot Ankle Surg 36(4):272–278. Discussion 330
112. Hunt NA, Liu GT, Lavery LA (2011) The economics of limb salvage in diabetes. Plast Reconstr Surg 127:289S–295S
113. Mulder G, Lee DK (2009) A retrospective clinical review of extracellular matrices for tissue reconstruction: equine pericardium as a biological covering to assist with wound closure. Wounds 21(9):254–261
114. Marston WA (2004) Dermagraft®, a bioengineered human dermal equivalent for the treatment of chronic nonhealing diabetic foot ulcer. Exp Rev Med Dev 1(1):21–31
115. Boateng JS, Matthews KH, Stevens HN, Eccleston GM (2008) Wound healing dressings and drug delivery systems: a review. J Pharm Sci 97(8):2892–2923
116. Parani M, Lokhande G, Singh A, Gaharwar AK (2016) Engineered nanomaterials for infection control and healing acute and chronic wounds. ACS Appl Mater Interfaces 8(16):10049–10069
117. Monecke S, Ehricht R (2005) Rapid genotyping of methicillin resistant Staphylococcus aureus (MRSA) isolates using miniaturised oligonucleotide arrays. Clin Microbiol Infect 11:825–833
118. Heller MJ (2002) DNA microarray technology: devices, systems, and applications. Annu Rev Biomed Eng 4:129–153

119. Agency for Healthcare Research and Quality. NCQA's the essential guide to healthcare quality, Chapter 1. p. 8. https://www.ncqa.org/Portals/0/Publications/Resource%20Library/NCQA_Primer_web.pdf. Accessed 1 April 2017
120. (2007) [Management of diabetic foot infections. Long text. Société de Pathologie Infectieuse de Langue Française]. Med Mal Infect 37:26–50
121. Agence Française de Sécurité Sanitaire des Produits de Santé (2004) Prescription des antibiotiques des antibiotiques par voie locale dans les infections cutanées bactériennes primitives et secondaires. Agence Française de Sécurité Sanitaire des Produits de Santé, Paris. http://agmed.sante.gouv.fr/pdf/5/rbp/dermreco.pdf
122. Lipsky BA, Hoey C (2009) Topical antimicrobial therapy for treating chronic wounds. Clin Infect Dis 49:1541–1549
123. Sotto A, Lemaire X, Jourdan N, Bouziges N, Richard JL, Lavigne JP (2008) In vitro activity of ertapenem against strains isolated from diabetic foot infections. Med Mal Infect 38:146–152
124. Sotto A, Bouziges N, Jourdan N, Richard JL, Lavigne JP (2007) In vitro activity of tigecycline against strains isolated from diabetic foot ulcers. Pathol Biol (Paris) 55:398–406
125. Goldstein EJ, Citron DM, Merriam CV, Warren YA, Tyrrell KL, Fernandez HT (2006) In vitro activity of ceftobiprole against aerobic and anaerobic strains isolated from diabetic foot infections. Antimicrob Agents Chemother 50:3959–3962
126. Goldstein EJ, Citron DM, Merriam CV, Warren YA, Tyrrell KL, Fernandez HT (2008) In vitro activities of doripenem and six comparator drugs against 423 aerobic and anaerobic bacterial isolates from infected diabetic foot wounds. Antimicrob Agents Chemother 52:761–766
127. Papazian HZ (1977) An overview of the podiatry service and podiatry residency program at the New England Deaconess Hospital. Hosp Podiatr 12(10):7–9
128. Wallace G. Are you providing quality healthcare? Podiatry Today 29(4). http://www.podiatrytoday.com/are-you-providing-qualityhealthcare. Accessed 1 April 2017
129. Hamburg BA, Inoff GE (1983) Coping with predictable crises of diabetes. Diabetes Care 6(4):409–416
130. Jacobson AM, Weinger K (2000) Psychosocial complications in diabetes. In: Leahy J, Clark N, Cefalu W (eds) Medical management of diabetes. Marcel Dekker, Inc., New York, NY, pp 559–572
131. Weinger K, Welch G, Jacobson A (2002) Psychological and psychiatric issues in diabetes mellitus. In: Poretsky L (ed) Principles of diabetes mellitus. Kluwer Academic Publishers, Norwell, MA, pp 639–654
132. Vileikyte L, Rubin RR, Peyrot M, Gonzalez JS, Boulton AJ, Ulbrecht JS, Cavanagh PR (2009) Diabetic feet. Br J Gen Pract 59:290
133. Jeffcoate WJ, Lipsky BA, Berendt AR, Cavanagh PR, Bus SA, Peters EJ et al (2008) Unresolved issues in the management of ulcers of the foot in diabetes. Diabet Med 25:1380–1389
134. Bus SA, Valk GD, van Deursen RW, Armstrong DG, Caravaggi C, Hlavácek P et al (2008) The effectiveness of footwear and offloading interventions to prevent and heal foot ulcers and reduce plantar pressure in diabetes: a systematic review. Diabetes Metab Res Rev 24(Suppl 1):S162–S180
135. Alexiadou K, Doupis J (2012) Management of diabetic foot ulcers. Diabet Ther 3(1):4
136. Das S, Baker AB (2016) Biomaterials and nanotherapeutics for enhancing skin wound healing. Front Bioeng Biotechnol 4:82
137. Kılıçoğlu Öİ, Demirel M, Aktaş Ş (2018) New trends in the orthopaedic management of diabetic foot. EFORT Open Rev 3(5):269–277
138. Tsourdi E, Barthel A, Rietzsch H, Reichel A, Bornstein SR (2013) Current aspects in the pathophysiology and treatment of chronic wounds in diabetes mellitus. Biomed Res Int 2013:385641
139. Silver S (2003) Bacterial silver resistance: molecular biology and uses and misuses of silver compounds. FEMS Microbiol Rev 27(2-3):341–353

140. Boucher W, Stern JM, Kotsinyan V, Kempuraj D, Papaliodis D, Cohen MS, Theoharides TC (2008) Intravesical nanocrystalline silver decreases experimental bladder inflammation. J Urol 179(4):1598–1602
141. Thirumurugan G, Veni VS, Ramachandran S, Seshagiri Rao JV, Dhanaraju MD (2011) Superior wound healing effect of topically delivered silver nanoparticle formulation using eco-friendly potato plant pathogenic fungus: synthesis and characterization. J Biomed Nanotechnol 7(5):659–666
142. Tian J, Wong KK, Ho CM, Lok CN, Yu WY, Che CM et al (2007) Topical delivery of silver nanoparticles promotes wound healing. ChemMedChem 2(1):129–136
143. Leu JG, Chen SA, Chen HM, Wu WM, Hung CF, Yao YD et al (2012) The effects of gold nanoparticles in wound healing with antioxidant epigallocatechin gallate and α-lipoic acid. Nanomedicine 8(5):767–775
144. Chen WY, Chang HY, Lu JK, Huang YC, Harroun SG, Tseng YT et al (2015) Self-assembly of antimicrobial peptides on gold nanodots: against multidrug-resistant bacteria and wound-healing application. Adv Funct Mater 46:7189–7199
145. Steffy K, Shanthi G, Maroky AS, Selvakumar S (2018) Enhanced antibacterial effects of green synthesized ZnO NPs using Aristolochia indica against Multi-drug resistant bacterial pathogens from Diabetic Foot Ulcer. J Infect Public Health 11(4):463–471
146. Zhang F, Chan SW, Spanier JE, Apak E, Jin Q, Robinson RD, Herman IP (2002) Cerium oxide nanoparticles: size-selective formation and structure analysis. Appl Phys Lett 80(1):127–129
147. Sudarshan TS (1996) Review of "The Encyclopedia of Advanced Materials" Edited by David Bloor, Richard J. Brook, Merton C. Flemings, and Subhash Mahajan Senior Advisory Editor Robert Cahn. Mater Manuf Process 11(6):1059
148. Shalaby TI, Fekry NM, Sodfy AS, Sheredy AG, Moustafa ME (2015) Preparation and characterisation of antibacterial silver-containing nanofibres for wound healing in diabetic mice. Int J Nanoparticles 8(1):82–98
149. Singla R, Soni S, Patial V, Kulurkar PM, Kumari A, Mahesh S et al (2017) In vivo diabetic wound healing potential of nanobiocomposites containing bamboo cellulose nanocrystals impregnated with silver nanoparticles. Int J Biol Macromol 105:45–55
150. Li Y, Tian Y, Zheng W, Feng Y, Huang R, Shao J et al (2017) Composites of bacterial cellulose and small molecule-decorated gold nanoparticles for treating Gram-Negative bacteria-infected wounds. Small 13(27):1700130
151. Xie Z, Paras CB, Weng H, Punnakitikashem P, Su LC, Vu K et al (2013) Dual growth factor releasing multi-functional nanofibers for wound healing. Acta Biomater 9(12):9351–9359
152. You C, Li Q, Wang X, Wu P, Ho JK, Jin R, Zhang L, Shao H, Han C (2017) Silver nanoparticle loaded collagen/chitosan scaffolds promote wound healing via regulating fibroblast migration and macrophage activation. Sci Rep 7(1):10489
153. Zhang Y, He H, Gao WJ, Lu SY, Liu Y, Gu HY (2009) Rapid adhesion and proliferation of keratinocytes on the gold colloid/chitosan film scaffold. Mater Sci Eng C 29(3):908–912
154. Gopal A, Kant V, Gopalakrishnan A, Tandan SK, Kumar D (2014) Chitosan-based copper nanocomposite accelerates healing in excision wound model in rats. Eur J Pharmacol 731:8–19
155. Sun G, Zhang X, Shen YI, Sebastian R, Dickinson LE, Fox-Talbot K et al (2011) Dextran hydrogel scaffolds enhance angiogenic responses and promote complete skin regeneration during burn wound healing. Proc Natl Acad Sci 108(52):20976–20981
156. Ma YQ, Yi JZ, Zhang LM (2009) A facile approach to incorporate silver nanoparticles into dextran-based hydrogels for antibacterial and catalytical application. J Macromol Sci A Pure Appl Chem 46(6):643–648
157. Păunica-Panea G, Ficai A, Marin MM, Marin Ş, Albu MG, Constantin VD et al (2016) New collagen-dextran-zinc oxide composites for wound dressing. J Nanomater 2016:5805034
158. Mohandas A, Sudheesh Kumar PT, Raja B, Lakshmanan VK, Jayakumar R (2015) Exploration of alginate hydrogel/nano zinc oxide composite bandages for infected wounds. Int J Nanomedicine 10(Suppl 1):53

159. Akturk O, Kismet K, Yasti AC, Kuru S, Duymus ME, Kaya F et al (2016) Collagen/gold nanoparticle nanocomposites: a potential skin wound healing biomaterial. J Biomater Appl 31(2):283–301
160. Vasconcelos A, Gomes AC, Paulo AC (2012) Novel silk fibroin/elastin wound dressings. Acta Biomater 8(8):3049–3060
161. Kawabata S, Kawai K, Somamoto S, Noda K, Matsuura Y, Nakamura Y, Suzuki S (2017) The development of a novel wound healing material, silk-elastin sponge. J Biomater Sci Polym Ed 28(18):2143–2153
162. Marques AP, Reis RL, Hunt JA (2002) The biocompatibility of novel starch-based polymers and composites: in vitro studies. Biomaterials 23(6):1471–1478
163. Mendes SC, Reis RL, Bovell YP, Cunha AM, Van Blitterswijk CA, De Bruijn JD (2001) Biocompatibility testing of novel starch-based materials with potential application in orthopedic surgery: a preliminary study. Biomaterials 22:2057–2064
164. Azevedo HS, Gama FM, Reis RL (2003) In vitro assessment of the enzymatic degradation of several starch-based biomaterials. Biomacromolecules 4(6):1703–1712
165. Sinha VR, Kumria R (2001) Polysaccharides in colon-specific drug delivery. Int J Pharm 224(1–2):19–38
166. Gomes ME, Sikavitsas VI, Behravesh E, Reis RL, Mikos AG (2003) Effect of flow perfusion on the osteogenic differentiation of bone marrow stromal cells cultured on starch-based three-dimensional scaffolds. J Biomed Mater Res A67(1):87–95
167. Villanueva ME, Diez AMR, González JA, Pérez CJ, Orrego M, Piehl LL et al (2016) Antimicrobial activity of starch hydrogel incorporated with copper nanoparticles. ACS Appl Mater Interfaces 8(25):16280–16288
168. Ansari MA, Badrealam KF, Alam A, Tufail S, Khalique G, Equbal MJ et al (2020) Recent Nano-based Therapeutic Intervention of Bioactive Sesquiterpenes: Prospects in Cancer Therapeutics. Curr Pharm Desi 26:1138–1144
169. Pottoo FH, Sharma S, Javed MN, Barkat MA, Harshita, Alam MS et al (2020) Lipid-based nanoformulations in the treatment of neurological disorders. Drug Metab Rev 52:185–204
170. Ansari MA, Thiruvengadam M, Farooqui Z, Rajakumar G, Jamal QM, Alzohairy MA et al (2019) Nanotechnology, in silico and endocrine-based strategy for delivering paclitaxel and miRNA: Prospects for the therapeutic management of breast cancer. Semin Cancer Biol. https://doi.org/10.1016/j.semcancer.2019.12.022
171. Pottoo FH, Barkat MA, Ansari MA, Javed MN, Jamal QM, Kamal MA (2019) Nanotechnological based miRNA intervention in the therapeutic management of neuroblastoma. Semin Cancer Biol. https://doi.org/10.1016/j.semcancer.2019.09.017
172. Ansari MA, Chung IM, Rajakumar G, Alzohairy MA, Alomary MN, Thiruvengadam M et al (2020) Current Nanoparticle Approaches in Nose to Brain Drug Delivery and Anticancer Therapy-A Review. Curr Pharma Des 26:1128–1137
173. Gainza G, Pastor M, Aguirre JJ, Villullas S, Pedraz JL, Hernandez RM et al (2014) A novel strategy for the treatment of chronic wounds based on the topical administration of rhEGF-loaded lipid nanoparticles: in vitro bioactivity and in vivo effectiveness in healing-impaired db/db mice. J Control Release 185:51–61
174. Sandri G, Bonferoni MC, D'Autilia F, Rossi S, Ferrari F, Grisoli P et al (2013) Wound dressings based on silver sulfadiazine solid lipid nanoparticles for tissue repairing. Eur J Pharm Biopharm 84(1):84–90
175. Küchler S, Wolf NB, Heilmann S, Weindl G, Helfmann J, Yahya MM, Stein C, Schäfer-Korting M (2010) 3D-wound healing model: influence of morphine and solid lipid nanoparticles. J Biotechnol 148(1):24–30
176. Gokce EH, Korkmaz E, Dellera E, Sandri G, Bonferoni MC, Ozer O (2012) Resveratrol-loaded solid lipid nanoparticles versus nanostructured lipid carriers: evaluation of antioxidant potential for dermal applications. Int J Nanomedicine 7:1841
177. Küchler S, Radowski MR, Blaschke T, Dathe M, Plendl J, Haag R et al (2009) Nanoparticles for skin penetration enhancement–a comparison of a dendritic core-multishell-nanotransporter and solid lipid nanoparticles. Eur J Pharm Biopharm 71(2):243–250

178. Küchler S, Herrmann W, Panek-Minkin G, Blaschke T, Zoschke C, Kramer KD et al (2010) SLN for topical application in skin diseases—characterization of drug–carrier and carrier–target interactions. Int J Pharm 390(2):225–233
179. Chu Y, Yu D, Wang P, Xu J, Li D, Ding M (2010) Nanotechnology promotes the full-thickness diabetic wound healing effect of recombinant human epidermal growth factor in diabetic rats. Wound Repair Regen 18:499–505
180. Das S, Singh G, Majid M, Sherman MB, Mukhopadhyay S, Wright CS et al (2016) Syndesome therapeutics for enhancing diabetic wound healing. Adv Healthcare Mater 17:2248–2260
181. Motawea A, Abd El-Gawad AE-GH, Borg T, Motawea M, Tarshoby M (2019) The impact of topical phenytoin loaded nanostructured lipid carriers in diabetic foot ulceration. Foot 40:14–21
182. Jayakumar A, Radhakrishnan EK (2020) Nanotechnological approaches to manage diabetic foot ulcer. In: Rai M (ed) Nanotechnology in skin, soft tissue, and bone infections. Springer, Cham. https://doi.org/10.1007/978-3-030-35147-2_8
183. Blecher K, Martinez LR, Tuckman-Vernon C, Nacharaju P, Schairer D, Chouake J et al (2012) Nitric oxide-releasing nanoparticles accelerate wound healing in NOD-SCID mice. Nanomed Nanotechnol 8(8):1364–1371
184. Han G, Nguyen LN, Macherla C, Chi Y, Friedman JM, Nosanchuk JD, Martinez LR (2012) Nitric oxide-releasing nanoparticles accelerate wound healing by promoting fibroblast migration and collagen deposition. Am J Pathol 180(4):1465–1473
185. Kasiewicz LN, Whitehead KA (2019) Lipid nanoparticles silence tumor necrosis factor α to improve wound healing in diabetic mice. Bioeng Transl Med 1:75–82
186. Kasiewicz LN, Whitehead KA (2016) Silencing TNFalpha with lipidoid nanoparticles downregulates both TNFalpha and MCP-1 in an in vitro co-culture model of diabetic foot ulcers. Acta Biomater 32:120–128
187. Kim H, Yoo H (2013) Matrix metalloproteinase-inspired suicidal treatments of diabetic ulcers with siRNA-decorated nanofibrous meshes. Gene Ther 20:378–385
188. Randeria PS, Seeger MA, Wang XQ, Wilson H, Shipp D, Mirkin CA et al (2015) siRNA-based spherical nucleic acids reverse impaired wound healing in diabetic mice by ganglioside GM3 synthase knockdown. Proc Natl Acad Sci U S A 112:5573–5578
189. Chakraborty SP, Sahu SK, Mahapatra SK, Santra S, Bal M, Roy S, Pramanik P (2010) Nanoconjugated vancomycin: new opportunities for the development of anti-VRSA agents. Nanotechnology 21(10):105103
190. Lin YH, Lin JH, Li TS, Wang SH, Yao CH, Chung WY, Ko TH (2016) Dressing with epigallocatechin gallate nanoparticles for wound regeneration. Wound Repair Regen 24(2):287–301
191. Vellayappan MV, Jaganathan SK, Manikandan A (2016) Nanomaterials as a game changer in the management and treatment of diabetic foot ulcers. RSC Adv 6(115):114859–114878
192. Li M, Zhao Y, Hao H, Han W, Fu X (2015) Mesenchymal stem cell-based therapy for non-healing wounds: today and tomorrow. Wound Repair Regen 23:465–482
193. Hamdan S, Pastar I, Drakulich S, Dikici E, Tomic-Canic M, Deo S, Daunert S (2017) Nanotechnology-driven therapeutic interventions in wound healing: potential uses and applications. ACS Central Sci 3(3):163–175

Correction to: Nanotechnology and Diabetic Foot Ulcer: Future Prospects

Mohammad Azam Ansari, Khursheed Ali, Zeba Farooqui, Hanan A. Al-Dossary, Mohammad Zubair, and Javed Musarrat

Correction to:
Chapter 20 in: Mohammad Zubair et. al., Diabetic Foot Ulcer: An Update, https://doi.org/10.1007/978-981-15-7639-3_20

The book was inadvertently published with an incorrect spelling of the author's surname name in Chapter 20 as Mussart whereas it should be Musarrat. This error has now been corrected with this erratum.

The updated online version of this chapter can be found at
https://doi.org/10.1007/978-981-15-7639-3_20

M. Zubair et al. (eds.), *Diabetic Foot Ulcer*,
https://doi.org/10.1007/978-981-15-7639-3_21

GPSR Compliance

The European Union's (EU) General Product Safety Regulation (GPSR) is a set of rules that requires consumer products to be safe and our obligations to ensure this.

If you have any concerns about our products, you can contact us on ProductSafety@springernature.com

In case Publisher is established outside the EU, the EU authorized representative is:

Springer Nature Customer Service Center GmbH
Europaplatz 3
69115 Heidelberg, Germany

Batch number: 10726133

Printed by Printforce, the Netherlands